YOUR HEALTH AT RISK

By the same author:

The Last of the Green-Toed Fruit-Bats: A Fairy-tale for adults
The Mile-High Staircase

About the author:

'Finding oneself a complete physical wreck "concentrates the mind" most wonderfully,' says Toni Jeffreys, who has been close to death three times in her life.

In her childhood she battled against Tuberculosis for several years. It was a battle she won but it left her in weakened health. However, in 1974 she graduated PhD from the University of Auckland and thereafter held several responsible positions, including that of Senior Researcher for the Australian Royal Commission on Human Relationships.

In 1977 Jeffreys became bedridden long term with severe ill-health. But despite this handicap, in 1980 she founded the Australian and New Zealand Myalgic Encephalomyelitis Society Inc, for people with '20th-century illnesses'; wrote her first book, *The Mile-High Staircase*, published by Hodder & Stoughton in 1982, and another, *The Last of the Green-Toed Fruit-Bats: A Fairy-Tale for Adults*, in 1989.

Your Health at Risk represents over 20 years of knowledge acquired in the course of studying health literature – orthodox medical, unorthodox medical, natural and traditional – and through her experiences helping others to recover from poor health.

Her conclusion: 'One can scarcely be healthy today without considerable knowledge of the hazards that surround us. Avoiding them is the first step to good health. And that knowledge should be available to all of us.'

YOUR HEALTH AT RISK

WHAT DOCTORS AND THE GOVERNMENT AREN'T TELLING YOU

Toni Jeffreys PhD

Thorsons

While the author of this work has made every effort to ensure that the information contained in this book is as accurate and up to date as possible at the time of publication, medical and pharmaceutical knowledge is constantly changing and the application of it to particular circumstances depends on many factors. Therefore it is recommended that readers always consult a qualified health practitioner for individual advice. This book should not be used as an alternative to seeking specialist advice, which should be sought before any action is taken. The author and publishers cannot be held responsible for any errors and omissions that may be found in the text, or any actions that may be taken by a reader as a result of any reliance on the information contained in the text, which is taken entirely at the reader's own risk.

Thorsons
An Imprint of HarperCollins*Publishers*
77–85 Fulham Palace Road,
Hammersmith, London W6 8JB

The Thorsons website address is: www.thorsons.com

First published 1998 by Howling At The Moon
Publishing Ltd, Auckland

This revised Thorsons edition published 1999

1 3 5 7 9 10 8 6 4 2

© Toni Jeffreys 1998, 1999

Toni Jeffreys asserts the moral right to
be identified as the author of this work

A catalogue record for this book
is available from the British Library

ISBN 0 7225 3925 8

Printed in Great Britain by
Creative Print and Design (Wales), Ebbw Vale

To the women and men of the medical profession who seek a better way;

To pay my respects, with love, to Dr Carl Pfeiffer, US, whose brilliance and kindness saved thousands of lives.

To Dr Orion Truss of Alabama, US, whose tenacity in opposing his less enlightened fellows saved at least one life ... mine.

To Dr Ann Cowie of Auckland, New Zealand, who long ago became a different kind of doctor.

And to all those struggling to be well.

'When I pluck a blade of grass, a distant star trembles.'

This Earth, our Planet, our Home,
A Treasure briefly lent us,
all gift-wrapped up in shining stars and drifting clouds.

Unwrap the Gift and Marvel.
Marvel at forest and field, birds and flowers.
Bring your Wonder to Everything that Lives.

For the Miracle that is Life Shines in All of us.
Can we not Find a Way to Live in Joy?

T J

CONTENTS

INTRODUCTION

In July of 1997, the World Health Organization predicted a tremendous upsurge in deaths from heart disease and cancer. In May of 1998 it reiterated this and predicted that in the US deaths from cancer would soon surpass those of heart disease, now responsible for approximately half that country's deaths, as it is in most countries. Presumably these calculations are based on the exponential growth we have seen in the past. We cannot delude ourselves that the rest of the English-speaking world is not a part of this prediction. As Alistair Cooke would say, 'Don't ignore what's going on in America, for there lies our future.'

A difficult time ahead for most of us seems inevitable. But it is my contention that these premature deaths are, always have been, and will always be **almost entirely unnecessary**. It is now long past time we ceased resting on a failing 'disease-care' system. We must concentrate on preventive measures, the fence at the top of the cliff. Moreover, there is no country in this world that can afford the ever-escalating price of 'high-tech medicine', that frail and ill-equipped ambulance at the bottom of the cliff.

Our daily lives are constantly bombarded with media messages about the wonders of modern medicine, and how much longer we are all living. The facts are quite different!

Health care in the US costs annually close to a trillion dollars. But despite this vast expenditure, it is generally believed that every third person is allergic to something; every fifth person is depressed or suffers from some mental problem. In America every 30 seconds someone dies of a heart attack, and every 55 seconds someone dies of cancer. Barring accidents, [cancer] has now become our number one child killer.[1]

The figures are almost as bad in other English-speaking countries. Significantly, the incidence of heart disease in women, which used to be lower than for men, is now surpassing it.

Is this state of affairs an inevitable part of life? It is not. A man aged 45 in 1900 had a life expectancy of 69 years; in 1980 it was 74, a mere five additional years,[2] gained primarily through the use of antibiotics. And those five years gained tend to be fraught with ill-health, whereas the chances are that the earlier man would more than likely have been carried off by influenza, 'the old people's friend,' or died peacefully in his sleep. His last few years may have been better.

Here is health scientist Dr Joseph D Campbell, BSA, MSc, PhD, on the state of health in the US and Canada:

A hundred years ago cardiovascular/heart disease was virtually unknown; now it is our number one killer. Cancer, our present number two cause of death, was responsible for only 3.4% of all deaths; now it is one out of every four for men and one out of five, for women. Our third most prevalent cause of death is diabetes; it was very rare a century ago; now it is one out of every 20. Alzheimer's Disease was also extremely rare; now it is the fourth leading cause of death. Moreover, all of the above killers are striking at younger and younger ages.[3]

Another expert in the field, Dr Jeffrey Bland PhD, says a similar thing:

Not only has life expectancy after age 40 in this country increased very little in recent years, but the American work force is plagued by absenteeism and reduced productivity as a consequence of chronic health problems. Despite tremendous expenditure on health care, many childhood illnesses, several types of cancer, and maturity onset diabetes are all on the rise. Most disturbing of all, the number of years the average person lives in a state of good health has not changed over the past 20 years. Today, an American can expect to be healthy only 80% of his or her lifetime.[4]

One thing we must be aware of, is that the present trends started long before 1945, which was the year antibiotics came into general use. Because one of the many excuses we hear for the appalling health of Westerners is: 'Well, we die of these things, we get these diseases because we're living longer.' But we should be aware that some years before the antibiotics came in, as we will see in the first chapter on the myth of cholesterol, a new kind of heart attack was in evidence in the 1930s. For 70 years it has been a mystery to most.

The most recent startling statistic that the people of little New Zealand have to come to terms with, is the fact that New Zealanders not only lose 12,000 people every year to heart disease, but we have 25% more of this heart disease than do Australians.[5] And when we determine the reasons for this difference we will have solved the riddle of heart disease itself. This subject will be dealt with in the first few chapters.

In addition to the more familiar chronic diseases, there are the newer '20th-century diseases', the diseases of a hundred names affecting hundreds of thousands of people and ever-increasingly. In New Zealand these illnesses are known as Tapanui Flu or ME (Myalgic Encephalomyelitis); in the UK they are also known as ME; in the US and elsewhere as Chronic Fatigue Syndrome and Chronic Fatigue Immune Dysfunction Syndrome; in Canada they also carry the name 'Nightingale's Disease', after Florence Nightingale; they have also been called Icelandic Disease, Environmental Illness, Multiple Chemical Sensitivity Syndrome, Gulf War Syndrome, the repercussions of Agent Orange, and numerous other names found all around the globe.

The main point to emphasize is that except in rare cases where there are genetic problems, there are always logical environmental reasons for poor health. And when we understand the reasons we will know that this type of poor health need not happen to any of us.

As we draw near to the close of the 20th century, I cannot help wondering how those to come in the middle of the 21st century will look back upon *our* century. That is, if there are any people left to do so!

It is my belief that in the area of health, both the health of our planet and the health of our bodies, future generations will regard the people of this century as having made good progress in a few areas, especially in the first half of the century. For we had virtually overthrown most of the old handicaps of superstition and ignorance. Under improved sanitation and nutrition for greater numbers, the old infectious diseases were slowly being conquered. Moreover the scientific method, for all its deficiencies, if used honestly and well could have led us to a far braver world than the one we have today.

But in the second half of the century, despite truly amazing advances in technology, in this matter of health future historians will see that it has been a time of missed opportunities, of wrong turnings and, worse still, one of unprecedented and possibly incurable damage to our home, the planet.

It has in fact been a disaster in these terms. To symbolize that disaster we should be aware that we could send a man to the moon and he could walk upon it, but we could not prevent that same man from having a heart attack at 43.

The reasons for the disaster lie in a combination of factors: Most of us, including our medical advisors, live by fallacious ideas about how both the mind and the body function. Combine that with enormous pressures from commerce and our entirely human love of ease. And in that combination has lain the recipe for certain disaster in human health and well-being.

The problem was *not* that we did not produce our share of geniuses, brilliant innovators in this field who saw 'the truth' or a better way. They tried and tried to tell us. The luminous Rachel Carson[6] comes to mind immediately. The problem has been that they could not make themselves heard.

At the halfway mark, in 1950, Albert Einstein, who also possessed one of the greatest minds of our century, looking at the way things were going, at Stanford University addressed the American Medical Association thus: *'You look like scientists. You talk like scientists. You use scientific methods. But you are not scientists.'*[7]

By the end of the century it is quite clear, judging by the nightmare that has been the inevitable result of our 'health care system', that that verdict has been proved absolutely correct. And in this book we will be looking at the reasons why he was right. For he understood that the medical paradigm of our century, the basic approach or world-view concerning health, was unscientific and basically unsound, and therefore almost anything medicine did could not be scientific. I would submit that the results speak for themselves.

All through history, ignorance, greed, corruption and pride have nearly always overshadowed questions of human health. The second half of our century has not in the least been free of these evils. In fact they have perhaps influenced and shortened the course of millions of human lives on a scale never before seen in human history.

The latest research on longevity (who lives longest, who is healthiest) comes from the US. Epidemiologists at the Harvard School of Public Health in Boston, and the federal Centers for Disease Control and Prevention in Atlanta, Georgia, have found unexpectedly large and significant differences in longevity, with some groups showing an average life expectancy in the early fifties, others in the sixties age groups, and others into the late seventies. Also, in comparison with other countries it was found that Japanese women have life expectancies into their eighties, the highest in the world. Future research will be directed towards finding out why these differences exist.[8] But there are many indications in this book.

These days, the maintenance of good health, or the restoration of lost health, is not merely a question of adding good exercise, good food and possibly supplements, helpful though they can be. Health today is a matter of first subtracting that which is harmful from our lives. It is as though we live in a minefield, and if we wish to be healthy we must learn to avoid the dangers all around us. I have seen some remarkable transformations, 'rejuvenations', from this kind of avoidance. Once one has mastered the difficult task of avoiding the health hazards, the minefield, then it is time to consider the 'addition' part of the health equation. I have frequently touched on this at the end of the chapters in this book, but to do this truly well will take another book.

This book concerns the land mines and how to avoid them.

I have been studying health for the last 20 years, without either the benefits or biases of specialist qualifications. Many of the facts that worry me have been aired in professional medical journals and elsewhere, many times and in many different ways. Numerous people have tried to tell their fellows in many carefully written books and journals. But the majority of people do not yet appear to be aware of the dangers we share in daily living.

I have written this book, in this particular way, because I believe people have a right to know the truth, especially when it comes to their health, their very lives, their right to live peacefully and happily, free of gross disease and suffering. And because I believe that **knowledge is the best form of health insurance**. Moreover, the very survival of the human race and our planet may depend upon our awareness of what is and what is not healthy. **And in that awareness also lies our hope of better things to come in the future.**

I should like to thank all those whose research and writing made this book possible. In addition, my thanks for assistance go to Dr Mike Godfrey, who looked over the chapters on mercury amalgam and root canals; to the late, very great Dr John Colquhoun for looking over the chapter on fluoride; to Irwin Alber for our discussions on vaccinations; to Judith Lopez of San Francisco for checking on AIDS; and I most heartily thank Dr Wayne Martin of Fairhope, Alabama, for sharing with me his invaluable insights and research into heart disease and cancer. I should also like to thank my friend Helen, and Meriel Watts, for information on pesticides.

I am grateful to my son David, for assisting with his computer skills, and a willing friend, Andy C., who nobly came to my rescue when equipment failed. Also thanks are due to my friends Glenda Leader and Patricia Davies for helping me track down some lost references, which are like a handful of sand in the pocket. Some grains do slip through the seams. Heartfelt thanks to Barbara Vesey, our patient and vigilant editor, for rounding up numerous deliquent footnotes. The always helpful librarians at the East Coast Bays warrant a mention, especially Lillian Grant.

And most thanks of all to my dear Noel, for his patience and his understanding of my need to write this book.

Most of the data I use comes from the United States, for several reasons. More data are collected there, and what happens in the US is also happening elsewhere in the so-called 'developed' world. The Americans have both the best and the worst of most things.

Also I use primarily American data because, through the magnificent *Townsend Letter for Doctors*, (now, *and Patients*),[9] a trail-blazer if ever there was one, a journal for people who hate lies as much as I do, I personally have greater access to American research than to any other.

For clarity's sake, this book will be the most rewarding if the chapters are read in the order of presentation.

Disclaimer: Any material in this book touching on health is for information purposes only and should be acted upon only with the advice of one's qualified health advisors!

1: CHOLESTEROL

'It's that evil cholesterol and saturated
fats that cause heart disease.'

Perhaps the most whopping lie, the most enduring confidence game of the second half of the 20th century has been what Professor Edward R Pinkney MD (former editor of the *Journal of the American Medical Association)* and Doctor Russell L Smith PhD call 'The Cholesterol Conspiracy'. In 1991 they produced a book with this title.[1]

Cholesterol is a substance found in animal fats. We are animals. Cholesterol is also found in most body tissues. The truth is we need a certain amount of it to be healthy. In fact, our livers go to a great deal of trouble to make the stuff, so it must be important to us. In fact, cholesterol is found in all cell membranes, in all tissues, and is the raw material for bile salts, vitamin D and our vital adrenal and steroid hormones, without which there is no sexuality, let alone reproduction.[2] Cholesterol is also a potent antioxidant. When we ingest too many harmful free radicals, cholesterol floods into the blood to take care of the problem. It promotes the health of the intestinal wall and protects against cancer of the colon. It also plays an important role in the development of the brain and nervous system.[3] In fact cholesterol is an essential nutrient, a precursor to the stress hormones cortisol and DHEA (the 'Mother' of all hormones). It is thus indispensable. Dr Alan R Gaby MD says that if serum cholesterol levels are low, 'the body's ability to adapt to physical and psychological stresses may be impaired'.[4]

In short, our bodies need cholesterol to live. It is not 'a killer'. Moreover, people in many other cultures consume far more cholesterol, more saturated fats than do we in the West, and they have less heart disease.

There is so much evidence that the prevailing ideas about cholesterol and saturated fats are nonsense, that it is clear that our observers from the middle of the next century will be more than incredulous of the fact that the nonsense was perpetuated for almost five decades.

If we consider only this:

We are evolutionarily evolved to cope with animal fat and have been eating this for hundreds of thousands of years. But doctors argue that the cause of heart disease is the lack of unsaturated (or vegetable) fats, such as corn oil, safflower and sunflower. It does not make sense. Before the modern hydraulic press and the new solvent processes were developed, we had little access to these plant oils. How can this present epidemic be caused through a lack of something we have always lacked?[5]

The myth about cholesterol goes back to the 1950s. Cholesterol in very small amounts was nearly always found in damaged Western hearts at autopsy, and from this came the mistaken idea that cholesterol is the main cause of heart disease. This despite the fact that the plugging of an artery involves 95% calcium and only 0.5% cholesterol.[6] The rest of 'the clog,' the arterial plaque, consists of fibrin, triglycerides, ceroids and sometimes blood platelets. Then it was found that cholesterol levels could be reduced by eating unsaturated vegetable oils. So this led to the massive effort to convince people to eat these oils in preference to the traditional fats and oils, and to persuade them to take the then hastily-burgeoning array of anti-cholesterol drugs.

It cannot be denied that the pharmaceutical companies have made enormous fortunes with their cholesterol-lowering drugs, as have the manufacturers of hydrogenated vegetable oils, fortunes which would not have been made without this idea that 'cholesterol is bad' or 'the conspiracy' Professor Pinkney and Dr Smith speak of.[7]

Rosetta Schuman, a health researcher of long standing, has done considerable work in this area. She cites Dr Ross Hume Hall, Professor Emeritus at McMaster University, who wrote a book called *Food for Nought*. On this subject Dr Hall said this:

It's just frightening what happens to these fats that people are taking, like the safflower oil and others. We're speaking now of the polyunsaturated oils which cause hardening of the arteries. They will lower cholesterol. But they lower cholesterol by driving it into the blood vessels. You'll get more hardening of the arteries with unsaturated fats than with saturated animal fats.[8]

Another eminent doctor echoed his sentiments. In 1956 Dr Paul Dudley White, cardiologist to President Eisenhower, was asked on television about the wonders of polyunsaturated oils. He said that he had begun his practice in 1921 and did not see his first case of MI (Myocardial Infarction, the kind of sudden death heart attack) until 1927. That is, before the 1920s, MI was extremely rare. Dr White maintained that people eating butter, lard and eggs did not get the new form of heart trouble, the sudden chest pain followed by death.

Parenthetically, we should here differentiate between two types of heart attack. The one that's been around for centuries in a very small way is known as Congestive Heart Failure, caused by atheroma or blocked arteries from a build-up of substances which should not be there. The result is a gradual blockage and slowing of the delivery of blood to where it is needed until the person involved is obviously in serious trouble. The other kind is Myocardial Infarction, MI, the sudden heart failure. This second and newer kind of heart attack, the MI, is probably caused by a blood clot. One's arteries could theoretically be 'clean as a whistle', but one could suddenly 'drop dead' from this rogue blood clot arriving in the wrong place at the wrong time. (This is generally the cause of younger people dying suddenly of 'heart trouble' which is really 'blood trouble'.)

In New Zealand we have in three years recorded nine deaths in young women from blood clots. They were all on the 'third-generation Pill' at the time, which association has caused the NZ government to advise against this drug for those with family histories of blood clots. I am inclined to believe myself that the cause may in addition to the predisposition be also a combination of this drug plus consumption of man-made fats and oils.

Another great doctor echoed Dr White's sentiments on vegetable oils. He was Dr T L Cleave, Surgeon Captain, formerly Director of Medical Research at the Royal Navy School in Britain. Of the drive against animal fats he said, 'For a modern disease to be related to an old-fashioned food is one of the most ludicrous things I ever heard in my life.'[9]

Supporting these views are the statistics on consumption of animal vs vegetable fats:

In 1920 the per capita consumption of animal fat in the US was 26 lb per year, while the per capita consumption of vegetable fat in that period was 11 lb per year. There were almost no MI heart deaths.

By 1989, with most forms of heart disease a serious nationwide problem, or rather 'epidemic', it was 10.5 lb of animal fat, vs 50.4 lb of vegetable fat.[10] (Also on this modern diet, Americans have never been more obese than they are today. Nor have the rest of us in the English-speaking world.)

In 1977 Dr Michael De Bakey, an internationally renowned heart surgeon, pointed out that only 30 to 40% of people with blocked arteries and heart disease have elevated blood cholesterol levels, and posed the logical question: 'How do you explain the other 60 to 70%?' Not long after, the Renfrew and Paisley survey found that there were about the same number of deaths among those with **low** blood cholesterol as among those with **high** serum cholesterol levels. And this was reported in the *British Medical Journal* in 1989.[11]

In Framlingham, USA, there have for decades been on-going long-term studies on the health of its citizens. The project's director, Dr William Kannell, declared he had found **'no discernible association between the amount of cholesterol in the diet and the level of cholesterol in the blood, regardless of how much or how little animal fat in the diet'.**[12] Cholesterol levels simply vary among individuals.

Following that, and much earlier evidence, should there not have been some attempt to re-examine the question? It is plain that modern orthodox doctors are saying one thing, but the more old-fashioned independents like Professor Hall, Dr White, Dr De Bakey, Dr Kannel and Dr Cleave have long been saying entirely another thing. When faced with a dilemma like this, if we want to find out the truth about anything we have to go back to the past and we have to look at the evidence from other cultures, the comparative statistics, the findings of epidemiology.

One hundred years ago there were far fewer deaths from heart disease in the West. A historical survey was done by Dr A U MacKinnon who studied the hospital records back to 1855 in a rural area of Yorkshire with a stable population level of 22,000 through time.[13] He found that between 1855 and 1900 there was but one death per year from Myocardial Infarction, known then as Coronary Thrombosis. (As noted, MI is the sudden heart attack, the chest pain followed by death.) Before 1900 most heart disease was classified as Congestive Heart Disease (CHD), probably caused by a weakness left over from childhood illness, or a gradual blockage. It was treated from around 1790 with digitalis. It rarely caused sudden death. The incidence of CHD has not increased at all since that day. However, by 1915 the deaths from the sudden MI kind had increased to five a year. And by 1983 they had increased to 43 per year in this stable population level.

In 1914 Dr Richard Cabot of the Harvard Medical School had published a paper, 'The Four Common Types of Heart Disease', revealing that in an analysis of 600 cases of heart disease by far the most common was rheumatic heart disease (a problem usually left over from rheumatic fever in childhood), at 46.3%. But by 1936 this situation had altered dramatically. The sudden heart attack (MI), the new kind of heart attack, was in first place. Something significant had happened between 1914 and 1936.[14] (We must here note again that antibiotics did not come on the scene till around 1945, so that the increase in MI cannot be attributed to the 'living longer because of antibiotics' theory.)

By 1956 there were 600,000 annual deaths from heart disease in the US, of which 90% were from MI. It was, in fact, an epidemic; an epidemic we still have with us today.

But to return to the historical record: There was another researcher, Dr Rodney Finlayson, who did a study in London hospitals similar to Dr MacKinnon's, going back to 1868, with identical results.[15] Even the great British medical journal, *The Lancet*, said that MI was almost unknown before 1926.[16]

It is clear that we must be doing something wrong. It is tempting to chalk up everything to 'psychological stress'. Are we to believe that pre-1920, an age of sharper, harsher class distinctions, more cruel gender distinctions, a period without social welfare, a period when war was almost ongoing in Europe and when at any time one's loved ones could be carried off by a virulent infection, that life was **less stressful** than now? Such a factor cannot be truly comparatively assessed, but it is my belief that life is probably less psychologically stressful now, but far more environmentally stressful – for example, in that we consume foods our bodies were not designed to cope with.

Before the 1920s the highly saturated fats – butter, lard and tallow – were eaten without fear. There was no margarine. Early in the century the margarine came in, and later the hydrogenated vegetable oils. And we must include as another possible influence in the increase in deaths, cigarette smoking, which had gradually become more common after 1910 when machine-made cigarettes arrived.

By the early 1950s, the full horror of what 20th-century food technology was doing to us should have been apparent. The evidence was there, as we have noted, in the gradually clogging arteries of older men and the sudden deaths among younger men 'in the prime of life'. But the people involved at that time jumped to entirely the wrong conclusion.

We have looked at the problem from the perspective of time. Now let us look at studies from other cultures:

Professor Stewart Wolf of Temple University supervised a study done in Roseta, Pennsylvania (US), where the population was 100% Italian immigrants still eating their traditional foods. That is, they ate a high-fat, high-cholesterol diet loaded with meatballs and cheese. They also used olive oil in great quantities, and olive oil is not unsaturated. What is important is that the people of Roseta **were actually found to have high serum cholesterol levels**. But despite the fatty food, despite their high cholesterol levels, they turned out to have **fewer than half the MI deaths of the rest of the country**.[17] Several other more recent studies have confirmed that those living on this 'Mediterranean diet' have lower incidences of both heart disease and cancer than do we in the English-speaking countries.

Recently I received a leaflet in the mail promoting a new grape extract, for the good of my heart. Here is what the leaflet said:

Scientists have long been intrigued by the phenomenon known as the French Paradox: The French diet is laden with saturated fat and cholesterol, yet the French have the lowest rate of heart disease of any Westernized society – nearly half that of the US. What's their secret to a longer, healthier life?

The leaflet went on to declare that it is the red wine the French drink that does it. This wine somehow counteracts the effect of all that fat and cholesterol. Therefore I should buy their new grape extract tablets.

There are two assumptions here: 1) that it **is** saturated fat and cholesterol that cause heart disease. And 2) that nobody but the French drink red wine. I would submit the leaflet is wrong on both counts. But anyway, if I must have red wine I prefer to have it in a glass, rather than in a tablet.

Of course more recent studies do indicate that drinking wine can benefit the heart, but they must be looked at with caution. Other studies indicate that alcohol can influence a tendency to more cancer in women. The main thing to be aware of is that saturated fat and cholesterol are not the causes of heart disease.

There are numerous other groups of people that positively wallow in saturated fat but have low rates of heart disease. A study similar to the Roseta study was done in 1970; it was called the Ireland Brothers Heart Study, comparing brothers living in Boston (US) and other brothers from the same family living in Ireland, a primarily dairy-farming nation.[18] The Boston brothers lived on a low-cholesterol diet – that is, low fat and using margarine and polyunsaturated oils. Meanwhile their brothers back in Ireland were pigging out on butter (a pound a week, approx 500 mg), plenty of cheese and eggs, etc. But when they added it all up, it was found that the butter-eating brothers in Ireland had fewer deaths from heart disease than their more cautious brothers in Boston.

Similar evidence came from Italy and from the Eskimos. The large quantities of fatty meats and fats consumed by Eskimos with their traditional diet produced no clogged arteries and no MI.

Two Polynesian island groups were compared, one with their traditional diet of highly saturated coconut fat, the other, a financially better off group which had Europeanized and whose members ate far fewer coconut fats. The latter group suffered from 25% hypertension (high blood pressure) in the males, while those wallowing in coconut fat had only 10% hypertension and no tendency to heart disease.

Then, in India, Dr S L Malhotra, head doctor for the Indian National Railway Systems, studied two different populations. There was a large vegetarian group eating polyunsaturated peanut oil and margarine in the south. This group had 15 times as many heart attack deaths as did the big butter-eaters in the north.[19] And this despite the fact that vegetarians generally fare better in heart disease statistics.

However, perhaps the most telling results came from the official American attempts to prove that the low-cholesterol diet was the way to go. Dr Wayne Martin tells the story, in his own inimitable style:[20]

Since 1956 there has been in place in the orthodox medical establishment the dogma, engraved in stone, that elevated cholesterol in food and blood causes heart attacks.

Part of this dogma is that saturated fats such as butter cause heart attacks while polyunsaturated fats such as in corn oil and margarine prevent deaths from heart attacks. A diet with low cholesterol, low in saturated fat was considered ideal. To establish this, first there was the Joliffe Anticoronary Study in New York City. Dr Joliffe was a diabetic and a vascular wreck. He looked to the standard Prudent Diet [this is Dr Martin's generic term for a low-cholesterol diet] for his salvation.

The control group was chosen because the members were big eaters of red meat with lots of cholesterol and saturated fat in their diet. The results of the Joliffe test were reported in 1966 as a great success. Serum cholesterol was reduced by 250 to 225 in the men on the Prudent Diet. Almost no mention was made of the fact that eight men on the Prudent Diet had died of heart attacks while none of the controls, eating all the 'wrong' things, had died. Then Dr Joliffe died of 'a vascular event', most likely a heart attack.[21] But it was reported that he had died of diabetes.

The reaction to this among the cholesterol orthodoxy was 'Well, if they could just get 500,000 or a million men on the Prudent Diet they could actually prove the point.' The result was the National Diet Heart Study. It was planned to a large degree by Dr Irving Page of the Cleveland Clinic. He had had a non-fatal heart attack. I met him at that time and he was absolutely convinced that the Prudent Diet would prevent him from having another heart attack. Before they got a million men involved in this huge test, they would start with 2,000. The results of this pilot test were reported in 1969 and there was no benefit at all from the Prudent Diet. The big million-man test was not undertaken 'for reasons of cost' and Dr Page died of a heart attack.[22]

Meanwhile a much better planned test was done in England by the Medical Research Council (MRC) in which the subjects had, like Dr Page, survived a heart attack. As with the [US] National Diet Heart Study, there was no benefit whatever due to the Prudent Diet. This British test was reported in 1966.[23]

Dr George Meinig, DDS, FACD, sums it up: 'In spite of all you hear from the American Heart Association and others, three recent studies show that eating foods containing cholesterol has never been proven implicit in the cause of heart disease.'[24]

Moreover, none of these studies assessed the effects of the low-cholesterol, polyunsaturated fat diet on the men's sex lives, but it cannot have been good, for as mentioned it is cholesterol which is the basis of sex hormones. However, despite all the **known** disasters, the average doctor today still wants the entire population to live on a low-cholesterol diet; moreover, doctors do not live any longer than the rest of us. On the contrary, a recent study of American Medical Association member obituaries (as reported in the *Journal of the American Medical Association*) put their average age of death at 57.6 years, or 5.5% shorter than the average US citizen's.[25] This has been queried as unrepresentative by some. However, for whatever reasons doctors do not appear to live even as long as the average. (There is further mention of this in Chapter 32.)

What is very plain is that there can be no doubt that polyunsaturated oils reduce cholesterol levels. There is also no doubt that these low levels do **not** prevent heart attacks. In fact, around half of the people who die of heart attacks fail to show high cholesterol levels. These cholesterol levels just seem to vary among individuals.

Worst of all, there is plenty of evidence that lowering cholesterol levels actually increases the cancer risk. It was the evidence for this that caused a *British Medical Journal* editorial to pose the question, *'Do polyunsaturated fatty acids cause cancer?'* The implication was that they did.[26]

One hundred years ago fewer than 6% of us died of cancer. Today it is 24%, and ever-increasing, especially among women. According to Dr Martin, cancer patients almost invariably have **low serum cholesterol levels**, and he believes that cholesterol has an anti-cancer effect. It may even be part of our defence system against cancer.

Dr Martin also tells of an interesting aspect of cigarette smoking. 'By 1930 80% of men smoked cigarettes, but death from lung cancer was rare. Nowadays with only 30% of men smoking cigarettes, death from lung cancer is 16 times more frequent.' And he links the increase to the cancer-causing effects of polyunsaturated fats. 'It is my contention that it is the combination of cigarette smoke and a big increase in polyunsaturated fats in the diet that has caused the vast pandemic of lung cancer.'[27] It is also significant because the tar content of cigarettes was much higher in those early days.[28]

Dr Martin may well be right. A recent *New England Journal of Medicine* article records high rates of smoking in Japan, but low rates of lung cancer. In those who take in significant fish oil, and do not take in hydrogenated fats, lung disease is less than half of those who do the reverse.

Dr A E Dugdale of the University of Queensland has a special interest in medical costs. In an extensive study he found that reducing serum cholesterol in the population would add considerably to the costs of medical treatment. Because there would then be more deaths from the more costly-to-treat cancer.[29]

But anyway, since most of us would prefer to go out with a heart attack, rather than cancer, what is the point of doing anything that increases our chances of getting cancer?

But unfortunately there's more. Studies have shown that the lower the cholesterol, the more likely men are to die from suicide or violent death:

650 consecutively admitted psychiatric inpatients were interviewed concerning lifetime history of attempted suicide, and the results were correlated with serum cholesterol

measured at the time of admission. Among the men, those at or below the 25th percentile for serum cholesterol were 2.2 times more likely to have made a serious suicide attempt than were those above the 25th percentile. There was no association between serum cholesterol and attempted suicide among the women.[30]

Dr Hyman Engelberg MD, writing in the *Lancet*, postulates that the reason could be that low cholesterol contributes to a decrease in brain serotonin, with 'poorer suppression of aggressive behaviour'.[31] And, presumably, this would include aggression towards oneself.

Pritiken, an American engineer suffering from leukaemia who designed the famous Pritiken diet, was one person who succeeded in dramatically lowering his cholesterol levels. But his leukaemia got worse and he took his life. It would seem that cholesterol may also be protective of our mental stability as well as of our sex lives, owing to the role it plays in the production of hormones.

(Later in this book we will be looking at the effects of cholesterol-lowering **drugs** when we look at Chapter 27 on prescription drugs.)

Perhaps the salient fact is that despite all the evidence – that is, that *'MI deaths have increased in direct ratio to the consumption of polyunsaturated fats as oils and margarines,'*[32] in the English-speaking countries almost nothing has been done to warn us as to the dangers of these 'plasticized' fats and oils, either by our medical advisors or by our own governments. Quite the contrary. Doctors are still, at least as of May 1997 in New Zealand, appearing on television with the advice to eat margarine and polyunsaturated oils. Meanwhile, by contrast, in Europe governments are more concerned with the truth, and that concern is reflected in what is and what is not permitted to be sold to the consumer. The type of margarine we in New Zealand are exhorted to eat is forbidden in most of Europe.

It is this unnecessary ignorance, or carelessness as to the certainty of millions of unnecessarily premature deaths that appalls me. Here are quotes from more of the best of doctors, the few who seem to be aware, or to care about what is going on:

Dr George V Mann, MD has said, 'Saturated fats and cholesterol are not the cause of coronary heart disease. That myth is the greatest scientific deception of this century, perhaps of any century.'[33]

And Dr Stephen E Langer, MD posed the practical question, the one that should concern us all: 'How did medical science ever get sidetracked into recommending the avoidance of dietary cholesterol and saturated fat, a practice which fails to address the basic problem?'[34]

Dr Robert Crayhan, reviewing Dr George Mann's book, *Coronary Heart Disease: The Dietary Sense and Nonsense*[35] reported as follows:

Dr Mann points out that 33 clinical trials have failed to show that cholesterol and saturated fat intake or cholesterol-lowering medication protect against coronary heart disease. The financial cost of such tests has been hundreds of millions of dollars. According to Dr Mann, these false accusations are not just a misunderstanding. They are perpetuated by scientists who fear they will lose funding if they do not go along with this politically correct theory and manufacturers who want to cash in on the erroneous paranoia. And as long as the accusation lives on that dietary cholesterol and saturated fat are the villains, more taxpayers' money will be wasted in an effort to prove it, and more lives will be lost due to dangerous medications and ineffective prevention.[36]

Professor Pinkney would go one step further: He says, 'Hitler did it. He was not the first but he did it quite successfully. "It" being the big lie. What is even worse, the big lie about cholesterol may well kill millions of people ...'

As we noted, Smith and Pinkney called their book *The Cholesterol Conspiracy*. It is a conspiracy because it continues out of ignorance, laziness, uncaringness and, moreover, so that the English-speaking world can be kept safe for the billion-dollar fats and oils industry, not to mention the billion-dollar pharmaceutical industry. It is just one of the reasons why our late 20th century is alas, sad, mad and bad. And there is perhaps no better evidence that at least in the English-speaking world, *no one is looking after our health*, mental, physical or any other kind.

(See also, Thomas J Moore's *Heart Failure*, Harcourt Brace, 1989.)

P.S. It is generally a waste of time for your doctor to investigate your cholesterol levels when what is truly relevant is your clotting potential – that is, 'platelet aggregation.' If there is a good result then your intake of fats and oils is not too bad, or you're very young and 'getting away with it!' If you have 'sticky platelets' then you definitely need to look to altering this part of your diet. Take vitamin E, and read on!

⚠️

2: MARGARINE AND HYDROGENATED OILS

'Eat up your delicious margarine.
It's better for your heart.'

Yes, margarine is lovely. It spreads ever so nicely. Moreover, you can leave it lying around for months or even years and it won't 'go off'. Nor will any animal, insect or microbe come near it. And that should tell us something important: The animals, insects and microbes must know something we don't know.

What they know is that there's nothing good in margarine, nothing worth the trouble of eating. In fact it's bad news for health, whether human health or other life. And especially bad for the human heart. And so are all the hydrogenated vegetable oils bottled in clear plastic or glass you can buy in the supermarket.

But the New Zealand Heart Foundation not only says they're OK; it recommends them.[1]

The Heart Foundations all over the world are misinformed and there is evidence that this misinformation has killed millions 'before their time'.

The US Surgeon General's report for 1988 (and similarly more recently), concluded that 15 out of every 21 deaths (more than ⅔) among Americans involve nutrition; that is deficiencies, excesses or imbalances.[2]

One of the world's foremost experts on the subject of fats and oils, Dr Udo Erasmus PhD of Vancouver, Canada, consultant in fats and oils, who wrote the world best-seller *Fats That Heal; Fats That Kill*, agrees with the Surgeon General's conclusion, but adds the concept of 'toxicity' or body poisoning. He claims that all degenerative diseases are caused by malnutrition and/or toxicity in the body, that fats can be highly toxic to the body; moreover he believes that eating the wrong fats and/or not enough of the right fats, *kills prematurely over ⅔ of the populations of affluent industrialized nations,* what we think of as 'the West'. And he breaks this down as follows:

Cardiovascular (Heart) disease	43.8%
Cancer	22.4%
Diabetes	1.8% [3]

Unfortunately, he says, medical doctors (with whom many of us entrust our lives) study disease, not health, and therefore know little on the vital subject of nutrition and its effects. And this despite several important findings on the subject reported in medical journals. We will look at those findings soon. The reason for the doctors' ignorance in this area: 'Their curriculum includes little or no nutrition, lots on pharmaceutical drugs, and nothing about the effects of processing fats and oils on human health.'[4]

On reading this huge book on fats and oils, one is amazed that there is such ignorance about their importance. And yet it is a fact that some years ago, the Paris press had a screaming headline:

MARGARINE STANDS INDICTED

and the *London Daily Express* echoed:

THE FAT IN YOUR FRYING PAN CAN BE DEADLY![5]

And yet we are still eating the stuff. Only always trying to eat less fat, and feeling guilty when we do.

'FAT!' These days the very word makes us shudder. Because we've been conditioned to think of fat *only* as the substance which prevents the slim and gorgeous person we really are from coming to the fore. Or that it will damage our hearts.

But FAT is essential to the health of every cell in the body, all '63 trillions' (at a rough estimate) of them. Fat is basic to life.

Here are some of the vital functions of fat in the body:

1 Fats are an important building material in cell membranes – that is, the outer shell of all of our cells, the cells of which we are composed, where they have vital roles to play in communication with other cells and with transporting nutrients into the cells and waste materials out of them.
2 They are also to be found in the myelin sheaths – that is, the covering of every nerve in our body. When the fat metabolism goes wrong and these sheaths do not work, we may develop Multiple Sclerosis.
3 The liver uses fats to transport numerous vital substances in the blood around the body.
4 Fat is used as part of the substance which helps the blood to clot, preventing us from bleeding to death in many different situations.

5 As mentioned, fats are the basis of the body's steroid hormones which control many body functions, the cardio-vascular system, sex and reproduction, the central nervous system and the immune system.

6 And there are many other body processes which use fats.

7 Most important of all, the *brain needs fats*, both to develop and to function well all through life.[6]

We simply *must* have some fat in the diet. Dr Udo Erasmus, one of the world's foremost experts on the subject, claims that we need 15 to 20% of the diet in fats, good fats. It should be clear that if we do not get the fats we need, we are in trouble. But any old fat just will not do. It's got to be the right kind of fat or fats to do all of the above.[7]

In the 1960s, under the unfortunate impression that it was fat, any and all fat, that caused arteriosclerosis or clogged arteries and heart attacks, Nathan Pritiken, the engineer we looked at briefly in Chapter 1, devised a diet in which the fat content was reduced to a minimum of 7% of the calories. He also believed in vegetable oils or polyunsaturates, as available on the market.

Through his conviction and the force of his personality, thousands of people became devoted to what came to be known as The Pritiken Diet, which in combination with plentiful exercise was supposed to bring us all to the promised land of healthy happy slimness, clean arteries and longer lives. It did clean out the arteries, but it did not bring long life. Pritiken, poor fellow, now has the cleanest arteries in the cemetery. He had leukaemia, a cancer of the blood and died too young, but he did not die of a heart attack. He took his own life. According to Dr Erasmus, 'Diets low in fats are deficient in essential fatty acids which inhibit tumour incidence and growth.'[8]

Dr Wayne Martin, scientist and health researcher, writing in the *Townsend Letter for Doctors*, tells it 'like it is':

The problem of preventing heart attack deaths and cancer deaths are intertwined both for good and for bad. While most doctors are telling one and all to have polyunsaturated fats in the diet to prevent deaths from a heart attack, there is evidence that they are actually increasing cancer deaths among us.[9]

(See Chapter 1 on cholesterol for his full account of the heart disease and cancer fiasco.)

A recent report in the extremely respectable *Archives of Internal Medicine* (vol 158, 1998: pages 41–5) confirms Dr Martin's thesis. Polyunsaturated oils may increase a woman's risk of breast cancer by 69%; while olive oil, a monosaturated fat, may actually reduce this risk by 45%.

For one of the most worrying discoveries of all has been that processed polyunsaturated oils are immunosuppressive. That is, they suppress the immune system, our defence against cancer. What is more, they are even more immuno-suppressive than the drugs designed for the purpose. This means that they prevent our immune systems from doing their job. And their job is, of course, to prevent cancer and infections. This was reported in Britain's most influential medical journal, the *Lancet* in 1978.[10] Does your doctor know about it?

What this means is that it has been known since 1978; it has been recorded in Britain's foremost medical journal, that polyunsaturated fats and oils, those lovely safflower and sunflower oils in the clear glass bottles, will dampen down the immune system. And yet who has acted upon this knowledge? And which governments have ensured that all of us would know and have a choice in what we eat or don't eat?

Dr Joanna Budwig of Germany, pioneer scientist in the world of fats in relation to health and seven times Nobel Prize nominee, has said this concerning fat and disease:

'Anatomically speaking, heart infarction observation studies reveal nothing abnormal in the picture except for solid fat, which encircles the normally lean heart muscle, confining and disturbing the heart's action.'[11] That is, on autopsy after a death from heart failure everything looks normal, except for the fact that the heart muscle is surrounded by solid fat. She also speaks of 'isolated fat' found in rheumatic tissue, that is, in painful muscles.[12]

Worst of all perhaps, the invention of the electron microscope has made it possible to see that the only difference between cancerous cells and healthy cells is 'isolated fat'.[13]

It seems that when fats are rejected by the body tissues, they are isolated and deposited in places where fats are not normally found. It is easy to see why people have in the past, and even now, blamed 'fat' for all our problems. But there is far more to it than that.

In an earlier time, each family or group of families produced its own food and ensured that it was both nourishing and safe. Later, people got their fats from butter in the local dairy or their oil from someone who grew olive trees or other oil-bearing plants. The oil was simply pressed out as needed ('cold-pressing'). The housewife or other person, would pick up the supply daily or every few days, because it was highly perishable and people could taste the difference between fresh butter or oil and the rancid or dangerous kind. Or sometimes there would be an 'oil-beater' going from door to door with the fresh product. Either way, once obtained it was stored in a covered ceramic jar, kept in a cool dark place and quickly consumed.[14]

In this manner each part of the world developed its own special oil, depending on what was available, for example fresh coconut oil is the oil of choice in the tropics. And living on these natural oils, people experienced very low rates of heart disease. Similarly, the Eskimos, who despite the fact that their natural diet includes enormous amounts of saturated fats from animal sources, have very low levels of heart disease. The Japanese also have low rates of heart disease with their natural diet. But today, when these groups give up their traditional diets and move to 'the West', or take up Western foods, their rates of heart disease, cancer and so on gradually become the same as for the rest of us. [15]

Our food troubles began when we ceased to be agrarian people and began to live in cities. Even so, up until 1920 most of the fats eaten were saturated and came mainly from animal sources – butter, lard or tallow.[16]

But as cities got bigger and bigger, the problem of feeding the inhabitants was eventually resolved by what today we call food technology. That is, the food technologists devised ways of preserving and presenting food so as to keep it long past the normal 'shelf life' of foods. And therein lie many problems. Particularly in the area of fats and oils.

After 1920, the manmade, highly refined fats came in – margarine, corn oil, sunflower oil and all the other vegetable oils. And since that time cancer deaths have increased threefold, and deaths from heart attacks 35 fold.[17]

Once again, it is not FAT per se that is killing us, but the *kinds* of fat we are eating.

In 1929, the most important parts of fats and oils, that which are known as Essential Fatty Acids (EFAs), were discovered by two scientists, Mildred and George Burr. They are called 'essential' because they cannot be manufactured in the body, but must be taken in regularly in the form of fats or oils, just as certain vitamins, minerals and amino acids are essential for human health, and must be taken in regularly.[18] The chemistry of these EFAs is complex, but suffice it to say that they are of many kinds and that each kind serves different purposes in the body.

They are essential for human health. But recent surveys have shown that 80% of the US population is deficient in these EFAs.[19] There is no reason to believe that the percentage would be much better in other parts of the English-speaking world. Moreover, inadequate EFA intake, among other causes, may contribute to Attention Deficit Disorder and/or hyperactivity in children.[20]

Laboratory animals deprived of EFAs will exhibit the following problems:

- Normal growth fails to occur.
- Wounds do not heal properly.
- In females pregnancy is rare, and if it does occur, miscarriage will usually follow.
- Hair falls out and skin problems develop.
- The body loses water through the skin, creating a concentrated urine and thirst.
- The kidneys fail.

- The liver degenerates.
- The glands atrophy.
- The immune system breaks down, and infections are common.[21]

These EFAs are considered so important that in 1977 the World Health Organization in Geneva, with agreement of the United Nations and the FAO in Rome, made the following recommendation:

In the light of present knowledge, it seems prudent to recommend that future lines of research follow these requirements for EFAs, that it is desirable that they are not lost by commercial processing and that the problem must be addressed by law.[22]

That statement is a very polite way of saying that manufacturers of processed fats should be controlled by law. And that in fact is what has happened in Continental Europe. It has *not* happened in the English-speaking countries.

As far as studies go, apart from the Pritiken diet which reduced fats in the diet to below 10%, we have not done experiments on *humans* wherein EFAs were completely eliminated, for obvious reasons.[23] But it has been found that infants fed formulas low in EFAs become irritable. They also develop large appetites and dry, scaly skin. When sufficient EFAs are added to the formula, the infants' appetites reduce and the skin clears rapidly.[24]

Another expert in the field is Dr Michael Crawford, formerly head of the Department of Nutritional Biochemistry at the Nuffield Institute of Comparative Medicine in London's Institute of Zoology, and now at the Institute of Brain Chemistry and Human Nutrition at the Queen Elizabeth Hospital for Children in London. He has a special interest in the history of evolution, the development of the human brain and degenerative diseases. Dr Crawford has found that there are two kinds of fat, as far as our bodies are concerned: the fat for storage and the structural kind.[25]

Stored fat is the stuff we need for energy; and these are the fats that become highly visible, not just in the bay window, but also in diseased tissues at autopsy. It is generally the stuff the body is forced to store because it cannot do anything else with it once it has used what it needs for energy.

In terms of our evolution, Dr Crawford believes that it was *structural fats*, or the Essential Fatty Acids, in the form of a fish diet, that made possible Homo Sapiens through the development of our complex brains and central nervous systems.[26] So if we were told to *'eat up your fish; it's good for your brain,'* whoever told you this was absolutely right.

It is this structural fat we need for all the vital tasks in the body. And the different fatty acids all provide differing building materials for different jobs in the body. For example, the outer sheaths of the nerves need saturated fats (from animal products) for rigidity, while it is unsaturated fats (from vegetable sources, but not the commercially made hydrogenated variety) that are needed for the softer linings of the arteries.[27]

Of the whole body, the brain has the greatest need for the right kind of fats. It is said that less than half of our brain development occurs during foetal life. And that this development must continue on throughout life. It is therefore of the utmost importance that pregnant and nursing women have the right kind of diet. What they need are the EFAs. 'Many authorities recommend that pregnant and nursing women consume fatty fish two to three times weekly and/or add a minimal amount of flax seed oil to their diets to insure adequate intake of EFAs.'[28] And as we have noted, 'good' fats should be around 15 to 20% of the calories in our diets. But studies have shown that 'American mothers produce milk that often has only one fifth to one tenth of the Omega 3 (the fish-oil fatty acid) content of the milk that well-nourished, nut-eating Nigerian mothers provide their infants.'[29]

In March of 1991, the US Mayo Clinic reported on a study of 19 'normal' pregnant women on 'normal' diets, a study which found all were deficient in the EFAs.[30] (It is also said that premature infants need more of the EFAs from fish oil, for it is they who are most at risk in their brain development.) Unfortunately, manufactured infant formulas are almost completely devoid of EFAs, as they contain the fairly useless and damaging refined products. In fact Dr Joseph G Hattersley believes there is an association between these marketed infant formulas and a percentage of crib deaths (SIDS).[31] According to Dr Finnegan, 'There are many serious consequences of generation after generation having diets deficient in an element essential for normal development of the nervous system.'[32] These dangerous and abnormal fats are not, of course, the only possible cause of SIDS. There are several, and we will look at them later.

We have in our time already seen the effects of not consuming sufficient EFAs and taking in the wrong kinds of fats. We have seen it in the sudden deaths and the clogged arteries so common today. And in the rise of Multiple Sclerosis we are already seeing signs of nervous system deterioration. For everywhere in the world the rise of MS follows the rise in heart disease, Alzheimer's Disease and mental ill health.

A lack of EFAs is also believed to be implicated in arthritis and cancer, other degenerative diseases and skin diseases.[33] With the majority of people these days being deficient in the EFAs, we must therefore ask the question: What is happening to our children's brains? Not to mention the rest of us? 'The frightening news is that for the past three generations ... the majority of the people in North America have not been given adequate nourishment for complete brain development.'[34] One can assume that this would also be true of the UK and some of the Commonwealth countries.

But it is not only that EFAs are essential to health in many ways, it is also that one is *never really satisfied* unless there is a certain level in the diet. For, as noted, we should have 15 to 20% of the calories or kilocalories in fats and oil, of the right kind.[35]

Here is what happens to conscientious dieters: Under the current misinformation about the role of fats in our health, they cut their fat intake back to the minimum. In addition they are probably not getting the right fat when they do eat it. They try very hard not to cheat. But their bodies, desperately needing the EFAs to do the thousands of things they are needed for, keep screaming out, 'More food!' 'More food!' So the hapless dieter keeps getting the message in the form of 'I'm hungry! I'm hungry!' So they gorge on anything but fat in the attempt to stem the *'I'm hungry!'* message. But no matter how much they eat, so long as the EFAs are missing they will still essentially be hungry, a situation reminiscent of the Mad Hatter's tea party. And they cannot be healthy. It is likely that most reducing diets fail because there is not enough fat in them.

A most interesting point is that when animals are to be **fattened** for market, the fat is eliminated from their diets, and cereals are greatly increased.[36] But this is precisely what **we** usually do when trying to **lose** weight! Fat actually burns off fat.

To look at what has happened to our fats since early in our century, first we must consider the desire on the part of manufacturers to make as much money as possible. To do this they use the cheapest materials available and the cheapest processes. They then are in a position to price their products well under that of the equivalent 'natural' product and thus to drive it out of the market. They did this for some decades. However, on capturing much of the market they then let the price rise until it reaches the level of the 'natural' product, the real fat. At least in New Zealand that is the case.

But food is not 'a product', or should not be. It is essential for health, for life itself. It should be rigorously controlled.

And here is what has happened to our precious EFAs:

In order to produce fats and oils which will not age, go rancid, 'go off', food manufacturers subject them to enormous heat, sometimes up to 1000°F. During this intense heating, hydrogen is bubbled through the oil and forced under pressure into the boiling fat molecules, as one account would have it, 'in the presence of nickel, aluminium or other heavy metal'.[37] A small amount of these metals are retained in the fat and are, of course, toxic to the human body.

Through these and other processes the oils are 'hydrogenated' 'deodorized', 'winterized', 'bleached' and 'refined'. And under these processes, especially the enormous heat and pressure, most of the naturally-occurring nutrients we need are lost: almost all of the vitamin E, lecithin, beta-carotene and the Essential Fatty

Acids. For there is no way these fats and oils can be subject to such heat and pressure, so altered, without losing vital nutrients.[38] (And most of these are the nutrients we need to prevent heart attacks and cancer.)

Once the fat or oil is 'hydrogenated' it will last indefinitely. The margarine is packaged attractively in plastic tubs; the oil is placed in clear glass or plastic bottles. And if they remain just so, sitting in the kitchen in all weathers, just what will happen to them inside our bodies?

In particular, the harder fats, the margarine, will remain firm in the body also. Scientists who have studied these effects speak of the 'stickiness' of margarine in the body. This 'stickiness' makes for 'sticky blood platelets', 'thick' blood, one of the worst initiators of clots and heart disease. And that is why so many of us are on drugs to 'thin' the blood. They also instigate fatty deposits in the arteries, liver and other organs. They change cell membranes for the worse by making our cells more permeable, so that undesirable substances can penetrate.[39]

Worst of all, the process of hydrogenating fats creates entirely 'new' molecules forced into shapes they were never designed to be in.[40] They are, in effect, poisonous to the body. And the name of the monster which emerges from these fortune-making fat factories is **Trans Fatty Acids**. 'Trans', the name for these Frankenstein fats, was a term dreamed up somewhere near the laboratory. It is yet another example of the subversion of the language for commercial reasons. For 'trans' implies positive things like 'transformation', 'transfiguration'. Whereas in truth the fat has not been transformed, it has been **deformed**.

Trans Fatty Acids (TFAs) can be seen as deformed monsters let loose upon the world. There were no such things in existence before modern food technology. And therefore our bodies were not designed to cope with them. It is as though these deformed molecules are maverick keys that do not open doors. Worse, just as we can sometimes get the wrong key in a lock but it will not turn, they do this and then prevent any good fat molecules from gaining entrance and permitting the body to function normally, or as it would with real molecules. And as we have seen, the metabolism of fats affects each and every organ in the body.[41]

Thus it is that the TFAs have been found to be a major cause of heart disease and cancer, for they do not fit in the body at all.[42] And what the body has to do with substances it cannot use is 'stash 'em in the arteries' and elsewhere. They become a part of our blood and all our cells.

It is said that early in the Second World War the country of Norway had almost all of its margarine stocks confiscated by the Germans as part of the 'spoils of war'. In this case the booty was not well named, for it would never spoil. And by the end of the war Norway had one-third the rate of heart attacks it usually did. But after the war the margarine came back, of course, and gradually the rate of heart attacks increased to the 'normal' rate.[43]

An important study, confirming that margarine and refined cooking and salad oils contribute to heart disease and cancer, was conducted in the Netherlands by two Dutch scientists and in 1990 was reported in the most esteemed of all American medical journals, *The New England Journal of Medicine*,[44] and also in the *Journal of Lipid Research* in 1992.[45]

In April 1995, a Danish Nutrition Council report commenting on this and other studies suggested that it is the trans fatty acids in margarine that are responsible for arteriosclerosis, rather than the much-maligned saturated animal fats.[46] In Europe today, trans-fats are severely restricted. Some countries permit no more than 0.1% in food products. In contrast, margarines in the English-speaking countries may contain up to 30 to 50%. The only margarine that is used, or permitted on the European continent, is a much more expensive version made of coconut and olive oils, quite different in food value from the stuff permitted in most English-speaking countries. In fact in Denmark and Holland, the kind of margarine sold in the US and New Zealand, Australia and other English-speaking nations is outlawed, and *anything* with TFAs in it must state the levels on the label.[47]

But perhaps the most conclusive study on the effects of margarine and hydrogenated oils was carried out at the Harvard School of Public Health where 85,095 nurses were studied over a period of 13 years. The study was actually set up to prove that margarine and hydrogenated vegetable oils were safer for the heart! But instead they found the complete reverse. Those who consumed the highest intakes of TFAs had the highest rates of heart disease. Reporting in the most prestigious of British medical journals, the *Lancet*, Dr Walter Willet MD concluded that the Danish and the Harvard studies had together established an 'unequivocal causal relation between the TFAs and the risk of heart disease'.[48] Even the most conservative *Harvard Health Letter* referred to trans-fats as 'the new enemy'.[49]

Following the publication of these accounts in both of the world's most influential medical journals, and elsewhere, studies so emphatically damning of the consumption of margarine and hydrogenated oils, there is absolutely no excuse for the cardiologists who advise Heart Foundations around the world, or the average doctor, to continue exhorting people suffering from heart disease to eat this dangerous rubbish. For the effects on people of this 'advice', it amounts in my view to criminal negligence.

These were not the first warnings about these dangerous fats and oils. As early as 1956, the *Lancet* cautiously warned that:

... coronary artery disease becomes in part a preventable disorder, but at the cost of a complete revolution in our present-day dietary habits. The hydrogenation plants of our modern food industry may turn out to have contributed to the causation of a major disease.[50]

It has been a warning ignored for 43 years by governments and many doctors. Wayne Martin: 'The threefold increase in our consumption of hydrogenated polyunsaturated fat has over 90 years resulted in a 35-fold increase in heart attack deaths and a three-fold increase in cancer deaths.'[51]

The problem is that today it is difficult to avoid the TFAs. Their presence in the diet has increased 50-fold in the last 20 years. If you eat bought cakes, biscuits and cheese made from hydrogenated fats, commercially fried foods, most breads and a thousand other products, there it will be. Check the labels.

Dr Mary Enig, research associate in the Department of Chemistry and Biochemistry at the University of Maryland has studied Trans Fatty Acids for decades. She has analysed 600 foods for their TFA content, and after all those foods and all those years, she concluded that Americans eat 11 to 28 grams of TFAs a day, or up to 20% of their daily diet.[52]

As if all this were not enough, there is something else. In order to get that lovely 'butter' colour, there is a yellow dye added to margarine. For this, they often use cadmium, which is a toxic metal, alien to the body. What is more, cadmium interferes with the absorption of zinc, a mineral vital to our health, especially to the immune system.[53]

We need to buy fresh butter, and oils that have not been heated – that is, we need 'cold-pressed' oils in dark glass bottles. For even the best of olive oil will in time become full of dangerous free radicals in a clear glass bottle.

But perhaps the worst blow of all: Dr Finnegan claims that some unscrupulous health shop owners simply buy cheap processed oils from commercial sources and put their own 'cold-pressed' label on them. And naturally they cost more than the supermarket variety. So that even those of us aware of the need for cold-pressed oils can get 'conned' into buying more worthless dangerous oil.[54]

It looks as though in the absence of any serious policing in this highly critical area, we are all of us out on that vast and dangerous highway which is Food Consumerism, 'playing chicken' all the time with most of our purchases.

And when I say 'playing chicken', I mean quite seriously that we are gambling with our lives, or the length of them. But we must not fall into the error of blaming those who make these fats for the market. They are producing something people are led to believe they want and need, and make fortunes out of doing so. This is the way of the 'free market'. They cater to our love of ease. And they have so much money left over after producing their toxic fats that they can spend a king's ransom on 'image-making' and on lies to tell us how good margarine is for us. 'Staying Alive!' is the phrase that comes to mind.

That these lies are permitted in the face of overwhelming evidence that refined fats and oils are killers, will be one of the marvels of the next century. And they will surely have a great deal to marvel at. They will surely marvel at the fact that the knowledge of the dangers of trans-fats has been around for many years, but that the fat processors have succeeded in keeping it quiet.

With hopefully more enlightened food laws and practices in the future, we will then be looked back upon as incredibly naive and ignorant to have accepted this unbelievable exploitation for most of our century. 'How can it have happened?' will be the question asked. For just as we think of people who used leeches to bleed the sick as pathetically ignorant, so they will regard us. In fact leeches, and 'bleeding', in a small way, actually make a lot more sense than eating TFAs.[55]

The fault in the English-speaking countries must truly lie in the failure of 'medical science' to show sufficient interest in nutrition and to make known the facts about fat, and with governments who do not care enough about the health of their peoples to act in this regard, as have some governments in continental Europe.

As noted in the Introduction, we have the technology to put a man into space and to watch him walk on the moon. But we could do nothing to prevent that very man having a heart attack at 43.[56] It is my belief that that heart attack could have been prevented.

I did not plan to take so long to tell this story. But it is not a straightforward one. To summarize:

1 It is very bad advice to *'keep your fats low'*. We need 15–20% of our food to be in fat, good fat. Every cell in our body needs it. That is, we need the Essential Fatty Acids.[57]
2 If we attempt to lose weight without sufficient good fats and oils, we will always be hungry. We will fail.
3 The body cannot handle margarine and hydrogenated oils. Eating these fats will clog up our arteries, our hearts, probably initiate dangerous blood clots, cause cancer and impair brain development in our children and in ourselves. They are *killers*. And that is why sales are controlled or forbidden in Europe.

The evidence clearly shows that we can indeed prevent this epidemic if we will just look at it and act upon it. For the truth is very simple. All we have to do is choose the right fats and exercise care in their preservation and consumption and we can enjoy better health, that is, *if* we are able to get hold of them.

We must do it, moreover the future of the human race will depend upon the brains and the health of our children. It is therefore imperative that there be an awareness that our bodies are designed to utilize natural foods, foods that contain nutrients, foods that spoil. If they do not 'go off' it is time to start worrying about them. In other words, a longer shelf life for foods will diminish *our* shelf lives.

For the right fats to eat see the section on the next page entitled 'What Fats and Oils are Safe to Eat?'.

EMERGENCY ADVICE

Vitamin E reduces the stickiness of platelets: 800 iu per day.

Other nutrients for the heart: magnesium; B_6, garlic, onions, fresh ginger root, L-Carnitine, cayenne. And see the end of Chapter 5 for other suggestions.

WHAT FATS AND OILS ARE SAFE TO EAT?

1 *Butter* should be eaten in preference to margarine, but it must not be rancid. To this end, keep it cool or frozen. Avoid putting it into a dairy compartment, the so-called 'butter conditioner' which is really the 'butter warmer' or 'butter rancidifier'. Only small amounts as needed for the next day should be put into the warmer parts of the refrigerator or left out at room temperature. Yellow outer bits should be discarded. In cooking, butter should not be heated to the smoking point, but at least it will not form TFAs when heated. Our ancestors ate butter for centuries without apparent harm, in fact many long-lived groups did.

2 *Olive oil* is wonderful! It is probably in part responsible for the low rates of heart disease and cancer in the Mediterranean peoples and other groups who consume it.[58] That and the equally health-bringing and marvellous garlic. But it must be bought from a trustworthy source, must preferably be in a dark glass bottle or tin, and should have on the label the words 'virgin' and 'cold-pressed'. Buy it in small quantities if possible. Once opened, keep it in the refrigerator. If it should become too hard to pour, it can be softened by placing it in warm (not hot) water. But it can remain fresh for some time out of the refrigerator if kept in a cool dark place, depending on how old it was when bought.

3 *Coconut oil* is an exceptionally fine oil. Dr Ray Peat of the International University of Mexico praises it highly and uses it extensively himself. It does not go rancid; it enables one to eat less as one can go longer without getting hungry. Unfortunately, hard to find in a pure form.[59]

4 *Flax seed oil* (linseed) is among the best. It must be bought in a dark bottle from the refrigerator section of a health food shop you can trust. It should bear an expiration date, as ideally should all fats and oils. It should be kept in the refrigerator. Dr Budwig has experimented with flaxseed oil for decades. She claims it is the best oil we can eat, that it contains the right balance of EFAs for human health. She also claims that a mixture of flaxseed oil and plain yogurt or cottage cheese (8 tablespoons in 100 grams, divided over the day) will over time dissolve hard deposited fats and thus cure cancer, heart disease and arthritis. She allows a little honey with it, and thus it can be

quite delicious. She claims to have turned around people in the last stages of cancer and heart disease with this mixture. If people are too ill even to eat, she puts flaxseed oil into the bowel.

5   *Evening Primrose Oil.* Taken as a supplement this is a most excellent oil and a source of EFAs, especially Omega 6. There has been much research done recently attesting to the value of EPO in most modern diseases. Keep in the refrigerator.

6   *Fish Oil,* taken either in the form of frequent oily fish or in capsules, contains EFAs necessary for a thousand processes in the body. A source of the essential Omega 3.

7   *Hemp Oil* is another first rate one, especially as it can readily be grown without pesticides. Hemp seeds can be ground into butter, a butter far superior to peanut butter, which is often full of carcinogenic aflatoxins. Also hemp fibre has numerous uses in textiles, rope and paper. However, government hysteria usually makes this one difficult to obtain and use.

8   *Tahini paste; nut and seed butters.* Spreads worth a try, provided the seeds and nuts are obtained without having been grown with pesticides and are not rancid. Should be kept in the refrigerator.

9   *Sesame Oil.* Used by many Asian groups for their stir-frying. Best for cooking when unrefined. But again, do not let it smoke.

Recommended Daily Intake of Flaxseed Oil[60]

¼ teaspoon for non-nursing infants 1 to 6 months
½ teaspoon for non-nursing infants 6 to 12 months
1–2 teaspoons for 1 to 2 year olds
2 teaspoons for children over 2 years
1–2 tablespoons for adults.

3: MILK

'Drink up your lovely milk; it's good for you
and it'll give you strong bones.'

If we look back once again to that 'idyllic' pastoral life we gave up to live in cities, the fresh unpasteurized cow's milk we had then was not truly suitable for us, being designed for calves, not humans, but it did contribute vitamins, minerals and enzymes to our health. It also had natural antibodies against bacteria. So even though it wasn't 'what nature intended' there were some nutrients we could use.

According to Dr Joseph G Hattersley MD, physician and medical researcher, back in 1929 the Mayo Clinic in the US used to cure patients with anaemia, high blood pressure, tuberculosis and many other diseases by feeding them with large quantities of raw milk.[1] Also, those areas of the world where dwelt people known for their good health and great longevity: the Caucacus mountains of Russia, the village of Vilcamba in Ecuador, and the land of the Hunza in northern India – all these people took in the whole unprocessed milk product. And there were many other healthy groups of people using fresh cow's milk.

But once we in the so-called 'developed world' left our individual family cows and the farms, milk began to be pasteurized – that is, boiled to 145°F for 30 minutes, to kill off any possible unwanted bacteria. And in the process most of those useful nutrients were killed off, particularly the enzymes without which milk is difficult to digest. The pancreas has difficulty replacing these enzymes. A lack of them can cause the pancreas to be overstressed, and sometimes this can initiate diabetes, especially in children.[2] The change was unfortunate in other ways also, because within two years there was a sudden rise in deaths from heart attack and stroke.[3] There was also an increased risk of cataracts, especially among people with diabetes.

But anyway, plain or pasteurized, the milk was different back then. It had large fat particles that drifted to the top of a clear glass bottle. This fatty layer on the top was called 'the cream', 'the top o' the milk' and doubtless other names. A Canadian friend tells me that in his childhood the kids used to bring in the milk all frozen stiff, used to pry off that creamy layer, pour maple syrup over it, and eat it like ice cream.

In our less rigorous New Zealand climate I remember 'the top o' the milk' being prized as something creamy to pour over the breakfast oatmeal porridge. With brown sugar it was a tasty treat. But it was a rare treat because the adults usually got to it first to put in their tea or coffee.

All this is largely the stuff of nostalgia now. In 1936 homogenization came to the US, a few years later to most other countries, to some many years later. Britain remains one of the few countries where un-homogenized milk can still be had. For the rest of us, there are fewer and fewer who remember what milk was like before it was 'homogenized'. Possibly the reason we have survived to remember it is that we gave up drinking milk about the time they started homogenizing it!

Homogenized milk has the fat uniformly distributed throughout the paler, thinner stuff. And whereas in those old nostalgic times, after the body had taken all the good stuff from the milk it wanted, the fat particles were too large to be dealt with so they passed harmlessly out; today we have those teeny tiny particles of fat which do not pass out of the body. Now they can go through the intestinal mucosa and into the bloodstream. So the body is confronted with yet another alien substance like margarine. What to do with it? Nothing else we can do but stash it in the arteries, the joints, the heart and so on. After all, we are not calves. We cannot really use that kind of fat.

By the 1950s, after the advent of margarine and homogenized milk, young men 'in the prime of life' were found to have arteries such as had never been seen before, except in much older men.

Undoubtedly these entirely abnormal fats in the arteries and elsewhere are among the several reasons why men are dropping dead younger and younger in our time, and why heart disease is also sharply on the increase among women, who have in the last decade been urged to increase the level of dairy to 'protect your bones'.

Above all there is that one overriding basic truth about cow's milk. It is not really designed for humans. And we humans (and mainly 'Westerners' at that) **are the only species** who drink any variety of the stuff past infancy. Of course your domesticated cat may actually drink it given the chance, but it will die sooner from doing so, just as we will.

Cow's milk is designed to fatten calves. It has way more fat (six times as much) as human breastmilk, which *was* actually designed for us. You should see how enormously calves grow in just a year! In fact, on this milk they double their weight in 47 days, and can weigh up to 1,000 pounds within a year. Dr Morton

Walker says that the milk industry claims whole milk is only 3.5% fat. But the 3.5% figure is based on weight, and most of the weight in milk is water. The amount of calories provided by fat in whole milk is actually 50%, over 14 times the quantity claimed.[4] He also says that 20% of Caucasians and 90% of Black and Asian people lack the enzyme lactase necessary for the digestion of milk. This lack will cause milk to be toxic to them, and cause cramps, bloating and diarrhoea. It can also be a problem in Polynesians. Then too, there's a lot of milk-related eczema in these groups.

As a young girl I spent over five years 'doing time' in boarding schools, and there we were encouraged to drink milk at every meal. Also the New Zealand Government, in its concern for our health (and for the milk surpluses) inflicted a pint of the stuff on us almost every school day. So no wonder most of my fellow boarders looked like fattened calves. All but me. They used to envy me my skinny body. But then I had tuberculosis and barely survived it.

But even more things have happened to milk since homogenization, at least in some parts of the world. In order to make more money out of cows, in order to get them to produce three times the milk they do normally, they are fed on a substitute high protein, a soy-based diet which produces abnormally large pituitary glands in the cows.[5] These cows are not therefore well, and need antibiotics to keep them going. In some countries the cows are also given hormones. The addition of these foreign substances cannot do anything for either the cows or their milk, or for those who drink it, but the practice earns more money for the dairy man, or more likely for the conglomerate which owns the farm. There are, in fact, some who speculate that the high fat content in milk and these additives are the possible reasons for the earlier onset of menstruation in girls in many Western countries.

One of the worst bits of news is that in terms of nutrients, homogenized *skim* milk is actually worse than plain homogenized milk, because without the butterfat the body cannot cope with what few vitamins and minerals remain after pasteurization and homogenization. Moreover, synthetic vitamin D, known to be toxic, is added to replace the natural vitamin D lost in the butterfat.[6]

Worse, nonfat *dried* milk contains oxidized or rancid cholesterol, which is the kind that promotes heart disease. And this dried milk is often added to whole milk. Dr Hattersley believes that it is this substance added to infant formulas that causes or contributes to crib death or SIDS.[7] (It is not, however, the only cause. We will be looking at another later on.)

So of course human breastmilk is best for human babies. It has everything nature intended for the survival and flourishing of the human race: the Essential Fatty Acids for the brain, the beginnings of immunity and all sorts of other nourishment for the tiny infant. (That is, of course, provided the mother is well nourished.)

Two studies reported in the *Lancet* establish that breastfed children have higher IQs and fewer nervous system dysfunctions than those fed commercially-made formulas.[8]

Commercially-made infant formulas will contain homogenized cow's milk, as well as those 'deformed' fatty acids, the TFAs. And the poor infant is designed to cope with neither. We should also recall (Chapter 2) that the Essential Fatty Acids (EFAs) are essential for brain development. An estimated 25% of today's children have some form of learning disability. The children raised on commercially prepared formulas are not getting their best start in life, to put it *very* mildly. If substitutes for human milk must be used, it is preferable to make one's own formula from the best ingredients. (See page 35 for two recipes.)

To be more specific, the following is a little list or summary of the health problems found to be related to the consumption of homogenized cow's milk:

1   Since 1992 there has been evidence for the allergenicity of milk, when it was found that a peptide in cow's milk causes histamine release in humans.[9] Milk therefore increases mucous production, and the development of allergies can lead to bedwetting, asthma, eczema, recurrent infections, abdominal pain, fatigue and depression.[10]

2   The American Academy of Pediatrics *recommends against* giving infants under one year whole cow's milk because it causes blood loss from the intestinal tract. This blood loss is directly linked to iron deficiency anaemia and it is estimated that over one-third of iron-deficiency anaemia is caused by gut bleeding due to cow's milk allergy.[11]

3   Also, based on a Finnish study, the American Academy of Pediatrics recommends against cow's milk because, as mentioned, studies in several countries have linked cow's milk to insulin-dependent diabetes, which often develops during childhood. Apparently the 'foreign' proteins in cow's milk cause the human child's body to make antibodies against them at an early stage. These antibodies then not only attack the protein, they also destroy the similar pancreatic cells that produce insulin. And hence diabetes.[12] However, another more recent study from the University of Colorado School of Medicine did not find this relationship between milk and diabetes in children.[13] So we must take our choice on these studies. It must always be remembered that in today's world there are very few disinterested (in the sense of impartial) 'scientific studies', which does of course make it difficult to choose. (Unfortunately it is often a case of 'he who pays the piper calls the tune.' And we cannot be certain who is calling the tune. If there are conflicting studies, sometimes one can decide by asking 'Cui Bono?' that is, 'Who stands to gain?' Not in this case, of course.)

4   In adults there is evidence for the devastation of the arteries and the implication of homogenized milk as a factor in heart disease, cancer, allergies, asthma, arthritis, autoimmune diseases and cataracts.[14] Dr Kurt A Oster MD, former Chief of Cardiology

at Park City Hospital, Bridgeport, Connecticut, and co-author of *The XO Factor*, believes that the milk fat enzyme Xanthine Oxidase 'initiates over 50% of all heart disease'.

In 1981 Dr Stephen Seely of the University of Sheffield reported on the results of an epidemiological study to assess heart disease in relation to homogenized milk. To do this, the amounts of milk protein in grams in the average daily diet were assessed in different countries: Finland had 30.4; Germany 14.1; Yugoslavia 8.1, and Japan 2.5. All the milk consumed in the Seely study had been homogenized.[15]

The heart attack rates were as follows: Finland had double the heart attack rates of Germany, four times the rate of Yugoslavia, and 10 times the rate of Japan.

Research shows that the key issue, the stuff that really does the damage in homogenized milk, is a substance known as Xanthine Oxidase (XO) in the milk fat. This is the substance that reaches the heart only through the consumption of homogenized milk. If the milk has not been homogenized (and the fat therefore has not been broken down into tiny particles), the Xanthine Oxidase cannot get near the human heart. But it is now found at autopsy in the diseased section of the heart and in the arterial walls of heart attack victims. For this XO destroys a substance called plasmalogen which makes up nearly a third of an arterial cell membrane.[16] Furthermore, it has been established that the XO comes from cow's milk and not from the patient's own body. Only the homogenization of milk makes it possible for XO to be absorbed into the human circulatory system.

And we cannot congratulate ourselves on avoiding these gruesome possibilities by drinking homogenized *skim* milk, as the XO is also very much present in this.

(At this gloomy point I must spread one tiny germ of joy for us cheese lovers. And that is that cheese does not count in at least *this* health problem. Because cheese is apparently *not* homogenized. And of course I do not refer to that extraordinarily hideous plastic cheese made from hydrogenated fat, which is unworthy of the name of 'cheese' and might better be employed for patching the roof. And, joy of joys, it is said that real cheese contains something magical which helps to prevent tooth decay. Altogether, excuses for me to wallow in it. Most plain yoghurt should also be safe, provided it is based on non-homogenized milk and made without the use of dried milk solids.)

Then there is that gross misinformation about homogenized milk, or even non-homogenized milk, that it will 'build bonny bones'. While dairy products do contain large amounts of calcium, most of the calcium never gets absorbed by the body, for it is difficult to use this source of calcium for the purpose of building bones. And the older we get the harder it is to absorb or use that calcium. In fact people who drink milk and take in lots of dairy in the hope of 'building strong bones' actually have the highest rates of osteoporosis, that is the inadequate kind of bone which will go crunch when you have a fall, or even go crunch *before* you fall. And these are breaks which are long and difficult to heal. Dr Nancy Appleton, author of *Healthy Bones*, maintains that there is a complex system of relationships among minerals which, if not in balance, causes bone loss.[17]

Consider the elephants and those wonderful horses with the big feet. They can pull enormous weights. They do this for years. Their muscles have to be powerful, their bones hard and tough. When did you last see an elephant or a Clydesdale horse drinking a glass of milk? What do they eat?

There are rules for building bones. There's not an entirely different set of rules for humans. We are animals too. Unfortunately humans often get things wrong. We get bad advice because someone wants to make money out of us. But we have subtle brains. How did they become so very milk-washed?

You may be tempted to say that you've never seen a cow with osteoporosis. But they probably get all the minerals they need from the grass. And also they are not foolish enough to drink their own milk past infancy. Moreover, as we have noted, this milk was designed for calves, infant cows only, certainly not for humans or infant humans.

The main issue is that in order to absorb the calcium in dairy products the body needs magnesium and other minerals. But dairy products contain very little magnesium. In fact there is nine times more calcium than there is magnesium in dairy products.[18] In prescribing these minerals, naturopaths today think in terms of 1:1 Ca:Mg, that is, equal amounts.

Without magnesium the body can use at best only 20 to 30% of the calcium in food or supplements. Magnesium also prevents the unusable calcium from becoming deposits that lead to arteriosclerosis, arthritis and kidney stones. For magnesium is the mineral which determines whether the substance that withdraws calcium from the bones or the one that deposits it takes precedence. And magnesium is only one of the minerals involved in calcium metabolism. Iron retention is also affected.[19] And there are 15 other minerals involved. Dr Nancy Appleton, PhD, author of *Healthy Bones: What you need to know about osteoporosis*, declares that 'excess calcium affects iron retention, magnesium depletion and causes other mineral imbalances'.[20]

Dr Sherry A Rogers MD, the brilliant environmental physician, also declares that it is dangerous to take in calcium without the necessary trace elements magnesium, boron, zinc, manganese and so on. That on its own, the calcium does not get put into the bone, but rather is laid down in areas of inflammation: the blood vessels of the heart and brain. And this calcification of blood vessels we call 'arteriosclerosis'. Remember (Chapter 1) that 'the clog' is 95% calcium. Also, by taking in calcium on its own we are accelerating the ageing process, as well as the many degenerative diseases that accompany it, like hypertension, diabetes, heart disease, arthritis and cancer.[21]

The PCRN, the American Physicians Committee for Responsible Medicine, recently issued a bulletin entitled 'Milk, No Longer Recommended or Required'. Dr Neil Barnard, MD, President of the PCRN, warns that athletes, especially body builders, would be wise to avoid dairy products:

The animal protein in cow's milk causes calcium wastage and calcium loss from the bone. In 1981 the *Journal of Nutrition* had more than one report demonstrating the negative effects the sulphur-containing proteins in dairy products had on calcium and bone ... Interestingly, plant protein does not seem to cause the same problems. If you look at the strongest known animals, the bull, oxen, horse, gorilla, and elephant, all with beautiful musculature and incredibly strong bones, they are all complete vegetarians. They have no need for tissue or dairy protein in their diets and yet support dense, strong muscles and bones.

It's true. As mentioned, I've never seen an elephant, or even a horse, drinking a glass of milk.

So today we have the Mad Hatter's tea party approach of most of the medical profession who, on the whole, advise women to take in more calcium, prescribing both more dairy and, in addition one of the vast numbers of calcium tablets the pharmaceutical companies convince them to prescribe, as seen in huge glossy advertisements in the medical journals. The result has been that the sales of both dairy products and these supplements have soared in recent years. (Even worse, they sometimes throw in fluoride tablets for good measure. More on this in Chapter 10.) But not knowing about the necessity for magnesium for a thousand different purposes in the body, those giving this advice can thereby create a serious imbalance in the very people they are trying to help. And of course the doctors then wind up prescribing *calcium blockers* for the ensuing heart disease.

If we were talking about Martians or The Dark Ages this just might be mildly amusing. But we are talking about our fellow human beings and their lives.

Coronary heart disease is today the leading cause of death in women in the US. Annually, 250,000 American women die of this; of these, 100,000 are considered 'premature deaths'.[22] Also these heart attacks, formerly considered primarily a 'male problem', since 1988 have actually been occurring in greater numbers in women than in men.[23]

Also, in susceptible women, taking in large amounts of calcium with too little magnesium can result in mood swings, anxiety, depression, irritability – all common symptoms we call PMS. Is it possible that a percentage of the recent increase in the numbers of women on anti-depressants and tranquillizers (the Prozac tribe) can be laid at the door of the modern 'Eat more dairy for your bones' advice? Meanwhile the PMS, the arthritis and the osteoporosis continue to escalate. Then too, there is also some research implicating magnesium deficiencies in ME (Chronic Fatigue Immune Dysfunction Syndrome), as reported in the *Lancet*.[24] While Dr Sherry Rogers advises that 'Calcium makes muscles contract, while magnesium makes them relax.'[25] Feeling tense? Need more Magnesium!

If we substitute soya milk for homogenized milk, women would find a more balanced drink, and also might find that they have scant problems with the menopause because soy is a phyto-estrogen (a plant-based estrogen). Menopause is primarily a Western problem, accelerated by magnesium deficiency. Incidentally, current research suggests that while soya products are good for women, they may not be safe for babies, children or men. (BUT also see soy in Chapter 15 on genetically-engineered food.)

Another thing, that all-engrossing craving for lovely chocolate is caused by a magnesium deficiency and other deficiencies, because chocolate is high in magnesium. So the more dairy we consume, the more the craving for chocolate. But this does not mean we should pig out on chocolate, for unfortunately it is full of TFAs, sugar and worse! It means we should eat more magnesium.

There are in fact much better ways of getting calcium and from more usable sources than dairy: nuts[26] (especially almonds), dark green leafy vegetables, beans, whole grains, brown rice, wild rice and millet all have generous quantities of usable calcium and magnesium.

Moreover, orange juice, pineapple juice, almonds and black beans all contain magnesium and calcium in perfectly balanced amounts that allow the calcium to be easily absorbed.

Strangely there is evidence that the more calcium we take in, the smaller the percentage that is actually absorbed.[27] And wonder of wonders, there is also research that shows that when we adapt to a low calcium diet we actually excrete less of the calcium and increase our absorption of it. For it is true that Japanese women, Indians, African women and others who take in *no dairy at all, actually have stronger bones than Western women with a high-calcium diet.*[28] As with the animals and their grass, so it is with us.

Dr Susan Brown PhD, author of *Better Bones, Better Body*,[29] also subscribes to the mineral imbalance concept of bone loss. She claims that osteoporosis is not a normal bone loss due to ageing, but is a degenerative disease caused by devitalized food, the loss of trace minerals and, in addition, chemical poisoning. For there is arsenic in almost all milk. Dr J Gordon Millichap MD, Professor Emeritus of Pediatrics and Neurology at Northwestern University Medical School in Chicago says: 'Cow's milk has an average of 30–60 parts per billion [ppb], and in the milk from cows that have grazed in arsenic-contaminated fields, it is up to 1,500 ppb.'[30]

Finally, according to the studies comparing vegetarians and meat eaters, the people with the strongest bones are generally those who do not eat meat. This is probably because the phosphorous from animal protein pulls calcium from the bones. And while we're looking at that, soft drinks contain quantities of phosphoric acid, especially cola drinks. And in a children's study it was found that the more cola drinks consumed the more calcium is to be found in the blood. This can also be related to seizures and other problems, as well as bone loss.[31] Children and adolescents who drink cola products and soda drinks are being set up for osteoporosis later in life.

We have noted that magnesium is the calming stabilizing mineral which can be decreased in availability by too much calcium, and the association between excess calcium and PMS, mental problems in women. This problem also, of course, affects men and children.

Dr Alexander Schauss, editor of the *International Journal of Biosocial and Medical Research*, has done extensive work on delinquent children and diet. He found that delinquent children consumed far more milk than children who were *not* delinquent. But researchers have not found this link in England, where the milk is not homogenized.[32]

If we must drink milk, we should if possible go back to fresh raw milk and obtain all those wonderful nutrients without the dangers.

There is something else very interesting and terrible about milk, and it has to do with colon or bowel cancer. It has been found that this type of cancer is almost directly proportional to the amount of beef one eats. Studies in different parts of the world have indicated this. For example, two places where beef consumption is very high are New Zealand and Scotland, so guess where the highest rates of colon cancer are found? Colon cancer is extremely low in Third World countries, but even industrialized Japan has very low rates.[33]

As far back as April 27, 1974, an editorial in the *Lancet* entitled 'Beware the Ox' noted the relationship between beef eating and colon cancer. Has anybody warned us about this? If not, why not?

In Chapter 2 we looked at that large Harvard Public Health study on the 85,096 nurses. Also gained from this study was the fact that any kind of red meat in the diet increased the risk of cancer 2.5 times.[34] So it has been reasonably well established that the more beef you eat the more likely you are to get bowel cancer. But here's the interesting part. No matter how much beef you eat, you don't get it unless you had cow's milk as an infant.

Dr Hugh Sinclair, Reader in Medicine and Human Nutrition at Magdalen College, Oxford had, long before the Harvard Nurses Study, already explained the phenomenon back in the 1950s.[35] And *who* has since taken note and acted upon it generally, for the good of humanity?

Apparently the immune system of an infant fed on cow's milk tries to react to it as a foreign invader because that is what cow's milk is, being basically unsuitable for human infants. But as there is so much of it, constantly coming, the immune system eventually gives up on it. It switches off.

Then later in life comes the beef with its similar molecules. And the immune system, having been deactivated in its attempt to protect the gut as an infant, is still deactivated, and fails to protect the adult from the similar molecules, and hence from cancer.[36]

Almost all of these horrors have been recorded in (supposedly) respectable medical journals. So how is it that we go on drinking this stuff? At least in this particular form?

Finally, while on this subject, there is, in my opinion, no such thing as 'Mad Cow Disease'. There are only mad human beings, misguided human beings, bad human beings, inflicting their mad and bad ways on the animals which get caught up in our lives.

EMERGENCY ADVICE

See page 35 for infant formulas that do not use homogenized milk.

P.S. I must tell my favourite dog story, because it is relevant to the subject of 'bones' and joints. There are a few breeds of dogs that develop paralysed back ends long before the end of their natural life spans, such as Labradors, Alsatians, etc. I encountered one such on a morning walk. Its owner was struggling along carrying the dog's back half in a towel. When I commiserated with him he said, 'Some people think I should have him "put down", but I wouldn't put down my grandmother just because her legs go on her.' He told me he was trying to get a special cart made, one where the dog's back half would be supported and would run along on wheels.

He obviously loved the dog dearly, so I went home and worried about that man and his dog. Next time we met I suggested he try feeding the dog fresh ginger root, because 'I've had a lot of luck helping people over their arthritis with ginger.' He looked sceptical. But I said, 'Well, he's a mammal too. It's worth a try.'

Two and a half weeks later that dog was running on the beach, albeit with a slight limp. Apparently it loved the ginger root, which had been chopped and put in with his normal food. No trouble getting it down him.

Perhaps ginger root could save millions in Guide Dogs for the Blind – who apparently suffer a great deal of stress to their back legs, long before the animals are anywhere near the end of their useful lives – and a lot of misery for both owners and dogs. Anyway, happy joints to both people and dogs!

For people, ginger root can be grated and taken in a tea. My favourite way to eat ginger root is to grate it on to a buttered rye wafer (or one spread with cream cheese.) Take in a teaspoon a day; more for severe arthritis. Fresh ginger is a pharmacy of helpful constituents, as is fresh garlic. With plenty of those two we can stay healthy!

TWO SAFE FORMULAS FOR INFANT FEEDING[37]

To be used if breastfeeding is not possible:

1. Milk-based Formula – makes 32 fl oz/900 ml

450 ml/2 cups raw organic milk, or cultured milk (e.g. buttermilk), not homogenized.
20 g/¼ cup whey
4 tablespoons lactose
1 teaspoon cod liver oil
1 teaspoon *unrefined* sunflower oil
1 teaspoon extra virgin cold-pressed olive oil
2 teaspoons coconut oil
2 teaspoons brewer's yeast
2 teaspoons plain gelatine
430 ml/1¾ cups filtered water
1 100-mg tablet vitamin C, crushed, or in powdered form.

Mix the gelatine with water and heat gently until the gelatine is dissolved.

Place all the ingredients in a very clean glass or stainless steel container and mix well. To serve, pour 6 to 8 fl oz (170 to 230 ml) into a very clean glass bottle, attach sterilized teat, and set in a pan of simmering water. Heat until warm but not hot to the touch. Shake the bottle and feed baby.

(NEVER never never heat infant formula in a microwave oven.[38])

2. Milk-free Formula – makes 32 fl oz/900 ml

800 ml/3½ cups homemade broth (beef, lamb, chicken or fish)
55 g/½ cup organic liver, cut into small pieces
5 tablespoons lactose
40 g/½ cup whey
3 tablespoons coconut oil

1 teaspoon cod liver oil

1 teaspoon *unrefined* sunflower oil

2 teaspoons extra virgin cold-pressed olive oil

1 100-mg tablet vitamin C, crushed

Cook liver gently in the broth until the meat is cooked through. Liquefy using a hand-held blender or in a food processor. When the liver broth has cooled, stir in remaining ingredients. Store in a refrigerator and reheat gently as needed.

4: ASPIRIN

'Just take an aspirin a day and it'll
prevent heart disease or a stroke.'

Dr Wayne Martin of Fairhope, Alabama scoured the medical literature to check
this one out:[1] Yes, aspirin does reduce those 'sticky platelets' somewhat. And it was
of course the 'sticky platelet' theory that, around 1980, began in part to accompany if not replace the disreputable 'cholesterol causes heart attacks' theory (see
Chapter 1). But what was actually causing those sticky platelets?

Dr Martin says that the first test of aspirin, that done to test its ability to prevent post-surgery blood clots, was done in Britain in 1971. It was thereafter
reported as useless in the highly esteemed British medical journal, the *Lancet* in
that year. The UK Medical Research Council then did 'a most exacting test of
aspirin in the prevention of post-surgery thrombosis (blood clots) in four major
hospitals'. Again aspirin was of absolutely no benefit, and this was also reported in
the *Lancet* for September 2, 1972 (page 441).

Then they thought they would see what aspirin would do to prevent a second
heart attack after a first one. A trial of 1,233 patients was undertaken. Then there
was a second trial of 1,682 patients. In neither case was there a statistically significant improvement in those on the aspirin. These trials were reported in the *British
Medical Journal* in 1974 and the *Lancet* in 1979.[2]

These dismal results were reinforced by a huge study in the United States. The
National Institutes of Health through the National Heart, Lung and Blood Institute
did a much larger study at a cost of $16 million, but with the same unrewarding
results for the prevention of heart attacks. And these results were reported in both
Science magazine and the *Journal of the American Medical Association* in 1980.[3]

In the American test the aspirin was not just a failure. The director of the
study, Dr Robert I Levy, reported that in addition to the fact that aspirin had

helped neither men nor women, it had also caused ulcer-like pain, inflammation and bleeding in the stomach and intestines. He concluded that heart attack patients should *not* be given aspirin on a sustained basis.

In the face of these results and this advice, one would have thought that that would have been the end of the theory 'aspirin prevents heart attack' – but not at all. About this time the majority of doctors in the US began to tell their patients to take aspirin as a preventive measure, no matter if they'd had a heart attack or not. Why, one wonders, in this age of instant communication and high technology are most doctors so behind with the information to be found in their own medical journals?

Meanwhile there were two tests set up to try aspirin in the prevention of thrombotic strokes (strokes caused by a blood clot in the brain). The first was reported in *Stroke* in 1977,[4] and the second, done in Canada, was reported in the *New England Journal of Medicine* in 1978.[5] In the latter test, aspirin appeared to have a slight positive benefit with men but not with women.

But because of the punishing 'side-effects', an editorial on the subject in the *Lancet*[6] advised doctors not to get everyone over 40 taking aspirin just yet. But, as Dr Martin reports, 'Doctors were like a dog with a bone it cannot eat but will not let go of.' One could perhaps add, **'in the absence of anything else to do'** and in the face of an epidemic of heart disease.

Then came two more major tests on aspirin, one in the US and the other in Britain. These two tests were to involve only doctors as test subjects, doctors who had never had a heart attack. The results of the English test was reported in the *British Medical Journal* in 1988.[7] There was no benefit whatsoever in the prevention of heart attacks.

However, the American test results from the Physicians' Health Study, as it was called, were reported in the *New England Journal of Medicine*[8] and were declared to be a complete success!

'And it was this last test which has been accepted as conclusive evidence that every one over forty should take an aspirin a day, or at least one every second day.'[9]

But when we examine the results of the Physicians' Health Study (PHS) we find that it indicated NO reduction in heart attack deaths attributable to taking aspirin. Also there was no reduction in deaths from any or all causes. There was also an apparent increase in the risk of bleeding strokes among the aspirin takers.

What *was* good about the PHS was that there was a 44% reduction in the number of first non-fatal heart attacks among the aspirin takers.

But sometimes the truth will out (one hopes sooner rather than later) to explain the PHS's contradiction with all the other studies. Eventually Dr James A Landauer of the Electrolyte Laboratories in Denver explained why the studies of aspirin in Britain and elsewhere showed no benefit to be gained from taking aspirin, whereas the Physicians' Health Study in the US showed a positive benefit, at least insofar as the prevention of first non-fatal heart attacks.

In the English tests aspirin alone was used. In the PHS test, *Bufferin* was used, probably to prevent the negative effects on the gut. And *Bufferin* contains a small amount of magnesium. Landauer then listed the many benefits to the heart magnesium can bring. There are several studies on this. Magnesium in fact has all the earmarks of a substance that can truly reduce deaths from heart attacks. It reduces the adhesion of platelets in a way that puts aspirin well in the shade. It is a powerful vasodilator and an anticoagulant; it prolongs clotting time. It has been shown to be a natural calcium channel blocker. It does several other things which are of positive value in heart disease. It has no acknowledged side-effects.

There is absolutely no doubt that the positive results obtained in the Physicians' Health Study were caused by the benefits of the magnesium which was combined with the aspirin. (However, see the postscript to this chapter.) How much better the results would have been had they given up on the aspirin and used a significant amount of absorbable magnesium such as magnesium citrate! Now that would have been a worthwhile trial. Unfortunately, when it comes to something 'natural', no one can make money out of it, therefore there is no money available to do trials on such natural substances.

But the concept of the efficacy of magnesium in preventing heart disease ties in nicely with the difference in heart attack deaths in hard water and soft water areas. Professor Henry Schroeder of Indiana University, a superb environmentalist, reported in the *Journal of the American Medical Association*[10] that heart attacks could be correlated with the degree of water hardness. In the US, nationwide, heart attacks are inversely proportional to water hardness (the harder the water, the fewer the heart attack deaths). And this is doubtless due to magnesium again. For there's a small amount of magnesium in hard water.

It would seem that doctors who tell patients to take an aspirin a day to prevent a heart attack are guilty of not reading their own medical literature. Because after all that, when aspirin was combined with another substance, dipyridamole, it reduced stroke deaths by 50%, heart attack deaths by 35% and cancer deaths by 25%. But when aspirin alone was given there were no reductions of any kind of deaths.

The extraordinary thing is that no one has done trials with magnesium alone or dipyridamole alone. For if they had done so, Dr Martin believes they would have 'hit the jackpot'. (Dr Martin himself takes both magnesium and dipyridamole on a daily basis as well as other supplements. He has long outlived most of his contemporaries.)

A more recent study from Britain indicates that a combination of aspirin and warfarin prevented 39% of fatal heart attacks. But the aspirin-alone studies showed scant reduction, and usually around 15% of the patients dropped out due to the adverse effects of the aspirin, mainly the stomach ulcers or the ulcer-like pain. Aspirin has other not so noticeable negative effects. It actually inhibits prostaglandins, a most important hormone which is known to prevent both cancer and heart attacks. But perhaps worse is the effect on the lungs. Dr Martin has, in his survey, homed in on this. In the long term aspirin can predate emphysema, or lung disease. And this was established in the work of Dr Timothy Gerrity of the University of Illinois College of Medicine, and reported in the *New England Journal of Medicine*.[11] According to Dr Gerrity, this happens because aspirin inhibits prostaglandin E1, necessary for the health of the cilia in the lungs. (The cilia are the hair-like brushes that sweep away all the 'gunk'.)

Aspirin will similarly also make asthma worse in about 20% of asthma patients.[12]

Warfarin may also take other kinds of tolls. There are far better ways of preventing heart attacks.

We are wont to think that aspirin always has to be 'safe' because it is 'natural', that is, it is derived from the bark of a willow tree, *Salix alba* (hence the generic name salicylic acid). But when we take 'aspirin' we are not getting the whole plant. The active constituent, the salicylic acid, has been isolated out and synthesized; so that the protective parts of the plant have been discarded; therefore the aspirin is not being taken 'as nature intended'. And the more we isolate, concentrate and synthesize the parts of a plant, the greater the chance of toxicity or side-effects. That is why whole herbs are generally so much safer.

But there are, of course, other hazards. As we have noted (see Chapter 2), margarine and vegetable oils contain unnatural TFAs. These isomers act very like aspirin in blocking the production of the beneficial prostaglandin E1. We know from the study on the over 86,000 nurses reported on in the *Lancet*,[13] that the more margarine the more heart attacks. (The test had actually been designed to prove that margarine and polyunsaturated oils were preventive of heart attacks. But in fact, the long-term study proved the exact opposite.)

Dr Martin also refers to studies which show that vitamin E prevents heart attack deaths. One was the nurses' study, and the other was among 55,000 male health care workers. In both studies heart attack deaths were reduced by 40% by the taking of 100 iu or more daily of vitamin E.

There is evidence enough that aspirin does not significantly prolong life expectancy, nor does it enhance the quality of life for stroke victims. In fact it can actually cause cerebral haemorrhage, which can lead to strokes. It can cause nausea and vomiting in as many as 20% of patients, also ulcers, liver damage and allergic reactions. Aspirin may deplete essential vitamins and minerals, especially iron.[14] This happens not only because it damages the lungs but because it 'changes haemoglobin so that it does not carry oxygen'.[15] Moreover, at least one observer has put forward the opinion that 'the prime cause of cancer is faulty oxygenation.'[16]

According to a 1997 *Townsend Letter* editorial, 'Aspirin is a popular treatment because it is cheap, not because it works.'[17]

There are other studies which show that magnesium, vitamin E, onion and garlic, fish oil, flaxseed oil, olive oil and evening primrose oil all are protective of the heart. So what is happening today? Many doctors are telling their patients to take aspirin, when in truth it will not reduce heart attacks and may even, as we have noted, have long-term adverse and most serious effects.

And this is because most doctors have no training in, and no inclination to use, the safer natural means of keeping their patients well. Therefore so many people are denied these cheaper, safer and more effective substances because of the prejudices of medicine against natural methods. It is a story which will **astound the future**.

PS A recent version of the publication of the organization established to help those suffering from diabetes in New Zealand (Diabetes New Zealand), *Breakthrough* (vol. 10, number 1, Autumn 1998), featured an article, 'An Aspirin a Day Keeps the Cardiologist Away', (pages 14–15).

This article, on the basis of the US Physicians' Health Study, recommends that people with diabetes take an aspirin a day to prevent heart attacks, both primary and secondary. But as we have noted, numerous other studies have found aspirin to be useless in the prevention of heart attacks. Only the US Physicians' Health Study, which used aspirin combined with magnesium, showed any benefit. Is it therefore kind to advise people with diabetes to take aspirin, which has the potential of wrecking their already over-stressed digestive systems, with long-term use their lungs, and perhaps predate many other chronic diseases, instead of advising them to take magnesium and vitamin E for their hearts?

But it gets worse: I consider my friend, Wayne Martin, as something of an expert on aspirin, simply because he has taken the trouble to search the entire medical literature on the subject. How many have?

He says that according to Nobel Laureate, Dr Bengt Samuelsson, of the Karlinska Institute, people with diabetes have difficulty making an enzyme, delta-6-desaturase (D-6-D); and it is this enzyme which converts the Essential Fatty Acid, linolenic acid, into PGE1, one of the prostaglandins essential to human health.

Prostaglandins are molecules derived from fatty acids, and found in all cell membranes (or should be). They regulate blood pressure, control gut mobility and hence influence digestion, and are also involved in the essential process of inflammation.[18]

The deficiency in D-6-D, within the context of our population-wide general deficiency in the EFAs (as described in Chapter 2), has serious repercussions for people with diabetes. Because it is this deficiency that ultimately causes people with diabetes to have a tendency to blindness, to suffer the loss of limbs through gangrene, and have higher rates of heart attacks and cancer.[19]

Aspirin, which interferes with D-6-D, has the potential to accelerate these problems.

Thus people with diabetes should in preference be advised to take various supplements, particularly GLA (Gamma-Linolenic Acid as a precurser to prostaglandin) which can be found in evening primrose oil or borage oil; fish oil, magnesium; vitamin E oil, magnesium and vitamin E, but NEVER ASPIRIN.[20] (I have also come across the idea that grape juice can serve the same purpose as aspirin in thinning the blood, without the potential harm. But it must be taken regularly.)

So where were the medical advisors to Diabetes New Zealand when this advice was to be proffered?

And one must ask whether this slick, expensive production, *Breakthrough*, with its recommendation to take aspirin, would have done this had Diabetes New Zealand received adequate funding from the government? For in my view, when we abandon these support organizations to business interests we leave them open to this kind of abuse. According to its credits page, *Breakthrough* is supported by both Lilly and Parke-Davis, huge pharmaceutical companies, both of whom stand to gain by sales of aspirin. I do not suggest that either of these companies played any role in the production of the magazine article, but I do believe that patient advocacy groups should be independent.

For many years I had the voluntary responsibility of editing a newsletter for a patient support group, an incorporated society, and never once would I accept advertising or sponsorship of any kind while it was in my care; for reasons that are quite clear from a look at the journal of Diabetes New Zealand.

⚠

5: HEART SURGERY

'A bypass operation is the best way
to treat heart trouble.'

Among the numerous failures in the treatment of heart disease we must number
bypass operations. There is no evidence that these massively complex, dangerous
and expensive treatments do anything to significantly help with the problem
in the long term. They do, however, enrich the thoracic surgeons and others
involved. In the US each such operation costs $50,000; it is at least a $35 billion-
dollar-a-year industry,[1] and it is said that some thoracic surgeons earn the
equivalent of a new car every day.

In New Zealand, where the commercial motives may be fewer, there are thousands of people waiting for, 'their lives dependent upon,' this dubious operation.

As far back as 1980 the *Lancet* published an article maintaining that the
bypass only rarely extended life or improved the quality of the short one remaining.[2] In 1988 the American Medical Association recorded in the *Journal of the
American Medical Association* that 44% of coronary bypass surgery was quite useless.[3] And that would have been a more than conservative estimate. Moreover, Dr
Charles McGee MD points to research which indicates that over 80% of bypasses
and angiograms are unnecessary.[4]

More recently, and with great fanfare, there was worldwide publicity about the
fact that, owing to technical progress, bypasses could now be done with less risk of
brain damage to the patient. But who, before this, was aware that there **was** a significant risk of brain damage with these operations? Lay-people have to find out
these things by such announcements. In truth, there can be numerous serious
sequelae to bypass operations, including death in at least 10% of operations.

In the normal course of life, it is of course difficult to find out the outcomes of
any medical procedure. In the case of surgery, there is always a great deal of 'media

hype', for the whole procedure is so dramatic. Don't we see it depicted as such, frequently, in the medical soaps? But attempt to find out exactly how many survive and for how long, and in what condition after a bypass in real life? Good luck to you!

How can there be other than doubts? In congestive heart disease the whole arterial system is on the way to being blocked. The bypass procedure takes care of one tiny portion, the worst bit of the moment. But even if the operation is 100% successful and the patient survives, it is only a matter of time before that bit is reblocked, or the system is blocked somewhere else that is vital. It is worse than knocking off the tip of an iceberg and leaving the rest. Because if one thinks one has solved the problem, then nothing else will be done. The problem remains, continues, worsens.

So it is a vastly expensive and pointless procedure, unless and only unless it is used in an emergency to tide over a heart victim till other more effective methods, such as clearing out *all the arteries* and correcting *the cause* of the problem, can be put into place.

Here's an important digression: Modern medicine rests on two phenomena (as do all the healing arts throughout time and space): the fact that most illness is self-limiting, and secondly, the placebo effect. In the first case, most illness, if graphed, follows a gentle curve – that is, a dip down below the comparatively level line of normality, then a climb back up to the line. This will happen without intervention of any kind. But most people visit their doctors at the bottom limit of the curve when it is about to climb up. Therefore the doctor, or other healer, will get the credit for the upward climb to normality.

In the case of the placebo effect, usually in about 50% of cases, following medical assistance or advice the brain will, under the influence of hope, desire and belief, produce endorphins and so on, to create better health or a temporary feeling of having better health. Faith healers rely heavily on this phenomenon, and in fact, if the sufferer is not too far below that line of normality, the placebo effect can actually restore health. However, in the case of more serious ill-health, the faith healer or the doctor can in some cases initiate positive feelings for even up to two weeks, which may be interpreted as a 'miraculous cure'; but then, in the absence of substantive healing there is the inevitable slump back to ill-health, with, in addition, feelings of disappointment, shame or extra exhaustion and illness, if the 'healing' has inspired activity beyond the true stamina of the ill individual.

In orthodox medicine there is a hierarchy among placebos. That is, capsules are more potent than plain pills; injections are very powerful, and surgery in all its grandeur and drama is the Granddaddy and the Hercules of all placebos. Following the bypass operation it has been found that over 90% will say they feel better after the procedure, or after recovering from it. But when objective means are used to test heart function, only 20% of these indicate any **actual** improvement; 60% show no improvement, and 20% are worse after the operation.[5] This 20% of actual improvement is not much to show for the enormous costs in human resources of this frequently performed dramatic procedure. Particularly when it is not getting to the cause of the problem, and treating only a tiny portion of that problem.

In 1961 the *Journal of the American Medical Association* published 'Surgery as Placebo: A quantitative study of bias' (1102–7). This was an account by the heart surgeon H K Beecher of a series of 'placebo operations' wherein the chest was opened up but the operation not actually performed. Beecher had found, following this, that this group did just as well as his groups who did get the operation.

And yet, after that study was reported, the charade went on, nay flourished.

Dr Ralph Ellis was an anaesthesiologist with a heart problem brewing up.[6] In 1982 he was Chief of Anesthesia in a Florida hospital, being in attendance at numerous open-heart surgery procedures.

At first he was enthusiastic about the good he presumed the open-heart operating theatres were doing. But as the patients came back and back again, he gradually became concerned about what the surgeons were doing. Could they be addressing the basic cause of the disease? Clearly they were not. Ellis says:

The bypass operation is a risky business even the first time. The chest must be sawn open. Then surgeons must graft healthy blood vessels on to the blocked arteries, rerouting blood to the heart ... Even the act of closing the chest can put a kink in some of the vein grafts. A graft can also shut down at the stitching site. It is impossible to tell until the next time you saw open the heart. And the second time is even riskier. Because then the heart is all enclosed in scar tissue and sticks to the breast bone.[7]

This is why an oscillating saw – the kind that can rip through plaster casts – is used the second time.

Ellis reports there were heart attacks, strokes and internal bleeding after the operations. 'We saw patients become permanent patients. We were even doing bypass grafts on 80 year olds.' In fact, some research indicates that one out of 20 does not survive the operation, which adds up to 15,000 to 20,000 deaths a year in the US. One-fifth of the survivors have (or had) at least minimal brain dysfunction, and kidney failure is another complication of bypass patients.[8] We do not hear about these things in the media, which generally prefer 'heroic' stories.

According to Dr Charles McGee M.D., author of *HEART FRAUDS*, there have been three major controlled studies, establishing that 'early surgery is unlikely to increase the prospect of survival.' Moreover, as mentioned, research shows that over 80% of bypasses and angiograms recommended were not even necessary. But patients are frightened into agreeing to them with terms like, 'You've got a "widow-maker" there,' or, 'You're living with a time-bomb.'[9]

As far back as 1977, Professor Eugene Braunwald, Professor of Medicine at Harvard Medical School, in an editorial accompanying one such study, pointed out that increasing numbers of patients were being operated on, not because of the presence of 'intractable angina', but because of the hope 'largely without objective supporting evidence at present, that coronary bypass surgery prolongs life'.[10]

Wayne Martin puts it all into historical perspective: 'Where coronary heart disease is concerned, the vast majority of our doctors are still wearing blood-caked frocked coats.'[11] (This refers to the standard dress of doctors in the last century, for all occasions in the practice of medicine, including surgery; and will be referred to again in greater detail in Chapter 32 on the medical profession.)

In 1984, our anaesthetist, Dr Ellis, developed chest pain himself, and tests showed a 98% blockage in a major coronary artery. He returned to his home in Kentucky and took up a less stressful way of life.

After two angioplasties (another clever and fairly useless procedure), Ellis was told he had to have a bypass or die. But having seen it so often, and having so many concerns about the procedure, instead he went to California to see Dr Julian Whitaker, author of the book, *Is Heart Surgery Necessary?* There he underwent chelation therapy and learned how to live and eat so that the problem would not recur. (Some of the preceding chapters in this book are good starters for this. And see the recommendations at the end of this chapter. Also, any of the books mentioned in this chapter will go into this more fully.)

The chelation therapy not only cleaned out *all* his arteries but it cost a tiny fraction of the cost of open heart surgery, which would have temporarily taken care of one tiny part of one artery. He is now very well.

Chelation therapy is a system whereby EDTA (ethylene-diamine-tetra-acetate), a substance which 'drags out' the unwanted stuff from the arteries and tissues (scours the plumbing, if you like) is dripped into the body intravenously, gradually over a period of weeks. Patients sit in comfortable reclining chairs and chat to each other during the procedure. It is, of course, not inexpensive, but it costs a tiny fraction of the price of heart surgery.

Chelation has been used for over 50 years *by orthodox medicine* and is approved for the removal of toxic metals from the body. It is actually FDA-approved (that is, approved by the ultra-conservative American Food and Drug Administration which virtually rules almost all health policy in the English-speaking countries) for lead, mercury, aluminium and cadmium poisoning. It is NOT approved by orthodoxy for heart conditions.

But in the past, during the process of receiving this chelation for heavy metal poisoning, so many patients felt better in other ways and found their heart disease symptoms clearing up (in fact objective measurements confirmed the improvement), that the brilliant few, those innovative doctors who have their patients' best interests 'at heart' (as it were) began to use it as a first-choice treatment for heart disease.

In one study of 22,000 chelation patients, 87% showed improvement with chelation,[12] even though many chelation patients are those for whom conventional drugs and surgery have failed and they are at 'the end of the line'. At the same time as they receive chelation, patients can be taught how to eat well and take care of themselves in the future so that it will not happen again.

As we noted in Chapter 1 on cholesterol, Rosetta Schuman claims that plugged arteries are 95% calcium and only .5% cholesterol, with 4.5% other substances.[13] So we need to attack the calcium deposits, and stop worrying about that .5% cholesterol.

Among the claims for the potential benefits of EDTA chelation are the following:

prevents cholesterol deposits
reduces blood cholesterol levels
lowers high blood pressure
avoids bypass surgery
avoids angioplasty
reverses digitalis toxicity
removes calcium from atherosclerotic plaques
dissolves intra-arterial blood clots
normalizes cardiac arrythmias
has an anti-ageing effect
reduces excessive heart contractions
increases intracellular potassium
reduces heart irritability
improves heart function
removes mineral and drug deposits
dissolves kidney stones
reduces serum iron levels
reduces heart valve calcification
reduces varicose veins
heals calcified necrotic ulcers
reduces intermittent claudication
improves vision in diabetic retinopathy

decreases macular degeneration

dissolves small cataracts

eliminates heavy metal toxicity

makes arterial walls more flexible

prevents osteoarthritis

reduces rheumatoid arthritis symptoms

lowers the insulin needs of people with diabetes

reduces Alzheimer-like symptoms

reverses senility

reduces stroke/heart attack after-effects

prevents cancer

improves memory

reverses diabetic gangrene

restores impaired vision

detoxifies snake and spider venoms.[14]

Well, if it does even half this, it should be used more widely. In fact, chelation has been used to clean out arteries for many years and in many parts of the world, so successfully that the best heart surgeons now use it instead of surgery. In fact, in New Zealand, the leading health insurance provider will pay 80% of the costs of chelation, because they are aware that they will be saving heaps in the long run. No insurance company would pay for it unless it were so. Moreover, unless patients are on their last legs and about to die anyway, chelation is, unlike the dangerous bypass operation, perfectly safe. But also, its obvious success threatens conventional medicine and the vast profits from heart 'procedures'.[15]

There are other procedures similar to the bypass operation. Early in 1998 a Canadian series (2,885 cases) revealed that an operation to clean out clogged arteries in the neck (carotid endarterectomy), can actually trigger the very strokes it is performed to prevent. Paradoxically, this is most likely to happen in those with minor blockages only. It is now recommended only for severe blockages, that is where over 50% of the area is blocked.[16]

One awaits the publication of such a series for the bypass procedure. We should know how many deaths occur at the time of surgery; how many are more disabled after surgery; and the average length of life after the procedure.

This should be compared with a similar series of people given chelation, supplements and dietary advice. The study should be supervised by those with no axe to grind. Whichever country does an honest study like this could perform a valuable service to the world, with the long-term possibility of saving many lives and billions of 'health' dollars. However, 'honest' is the operative word here.

The reason Dr Ellis had to go to California for chelation treatment was because this therapy had been driven out of Kentucky. On his recovery he attempted to do battle on behalf of the people of Kentucky so that they would have the same choice he'd had. But he came up against a brick wall. In fact the President of the Kentucky Board of Medical Licensure is a thoracic surgeon (that is, one who does bypass operations) with a vested interest in keeping chelation out of the state. Dr Ellis calls the situation 'Medical McCarthyism'.[17] But he continues his campaign to get more alternative treatments such as chelation therapy into Kentucky.

Ellis says, 'Patients have a right to nonsurgical treatment. This kind of medicine does not kill patients, nor maim them, which cannot be said for some of the so-called orthodox methods.'

It is interesting that surgical procedures are not required to pass anything like the reviews drugs are (such as they are). No 'double-blind' studies are required, or possible. (We noted that Dr Beecher's extraordinary effort has been ignored.) So there are scant opportunities for assessments. Surgical procedures are simply dreamed up and performed.[18] From then on a massive propaganda machine goes into action. We seldom hear about the failures, how many die in how brief a time after major surgery. (An exception would be the 'whistle-blown' warning about the deaths of 29 infants and young children following cardiothoracic surgery at Bristol Royal Infirmary in 1998).[19] Another example of blind faith in medicine would be breast cancer treatment, which for decades involved taking off the whole breast and the nearby lymph nodes as initiated in the 1920s. However, more recently it has been found that a lumpectomy only, just the removal of the breast lump does, just as well as the former way (by 'just as well' I also mean, 'just as badly'). And yet when driving out chelation and persecuting doctors who do it, the orthodoxy will say that chelation is 'unproven'. None so blind as those who do not want to see.

In any event, Dr McGee calls heart surgery 'a $35 billion a year waste', a huge chunk out of the US health care dollars.

In New Zealand we have people dying on the waiting lists for such surgery, apparently for want of it. But even if it could be established that this surgery is a good way to save lives, where is the justice in denying these people the alternatives – and far less costly alternatives at that – while they are waiting?

It is my belief that in the next century bypass operations will be looked back on as far worse than 'applying leeches' used to be regarded. However, today's heart surgeons enjoy colossal incomes based on the betrayal of the futile hopes of heart disease sufferers. Moreover, many of them contribute to the hounding and persecution of those who have far better answers to late-stage heart disease.

Dr Joseph Hattersley believes that[20] 'it is not unrealistic to hope that from the year 2041, people will read about the 20th century's epidemic of heart attacks and strokes, heart transplants, bypasses and the like with accounts of blood-letting and the iron lung – in medical history books.' I'd like to see it a whole lot sooner.

EMERGENCY ADVICE

Dr Hattersley has researched all the ways to avoid heart attacks and strokes, and he maintains that vitamin B_6 is the main supplement to do the job.[21] (One could also add magnesium, vitamin C, folic acid, flaxseed oil, garlic, vitamin E, lecithin, carnitine, CoQ10, gum guggul extract, inositol hexanicotinate, chromium, penterhine. And then there are excellent herbs for the heart: hawthorn, cactus grandiflores, lily of the valley, dandelion, ginkgo, black cohosh, lobelia, motherwort and arnica.)

Above all, as we have noted, one must of course avoid the technologized 'foods' which contribute to heart problems. According to Rosetta Schuman, long-time health researcher, 'The prime concern is the quality of the fat: whether it is natural, unrefined, and unheated; or hydrogenated and refined. This latter group causes heart problems.'[22] We must be aware that almost all bought baked goods contain hydrogenated fats and oils. Check the labels. You will probably end up making your own with butter. There is also the necessity to avoid smoking and homogenized milk, and to cut down on sugar, as we will see.

In the Introduction we noted that New Zealanders have 25% more heart disease than Australians, and I said that when we find the reason for this we would have the answer to heart disease itself. Possible explanations:

1   A significant proportion of the Australian population comes from Mediterranean countries such as Italy, Greece and Lebanon. In these countries they consume cold pressed olive oil; they do not eat hydrogenated oils. They also would disdain margarine; they do not drink milk. As in the Rosetta study they consume high levels of saturated fats. And it must be recalled that food habits are among the very last things to change when people move from one country to another, one culture to another. These people would therefore improve the heart disease statistics. Also the chances are they take fewer drugs.

2   More speculative: New Zealand, under New Right governments, now has more poverty than Australia, and heart disease tends to go with poverty and cheaper foods.

3   Also speculative: New Zealanders do not 'throw off the yoke' as do Australians. We are more polite and appear to be more vulnerable to sophistry: both the blandishments of advertising and the fallacious reasoning of governments and most doctors.

This political helplessness does not add to one's self-confidence in any way, including confidence in one's ability to make choices about one's own health.

6: MERCURY AMALGAM FILLINGS

'It must be OK to put mercury in our mouths.
Otherwise the dentists wouldn't use it.'

Unfortunately it is *not* OK. And they do, most of them.

This will probably be the one which will amaze those observers from the next century most of all. 'You mean they *actually* put the most toxic, the most poisonous (non-radioactive) substance on the planet, *in their mouths?*' (Of course there is plutonium. It could have been worse.)

In any event we can be sure that the governments of Sweden, Denmark, Austria and Germany would not be requiring the phasing out of mercury amalgam in people's mouths without good reason. In fact, the Swedish government will even pay for the removal of mercury amalgam fillings when a doctor decides it is a medical problem.[1]

Professor W William Hughes, School of Allied Health Professions, Associate Professor of Pathology and Human Anatomy, School of Medicine, Loma Linda University would remind us that there are over 5 million natural and man-made chemicals, over 80,000 synthetic chemicals in daily use, and the list is being added to every day.[2] So it's no use telling us that 'this little bit of mercury is of no consequence, a drop in the bucket.' For every day of our lives we are dealing with thousands of non-nutritious materials we were in no way designed to cope with, and nobody knows the synergistic effect of this cocktail, that is, what happens when they all get together.

Especially when the effects are cumulative. When we are trying to gauge the effect of mercury on the human brain, how can we know what contribution mercury has made when someone becomes mentally unstable? Was it the lack of minerals or Essential Fatty Acids before and after birth? Was it the mercury, also before and after birth, or both? Etc.

In the US in the last few years there have been numerous government blunders of colossal proportions (which have affected many in other parts of the world), for example the drug DES (Stilbesterol); Oraflex, the anti-arthritis drug; DDT the pesticide (in fact, of course, most pesticides); the Dalkon Shield; Norplant (against which 50,000 American women engaged in a class action suit[3]); Calcium channel blockers and silicon breast implants (Dow Corning now forced to pay out $3.17 billion[4]), to name just a few. All had received an official Food and Drug Administration stamp of approval before they were launched upon a trusting public.[5] I believe that mercury amalgam will one day join that list.

Enough studies have now been done to prove beyond doubt that the risks of using mercury in our mouths are totally unacceptable. If we were cars we would have been urgently recalled for removal of the dangerous part long ago. But since we are only human beings, and no one seems to be looking after us, we in the English-speaking countries have to wait to hear about it through the efforts of dedicated individual dentists, like Dr Hal Huggins of the US,[6] and hard-working pressure groups set up by people who know that mercury is poisonous to human health. Usually they do this because they have personally experienced the health problems associated with having mercury in their mouths, and are aware of the health improvements they experienced after its removal.

A study of 1,569 people showed a 63 to 97% resolution of the following complaints after removal of amalgam fillings: allergy, anxiety, bad temper, bloating, blood pressure problems, chest pains, depression, dizziness, fatigue, gastrointestinal problems, gum problems, headaches, migraine, insomnia, irregular heartbeat, irritability, lack of concentration, lack of energy, memory loss, metallic taste, multiple sclerosis, muscle tremor, nervousness, numbness, skin disturbances, sore throat, tachycardia (racing heart), thyroid problems, ulcers and sores in the oral cavity, urinary tract problems, vision problems.[7]

Mercury was used in medicine for some centuries, probably because 'it was there', long before it was used as part of a filling for teeth. It was used for everything from skin problems to syphilis. In Germany mercury was known as 'Quacksalber'. Paracelsus used it to treat syphilis, which earned him the name of 'Quack', and for a time all doctors became known as 'Quacks'. Eventually it was also used to classify dentists who used the 'Quacksalber'. But generally today doctors and others use the term only to describe those health workers they happen to disagree with. Mercury was, of course, 'Quicksilver' in Britain.

The mercury did attack microbes in the same way antibiotics do, but just as antibiotics force the microbes to mutate to survive, so does mercury. And when mercury is stored, you never get rid of it without some kind of chelation to remove it. So it forces all our microbes to become resistant, as well as having numerous other adverse effects we shall be looking at. In fact, it was the horrifying results of using mercury and other such toxic materials as 'medicines' that caused the brilliant doctor Samuel Hahnemann to give up medicine entirely, in disgust and anguish.

(He then created an entirely new healing modality, Homoeopathy, which is still the first healing method of choice in many countries, but which was largely driven out of the US by the American Medical Association early in the 20th century. It is of course coming back.)

During the 1960s, Mercurochrome, a mercury-based liquid used on the skin for various problems, was removed from the market because of concern over its dangerous toxicity.[8] But here is the unbelievable part: They did **that**, but permitted the continuance of its placement in our mouths.

There is no question that were mercury amalgam to be proposed today, the weight of scientific evidence as to its potential risk would preclude it ever being accepted for the use to which it is currently put.

Mercury amalgam fillings, cheaper and easier to work with than gold, were first introduced into Britain in 1819, and in France in 1826. There was at this stage grave concern, from both medicine and the American Dental Association, because the main constituent, mercury, was so poisonous. And doctors at that time were worried about the results, as seen in the following medical reports:

'Death caused by swallowing a large amalgam filling.' 'Mercurial poisoning.' 'Case of deafness probably caused by amalgam fillings.' 'Diseased eyes – amalgam fillings.' 'Acute mania attributed to an amalgam filling.'[9]

But before long, certain changes in medicine we will be looking at caused medicine to turn a blind eye; they 'dumbed down' on the subject. Mercury became acceptable.

An amalgam filling is usually made up of about half (or more) mercury (in fact it can be over 0.5 grams of mercury); the rest of it will consist of silver, tin, copper and zinc. Of course, amalgam fillings are not the only source of mercury in our environment. There is mercury in the water, in the air, in the diet, in fish, in latex paint and so on. But nothing compares with the released mercury from amalgam fillings, averaging up to 15 micrograms (mcg) per day. [10]

For, once your fillings are in, then eating, brushing your teeth, smoking, talking, gum chewing, teeth grinding (at night while asleep), and breathing through your mouth all release mercury vapour. Moreover, it takes an hour and a half after these activities cease for the mercury released to settle down again. So if you smoke, talk or eat frequently, you could be releasing mercury from the fillings a good deal of the time.[11]

Keeping in mind that the filling is half-mercury, it has been found that by the end of five years 50% of the mercury on the surface has washed out. In 20 years no measurable mercury can be found.[12]

Most of the damage comes from the vapour that has been released during chewing. In fact, subjects in tests using chewing gum actually had mercury vapour levels in their mouths higher than is permitted by the US National Institute of Occupational Safety and Health for air in the workplace. The vapour then goes directly to the brain and to the lungs where the blood picks it up and delivers it to various organs within 29 days. This has been established by several studies wherein radioactive mercury isotope mixed with dental amalgam fillings were placed in the teeth of adult sheep.[13]

A recent German study (February, 1997) conducted by Professor Kraus of Tubingon University took 17,500 people off the street and tested their saliva for mercury content, before and after chewing. It was found that chewing released up to 800 mcg of mercury per litre of saliva. We produce one to two litres of saliva per day and, significantly, it is illegal to have more than 2 mcg mercury per litre of water used for any purpose.[14]

In the US, if half a gram of mercury were to be found in a 10-acre lake, it would warrant the immediate issuance of a fish warning for that lake.[15] The average amalgam filling placed in our mouths contains that half a gram of mercury.

Also in the US, in 1994 the Minnesota Legislature banned the sale of running shoes with mercury lights in their heels as too dangerous to public health. Those little lights contained a half a gram of mercury.[16] So it's not safe in fishing lakes or in the backs of our shoes, but it's quite OK in our mouths? What will these facts say about our sanity to those observers from the next century? Is it that so many are brain-damaged by mercury that they cannot see the utter madness in all this?

Mercury also enters the bloodstream via the intestines. Perhaps the worst aspect is that mercury is attracted to sulphur, which is a part of the proteins in various hormones and enzymes. Mercury does this by replacing the hydrogen in sulphur-hydrogen bonds, thus inactivating the protein.[17]

Mercury toxicity can cause symptoms which affect energy and behaviour. It can affect the brain, the nervous system, the heart, digestion, the hormonal system, the immune system and the mouth. Symptoms will vary as the mercury seeks out each genetically weak area in our bodies.[18]

All forms of mercury have the ability to suppress immune function, and even to precipitate autoimmunity, as manifest in multiple sclerosis and other horrific diseases. There are also subtle mental/learning defects which can occur as a result of mercury exposure in utero and during breastfeeding.

Some of us may be aware of the reports of the disaster that occurred in the 1950s when mercury (industrial waste) was released into Minamata Bay in Japan. But how many of us have made the connection between that disaster and our fillings? In Minamata, that one small area, there were over 46 deaths; and out of 400 births there were 22 deformed and retarded infants.[19]

Numerous other studies have been done. At the University of Calgary Medical School it was established that after placement of mercury amalgam dental fillings in the teeth of pregnant animals, mercury from these fillings passed the placental barrier and accumulated in the foetus within 24 hours. Within 30 days there was a 50% impairment in the kidney of the foetus.[20] In recognition of these studies, the British government now warns that pregnant women should not have fillings installed or removed because of the risk that mercury vapour could cross the placenta and harm their unborn children.[21] However, they are not, as are Sweden, Denmark, Austria and Germany, requiring the phasing out of mercury amalgam.

A drug known as colchicine is the standard comparison used for chemicals that produce birth defects and chromosomal damage, because it is the strongest drug known to produce genetic damage. Methyl mercury from mercury/silver dental fillings is 1,000 times more toxic than colchicine. 'Methyl mercury is one of the most potent and insidious poisons in existence.'[22] We ourselves produce methyl mercury from mercury with the help of the bacteria in plaque, and other common microbial residents in the mouth.

Mercury has also been implicated in leukaemia,[23] in autoimmune diseases such as myasthenia gravis, mental illness and birth defects. Dr Keith W Sehnert MD, a researcher in this area, says on behalf of his research group, 'It is our conclusion that mercury toxicity is an autoimmune disorder.' That is, mercury toxicity can damage the immune system to such an extent that it can turn on the body it is supposed to be protecting.

Another shocker: In 1991, a University of Georgia study putting mercury fillings in the mouths of monkeys revealed that mercury induced resistance to antibiotics.[24] Perhaps this is one of the reasons behind the modern failure of antibiotics in some cases, because there is undoubtedly a build-up in the resistance of microbes from generation to generation. Moreover, mercury can actually create a unique kind of antibiotic-resistant bacteria.

Worse, there is also 'genetic susceptibility', in that mercury targets DNA through its attraction to the essential nucleic acid, thymine. Such binding produces a rigid strand of DNA which does not uncoil easily. According to Blesius et al., this finding makes a mockery of the concept of a 'safe threshold' for mercury, because even one mercury atom can interfere with the proper functioning of the genetic code.[25]

Perhaps worst of all, in 1991 medical researchers at the University of Kentucky found high levels of mercury in the brains of those who had died of Alzheimer's Disease; far higher levels than in those without the disease.[26]

If you're wondering how this could happen, and how your fillings are gradually losing you your marbles, here is Dr Mike Godfrey of Tauranga, New Zealand, on the subject:

Mercury vapour from mouth fillings to the brain does not have to go 'the long way around' as it has direct access through the roof of the nose because thousands of nerve endings come down through holes in the skull there; this is in fact how we have the ability to smell. Even an amoeba from a hot pool can squeeze through these holes to give one meningitis, so mercury vapour 'wouldn't even touch the sides'. Published in 1943 in Germany were the results of 63 autopsies where it was shown that the mercury levels in the brain 'above the nose' were over six times higher than in the rest of the brain. These areas include the pituitary and the 'limbic' brain (our central computer that controls every body function).

So! Ho HUM! This information was first published in 1943. Just who is looking after us, our precious brains?

In his fifties, Tom Warren was an insurance agent with 22 amalgam fillings and diagnosed Alzheimer's Disease. His wife was a pharmacologist. And between the two of them they refused to accept the medical verdict of 'incurable'. (Tom Warren says that he has found not one Alzheimer's sufferer who was given more than a cursory examination. At the onset of short-term memory loss they are diagnosed with Alzheimer's, sent to a psychiatrist and given psychotropic drugs to control their behaviour.)

Undeterred, Tom and his wife went on searching the medical literature and elsewhere but found no recorded recovery from Alzheimer's. And yet they persisted.

Eventually they worked out a solution to his problem that involved detoxifying Tom from the toxic metal and chemical poisoning damage he was suffering. He underwent chelation treatment (which eliminates toxic metals from the body) and others, and went on to recover completely. A CAT scan revealed that Tom Warren at the age of 53 had completely reversed his condition.

He continued to fine-tune his health, his brain, and went on to write a book, *Beating Alzheimer's: A step towards unlocking the mysteries of brain diseases: The Remarkable Story of How One Man Reversed the Devastating Symptoms of Alzheimer's Disease.*[27]

Today Tom Warren claims that he now thinks as clearly as he did at 40. He continues to take an interest in the problem and clearly has sufficient brain power to write brilliant articles on the subject in medical journals! He also lectures widely to anyone who will listen. He doesn't want others to lose their brains unnecessarily.

Tom believes that a deficiency in zinc is the main reason some of us store cadmium, mercury and lead in the brain. The brain is trying to get hold of some zinc, cannot find it, so latches on to the toxic metals coming its way. And, of course, the way we live there are plenty available.[28] (And as we will note, it is fluoride that negates our zinc intake.) If supplementing with zinc, I would personally recommend the organic variety as found in sunflower seeds, oysters etc., because some think that the inorganic forms of zinc can merely add to the problem of Alzheimer's Disease.

Tom says that in addition to the toxicity of mercury, the electrical current generated by the combination of metals and saliva within the oral cavity can cause up to 1,000 times more electrical activity in the brain than the brain is designed to run on. It is even possible that some people require pacemakers because of this effect. And Tom Warren is one of many who believe that cancer in the mouth can be caused by dental fillings.[29]

Root canal fillings are also in the brain-damaging category, and we will look at them in the next chapter. There are other reversible reasons or combinations of reasons why people develop Alzheimer's, and all should be investigated.

Tom Warren has, in his research, gathered up other health problems associated with mercury and toxic chemical poisoning which can give us clues to the origins of other problems and warnings as to future possible Alzheimer's. He lists:

1   Candida albicans overgrowth
2   H. pylori (*Helicobacter pylori*)
3   digestive problems and low stomach acid
4   excessive belching and flatulence
5   malnutrition
6   obesity
7   intolerance to alcohol
8   putrefaction, parasites, fungus, etc.
9   chronic fatigue
10 leaky gut syndrome
11 food allergies and chemical sensitivities
12 poisoning of the liver
13 dry, flaky skin
14 abnormal white cell blood count ranging from 10,000 to 22,000 mm^3
15 discolouration of the genital organs – jocularly known as '*Grey Penis Syndrome*'. But there is sometimes also a greyness in the testicles and arm pits. In women the insides of the lips of the vulva are grey where they should be pink. Also there can be that facial 'grey look'. After mercury detoxification, chelation, all these areas become light pink again.[30]

Hair analysis will also tell us if we have a mercury problem, and for all mercury problems it is worth trying the homoeopathic remedies Amalgam and Mercury in their mildest forms. However, self-dosing in this respect can be dangerous. It is best to see a qualified homoeopath to decide which one and in which potency for your unique situation. Be warned that the initial excretion can make one feel quite ill if the problem is severe. Also, chelation therapy is a traditional and, as we noted in Chapter 5 on bypass operations, the **orthodox medically-accepted way** of getting rid of heavy metals from the body.

The major effects of chronic mercury poisoning may perhaps make itself felt in gradually manifest mental symptoms, making it difficult to spot the source of the damage. The Romans had their lead to drive them mad; the British hat-making industry had its mercury. The phrase *Mad as a hatter* originated in the effects on the workers in the industry required to use mercury to stiffen the hats. We merely put it in our mouths and keep it there.

The estimates on the incidence of Alzheimer's Disease are: 10% of those over 65; 25% of those over 80; and 50% of those over 85. It is the fourth-ranking leading cause of death, with 350,000 newly diagnosed cases annually in the US.[31]

I always enjoyed the scene of the 'Mad Hatter's Teaparty' in *Alice in Wonderland*, but I cannot help seeing much of modern 'health care' practice in these terms. However, neither the sufferings of the 19th-century hat makers nor those of today's people with Alzheimer's and their families, nor the complete unconcern of most of 'modern medicine' with environmental factors in health, are anything to smile about.

The US Toxic Element Research Foundation in assessing the cumulative effects in the US of mercury amalgam poisoning puts the problem on a par with the Chernobyl tragedy. 'The magnitude of the crisis is not the few who have died from massive exposure, but rather it is the millions whose health will be eroded by the ongoing, small-dose poisoning.'[32]

For every day in the United States alone, half a million amalgam fillings are put into people's mouths.[33] Altogether it is routinely implanted in over 65% of the population, and this despite mercury being one of the oldest of recognized poisons. In fact, disinfectants, antiseptics, pesticides and insecticides all contain mercury *because it is so hostile to life*.

After several years of research, Tom Warren claims that 85% of the population has been poisoned to some extent by mercury amalgam.[34]

And what have our Dental Associations been doing in response to all these horrific findings, most of them from respectable scientific research? Despite the fact that they have never been able to offer scientific proof as to the safety of amalgam; despite, as noted, the fact that in Europe four governments have banned any future use of mercury in their people's mouths, governments in the English-speaking countries have done nothing, and our Dental Associations not only stall, but worse, actively persecute and harass dentists who speak out, or in the US who even let it be known to their patients that they replace amalgam fillings with any of the many alternatives available today.

In the US, one of the documents used by the American Dental Association (under Section WAC 246-816-160 [1]) proclaims:

the best currently available scientific research and information justifies the finding that it is unsatisfactory conduct for a dentist to advocate to a patient the removal of clinically serviceable dental amalgam restorations solely to substitute a material that does not contain mercury, unless the patient can be shown to be allergic to mercury.[35]

Any violation of the above injunction, by dentists, is officially classified as 'moral turpitude, dishonesty, and corruption' on the part of the dentist attempting to save his patient's health.

But World Health Organization toxicology experts have declared that no amount of mercury vapour in the body can be considered harmless.[36]

Despite all this the American Dental Association, and its counterparts in other countries, remain unmoved. Clearly they are in a position where they believe they cannot afford to change their minds. And as we will see over and over in this book, people's livelihoods and incomes usually take precedence over the health and the lives of others. Moreover, the ADA continues to spend large amounts of money to block local requirements that dental officers obtain an industrial waste discharge permit for mercury being discharged into the environment. Also huge sums are spent on the persecution of any dentists who fail to toe the line.

The saga of the harassment of Dr Hal Huggins DDS, undoubtedly America's most dedicated expert on the perils of modern dentistry, and others, will one day be told in full. It will bring no credit to the American Dental Association.

The most recent and startling development in the field of dentistry involves admissions on the information sheets now included by two amalgam manufacturers with their products. There is admission that amalgam is a health hazard in the words 'mercury poisoning – usually chronic'. And the contraindications (recommended restrictions on use) include: children under 7; under crowns or in root-filled teeth; pregnant and breastfeeding women; people with reduced kidney function; and people hypersensitive to amalgam. The listed adverse health effects from chronic inhalation and/or ingestion of the product include: tremor, fatigue, headaches, irritability, excitability, depression, insomnia, loss of memory, hallucinations, psychiatric disorders, mental deterioration and resentment of criticism. Lung (bronchitis), kidney failure, heart (chest pain, tightness, palpitations), colitis, dermatitis, blood disorders, infertility and birth defects were also cited as possible effects of mercury amalgam poisoning.[37]

These admissions are particularly serious because manufacturers do not admit to adverse health effects unless they have been established in law. They are there because the manufacturers seek to protect themselves from future lawsuits. Next time your dentist suggests an amalgam filling, ask to see the manufacturer's warnings which come with the product.

And what of the effect of mercury amalgam on dentists? The ones who handle this toxic material, breathe it in all their working days? A recent study shows that dentists have impaired memories, relative to other professional groups. It is also a fact that, among the professions, dentists have the shortest life expectancy, and the highest rates of suicide.[38]

Hal Huggins recently walked out onto the stage in Colorado Springs to address 350 doctors at a medical conference. His opening statement to the doctors was:

'You can thank dentistry for 80% of your business.'[39]

The Ziff brothers, both dentists, would agree:

Our purpose is to suggest that the medical profession rediscover mercury for what it is – an insidious poison, more toxic than lead or arsenic, that may be the greatest unrecognized disease aetiological factor in the history of modern medicine.[40]

We got into this monstrous situation because of the lack of a whole, or holistic view of the body and its workings, the false idea that the body can be carved up into bits and pieces, and each of the bits parcelled out to a specialist of some kind. But it is clear that an event in one part of the body can affect one or all of the other parts in the body, and the brain.

So in their rampant ignorance, the doctors left the mouth to the dentists, the dentists became what Mike Godfrey calls 'molar mechanics' who regarded the mouth as a disembodied entity, and left the question of health to the doctors. And in the process *a major catastrophe has fallen through the cracks* between the two professions.

When you try to add up all the damage from overheated oils and fats, the fluoride, the poisonous mercury in our mouths, the poisons in our environment, and the many other things discussed and to be discussed in this book, it is impossible to see exactly what is responsible for which health problem.

But each person studying any one health problem finds plenty to worry over, hence Hal Huggins' 80%. So all we can say is that each of these health menaces contributes to the whole load. And that it is no wonder that almost everyone over 50 has a chronic health problem and that many are slowly dying.

EMERGENCY ADVICE

1 If you think you have a problem with mercury in your mouth, you can either have future dental work done with non-amalgam replacements, or you can have them all changed over in one period of time. The latter is expensive, but the state of one's health, mental and physical should be the guiding precept. Either way, one needs to find a dentist experienced in its removal and its replacement with other substances. In looking for this good dentist, find out if he or she is concerned about the order in which they are removed. If that is not considered a problem, continue searching for one who really knows what is going on in the mouth. For example, the quadrant with the most negative charge should be removed first. Failure to remove them correctly can result in worsened health. If you are seriously ill in any way, do not have more than one filling removed at a time.

2 If you are concerned about the health effects of the stored mercury in your tissues (and it is said that we've all got it if we have four or more fillings) then you need to get it out. Take substantial quantities of vitamin C (preferably in the buffered or calcium ascorbate form). Try N-acetyl cysteine; and try intravenous chelation which will have the added bonus of cleaning out your arteries at the same time. Under best advice only, try the homoeopathic remedies (to be taken very carefully).

⚠️

7: ROOT CANALS FOR INFECTED TEETH

'A neat way of saving your teeth!'

Like most people, first thing in the morning I hasten to a window to see what sort of a day it is. And being very fortunate, I look out over the Hauraki Gulf, dotted with little islands, going out to the horizon as far as the eye can see.

If it is an overcast day, the islands in the foreground will be but dimly seen, shrouded in mist. But if it is clear and sunny I might see two layers of islands, while on a really superb day with perfect visibility I can see three layers back and more, the islands dotted in a blue-green sea.

So naturally I mark out the days as 'one-layer' days, 'two-layer' days, and so on. Life's a bit like that. There's always another layer behind! And unfortunately, so is trying to stay well in this rather insane 20th-century world of ours.

So you've got all the amalgam out of your mouth, and now your teeth are beautifully white or creamy where once they were a nasty black. You're either rapidly (or gradually) chelating out your stored mercury. All is going well.

But that's not the end of it. There's another layer behind. There are the root canal-treated teeth to consider. Because in these teeth the nerve has been removed. Your dentist did his best to clean out the infection and then sealed up that tooth. It looks just fine.

However, research has revealed, particularly the research of the brilliant Dr Weston Price,[1] that chances are the infection that caused you to have the tooth thus treated will still be there, lurking in the infinitely numerous and labyrinthine tubules of the now dead-tooth.[2] Dr Price also found that the medications used to sterilize the root canals have no effect against the bacteria found in dentine tubules. Moreover, that there was leakage of this bacteria into the bloodstream surrounding the tooth.[3]

The problem is that if there *is* an infection in that tooth and beyond, then because the nerve has been removed you won't feel a thing. Nor will an X-ray reveal any problem because there's bone all around the root, and sometimes something called 'condensing osteitis' around the tooth in question, a blurring of the outlines.[4]

This is precisely what happened to me. I was seriously ill and could not recover. Every possible cause of the chronic ill-heath was explored, to scant avail. Eventually I went to my dentist and asked him to remove my one and only root canal-treated tooth which had been there for over 20 years. I had nothing to go on but my reading, my intuition and a muscle test.

But my dentist was astonished, offended. 'Absolutely not. There's nothing wrong with that tooth.'

I argued and pleaded, to no avail.

'Well, look at the X-ray,' he said, bringing it out, 'Nothing wrong with that tooth.'

To cut a long story short, in the end I had to threaten to 'go elsewhere', whereupon he agreed to remove the tooth. When the tooth was extracted, my dentist in astonishment held it before my eyes. There was a mass of bright green pus around the top of it. In fact it was a beautiful shade of emerald green never seen before by me in my body, or anywhere else for that matter.

'Well ... you were right about that tooth,' he had the goodness to say.

And I went home, believing I had solved a problem.

BUT, **there's another layer behind that one.**

And this third layer is called (and only very advanced thinkers in dentistry today seem aware of it), CAVITATIONS. This means you can have infections in the places where you once had teeth. That is, in the bony parts in the cavities, and not just where the root-treated teeth have been, but in *any cavity*. Back in 1940 Dr Martin Fisher, Professor of Physiology at the University of Cincinnati, wrote, 'When a dentist removes a tooth he leaves 50% of the problem behind.'[5] That is, in any infected tissue left after extraction.

So when my dentist pulled that tooth, he should have thoroughly cleaned out the cavity to remove any traces of infection, in fact *all* tooth cavities should be scraped right back to the bone, or one will not get out all the infected material. And that is the only way to prevent further trouble unless one happens to have a Grade A immune system to the end of one's days, which hardly anybody has any more.

And because my dentist did not know to do that, I had another 10 years of illness. In fact, I continued to get abscessed teeth and had them removed rather than live with the time bomb that is a root canal-treated tooth. But eventually there were life-destroying infections in all the cavities. It was a long time before I found a dentist with the slightest interest in my teeth-health problems. And when I did find a good one he found fragments of amalgam left by careless others paid to get it all out. (I think I've had my amalgams 'out' three times for some teeth.) Worse, he found evidence on the X-ray, evidence that had been there for anyone to see for 30 years (even I could see it when he showed me) that cement from that one root canal-treated tooth had been pushed up into the sinus above. It is still there, because I've found no one game enough to take it out. And these are the sorts of things that can bring one years of poor health.

Tom Warren, author of *Beating Alzheimer's* fame, never ceases his investigations into all of the causes of 'losing one's marbles'. Inspired by his marvellous new brain, he is a tireless researcher, bless him!

He says that in the earlier part of our century, it was a Dr Frank Billings who was responsible for the focal infection theory in relation to teeth. That is, that 95% of all infections in the body come from decayed teeth and infected tonsils.[6] This theory, in a pre-antibiotic age, was apparently what caused the wholesale removal of tonsils in children and teeth in young adults, in the period before the Second World War. For these were considered a potent risk to life.

Anyway, whether Billings was right or wrong, back in those pre-antibiotic days, because any infection was life-threatening, Dr Weston Price, a brilliant dental researcher and author of *Dental Infections and Degenerative Disease*, was placed at the head of a team of 60 scientists and physicians working on a study of focal infections. This study established the fact that bacteria and toxins within the dentine tubules of teeth and cavities, and the area where an infected tooth had been removed, could spread to other parts of the body. But the method of transmission throughout the body had not yet been found.

Then the magical penicillin was discovered. And immediately that whole field of endeavour was simply dropped.[7] This was a grave misfortune for untold numbers of people to come. But who, in those days could have known that **there is no drug which can reach all of the dentine tubules?** And that as Tom Warren so aptly puts it, 'Having a little infection is like being a little pregnant.'[8]

For the hard truth is that today it is quite often *not an obvious, virulent or acute infection* that is the real problem. It is the chronic, niggling, undermining kind of infection one is not even aware of which is so dangerous, *accompanied as it is by the very serious problem of what it may do to us long term.*

Tom Warren tells an amazing story about a woman with a breast tumour who was sent to get an abscessed tooth removed before surgery to remove the breast.[9] (Good surgeons never operate if there is an infection present).

Apparently, immediately after the tooth was removed, and while there was still the lidocaine (the anaesthesia) in her body, she went on to have a full thermography X-ray in another part of the hospital. To the astonishment of all who looked at the X-ray result, there was 'plain to be seen' a thin white line running from the tooth site down the neck and to the tumour in the breast, then on down to the stomach.

The surgeon, on seeing the X-ray, wisely decided not to operate. And within four months the breast tumour had disappeared.

Tom Warren regards that moment when the X-ray showed a thin white line from the tooth to the tumour as seminal, a 'moment of truth' in the progress of Western medicine. For that line had delineated an exact meridian, as upheld in the Chinese system of acupuncture. And in that system every tooth has a separate acupuncture meridian running through all the major organs in the body.

Since that time several Western researchers have established the presence of the meridians using radioactive isotopes followed by gamma-camera imaging. Within six minutes after injecting a radioactive substance into a meridian it will have travelled 30 centimetres (approximately 12 inches). Injections into random points produce no such pathways. And these meridian pathways are totally independent of the known vascular networks.[10]

What it means to thee and me is that the teeth can affect any part of the body, including the brain. And according to Tom Warren, the guiding precept is: 'NO tooth is worth saving if it damages your immune system.'

How many women, I wonder, develop breast cancer because of unsuspected infections in their mouths? This story may offer in part the solution to something which has puzzled me for over 20 years. I was, in the late 1970s, working with health statistics at the Auckland School of Medicine. And I was extremely puzzled by one statistic I came across. All of the health problems, including cancer, were worst in the so-called lower socio-economic levels of society, except for one type of cancer, breast cancer. There was more breast cancer among middle-class women than among the so-called working-class women. And this is still very much the case today.

I have gone on puzzling over this one lo these many years, because this extraordinary reversal should give us some clues. Why, why? More invasive investigations (X-rays)? More deodorant use, and hence more aluminium absorbed close to the breast? Longer periods of bra wearing? (See Chapter 29.) What could it be? Because it has to be *something*. These things do not happen without good reason.

I now believe that differences in tooth care may possibly be one important factor. Because getting the kind of dental work we are discussing, that is root canal work, is expensive. Perhaps poorer women are more inclined to have a tooth extracted because it is cheaper. And thereby some are spared the horror that is breast cancer? For simple extraction is safer. The root-filled tooth is dangerous.

Another possible theory as to why middle-class women have more breast cancer: toxins, especially pesticide residues, tend to be stored in fatty tissues; they have been found there. And when there is a shortage of fatty tissue then the breast tissue will be used for this purpose, and such accumulations may cause the breasts to become cancerous, as in the Israeli experience to be looked at in Chapter 21 on pesticides. Thus thin women, like the late Linda McCartney, tend to have more breast cancer than fat women, a reversal of the case with most other cancers. And, of course, it is middle-class women who tend to be on the thin side.

(Cancer is probably never a question of A leads to X or B leads to X. Life is not that simple. And one of the problems with medicine today is that it looks at everything too simply. But ongoing infections from root-filled teeth and/or stored biocidal residues may constitute pre-disposing factors which pave the way for other factors to do their worst.)

It is significant that cancer specialists in some parts of the world will not treat patients till all mouth problems have been resolved. Examples would be the current or past Presidents of the German and Austrian Societies for Oncology. All have confirmed that every patient attending their hospitals has an early appointment with the hospital dentist to remove both all amalgam and any dead and/or root-filled teeth. These would be Dr Hans Nieper, Hanover Germany; and Dr/ Professor W Kostler, Vienna, Austria.

Dr Kostler says that it is a waste of time trying to help someone with cancer when their immune system is continuously being poisoned by their teeth.[11] Moreover, as with our lady with the breast tumour, it is apparently not uncommon to find a dead tooth (or cavitation following inadequate extraction) on the same acupuncture meridian as the cancerous organ. If we want to avoid cancer we must look to our teeth, among other things.

I would add to what Dr Kostler has said. The salutary truth about all this is that, in my opinion, it is of scant use trying to treat **any** sick person with **any** health problem until the teeth and gums have been treated fully. For if there is a problem there, success in treating the other health problem will be limited and short-lived, that is if there is any success. Unfortunately, as mentioned, most medical people leave any problem in the mouth to the 'molar mechanics.'

Dental detoxicologists (a rare and precious sub-species of the genus 'dentist'), who specialize in the removal of mercury-silver amalgam, infected root canal teeth and the cleaning out of cavitation infections, claim that there are at least 200 different specific diseases related to these infected socket areas. Dr Price in his research found that only 30% of those patients with root canal fillings remained in good health.[12]

Carl K Telleen DVM, BS, reiterates,[13] 'Bacteria can migrate from infected teeth or root canals to joints, skin, and to any organ in the body.'

According to the *British Medical Journal*,[14] the risk factors for heart disease appear to be as follows: Smoking, diabetes, high blood pressure and a heavy stress load. To that of course I would include the more recent knowledge: taking in the wrong fats and oils, and drinking homogenized milk, to name but two additional factors. But a percentage of heart attack victims do not appear to fall into these categories. From *A Cardiologist Looks at Gum Disease*:

Focal infections in the mouth from periodontal disease (pockets of pus in the gums around the roots of the teeth) were found to be more common in heart attack victims than among people of similar age and sex without heart attacks. Researchers speculate that bacterial toxins get into the circulation whenever food is chewed and pressure is thereby exerted on the gums and teeth. Bacterial toxins are known to have injurious effects on the lining of the blood vessels, and might help to set the stage for coronary artery narrowing.[15]

Dr C C Bass, Dean of Tulane University School of Medicine wrote some years ago in the *American Heart Journal*: '... health, welfare, and even life itself, of persons who have heart conditions which predispose to infection, may depend upon prevention and control of dental disease.'[16]

Another senior doctor, Dr Lester Burket, chairman of the Oral Medicine Department (later Dean) of the University of Pennsylvania Dental School, said in his textbook *Oral Medicine*, that in a case of gum disease, a mild one – if laid out flat, the total ulceration area of the gum disease would minimally cover a post card –

'If that were on a patient's leg or arm, he'd run to a doctor – but it's in the mouth – and he doesn't feel it ... so the condition goes on and on.' Dr Burket added that from this rather large area, bacteria and toxins enter the bloodstream whenever food is chewed ... and that these transient bacteria can affect the total health of a person.[17]

Also, from even the journal of the conservative American Dental Association we find: 'It is not uncommon to see oral hygiene, which obviously contributes to total body welfare, being totally ignored in a patient who has severe systemic (total body) disease. Germs in the bloodstream are carried throughout the entire body.'[18]

Dr Samuel Charles Miller, then Chairman of the Periodontal Department of NYU's School of Dentistry, homed in on the problem and observed that

focal infection from the gums affects all our systems, such as: 1. the nervous system, leading to neuritis; 2. the cardiovascular system, leading to endocarditis, myocarditis, pericarditis; 3. the respiratory system – contributing to everything from sinusitis to lung abscesses.[19]

According to Dr Victor Penzer MD, DMD, FASCD, whose beloved brother, Dr Edward Penzer MD, LFADA died in 1992 of acute infectious endocarditis (infection in the heart) subsequent to numerous chronic silent mouth infections occasioned by allegedly incompetent dental treatment of root canals, if great care is not exercised, bacteraemia and septicemia can follow careless orthodontic treatment. And, 'Any non-resorbable material within the connective tissues can become the focus of a disease. A human tooth, with or without root canal filling, would be such a non-resorbable substance.'[20] Victor Penzer mourns his lost brother the more acutely, because he believes the loss was unnecessary.

What I am attempting to convey in this chapter is not a new idea, an untested novelty in the field of human health. In the earlier part of this century when they yanked out healthy tonsils and teeth so unceremoniously one could say it was perhaps an over-reaction. But they were doing it for a reason. It is a grave pity that that hard-won knowledge, that crucial reason, was ignored after the antibiotics came in. These may be 'wonder' drugs, but they have had some dreadful repercussions. And this casualness about what goes on in the mouth is just one of them. For untold numbers of people have died unnecessarily prematurely since the Second World War and the discovery of potent drugs, because after that, what went on in the mouth was considered 'not a problem'.

Tom Warren records one case of a physician with Alzheimer's Disease who recovered his normal brain function within two hours after having 13 root canal-treated teeth removed.[21] Tom Warren has certainly proved that Alzheimer's Disease can be reversed. But it will not always be in the same way for every victim.

Hal Huggins, who is pioneering the path of rediscovering the dental wisdom of the past, says that the damage occurs because the microbes found in teeth and gums can convert from aerobic life-forms to deadly **anaerobic** microbes within the dentine. Dr Weston Price, the early researcher, had found that the prevalent bacteria was *streptococcus fecalis*.[22] They are thus indescribably, astoundingly toxic, and they are free to roam the body.[23]

If you will pardon the analogy, I cannot help but see this infectious material as travelling the body like those predatory, marauding hordes of Genghis Khan; raping, pillaging, torturing, exterminating and striking fear into the heart of every cell they encounter.

Dr Huggins, who has been reproducing some of the earlier experiments done by Dr Price, as mentioned earlier, has found that rabbits injected with just 3 mcg of the toxins found in root-filled teeth will die in exactly one and a half minutes.[24] Moreover, these toxins appear to be specific to specific diseases. For example, a patient suffering from severe kidney disease recovered after a root-filled tooth was removed. And when tiny sections of that infected tooth were implanted into 30 rabbits, all 30 rabbits died from acute kidney disease and kidney failure.

Dr Price had begun by removing a tooth from a patient confined to a wheel-chair suffering with severe arthritis. Within two days of embedding this tooth in a rabbit, it developed crippling arthritis and died in 10 days. But by that time the patient was out of the wheelchair and on the way back to health.[25]

Inasmuch as an X-ray cannot always tell us when a tooth is in serious trouble, nor can we feel it (the nerve having been removed), it seems that even the very fit should not risk root-filled teeth. And of course people with root-filled teeth who have chronic health problems *should get them out as soon as possible.* And get the cavities thoroughly cleaned out.

For it is my belief that these silent enclaves in our mouths, which send out marauding hordes of toxic microbes, are a major health problem in all Western populations, and may even be a factor in what we refer to as 'ageing'.

EMERGENCY ADVICE

If you think you have a problem in the mouth as above, there may be difficulty finding someone to assist. Do not risk trying someone inexperienced. In the meantime, while you're looking, use frequent dilute peroxide mouth washes, both before and after eating. Also, use hot sea salt mouth washes. Swish these mouth washes around the gums in the mornings and last thing at night, to stimulate and firm the gums.

8: AIR QUALITY

'The air is OK. I can breathe!'

Scientists analysing the air mixture in bubbles trapped in fossilized amber find it isn't all *Jurassic Park* in there.[1] They find also that back when the mammals evolved there was 30% oxygen in the air, about twice as much as most of us get today. And if we're living in a big smoggy city, the oxygen level could be down as low as 12%.

People are given oxygen in emergencies for good reason. It is the main element in our bodies. We are approximately 80% water, and water is mostly oxygen.

Apparently it takes around 5 minutes for carbon monoxide to fill a garage with lethal exhaust fumes, enough to kill any living occupant. According to Waves Forest:

Stretch the minutes to years, multiply that car motor by several billion, add in all the jet engines and industrial belchings, and how many years do we have before most of the ground layer of our atmosphere tastes like a garage? In some places it already does, and these spots are growing rapidly. The rains can only wash out so much of it.

At the same time, the planet's oxygen-producing forests have shrunk to the smallest size in recorded history, so now far less oxygen is being released back into the air, and less carbon dioxide is being absorbed and broken down. Half of the rain forests we came into this century with have been sent quite prematurely and rudely to that great jungle in the sky, along with vast wooded areas that used to occupy temperate zones ... But because the atmosphere is so vast, a severe imbalance between global production and global consumption of oxygen can exist for decades before the effects become obvious enough for humans to notice.[2]

But one of the present problems is that oxygen deficiency is a major cause of disease; it can happen also because of all the 'extra baggage' we're carrying around in our veins. For example, the pesticides, the heavy metals, the chlorine and the fluoride, the end-products of the TFAs, the Xanthine Oxidase from homogenized milk and a thousand other things. When the bloodstream contains too much rubbish, our overworked elimination systems have difficulty keeping up and there's not enough room for those precious oxygen molecules we need to stay well. The more debris, the less oxygen. Also disease organisms cannot survive in high oxygen levels, but they flourish in low levels.

EMERGENCY ADVICE

Waves Forest advises replanting the lungs of the planet on a massive scale. Till then, Hydrogen Peroxide, 35% Food Grade, 1–3 drops in a glass of water daily, can put oxygen back into our bodies. Chelation can get the rubbish out. Everyone plant a tree!

⚠

9: WATER QUALITY

'After they've treated the water
it's perfectly safe.'

There are several recent books published on the absolute necessity for people to have good, safe water. After oxygen, water (which is mostly oxygen too) is critical to life. We are, or should be, nearly 80% water, and that includes our brains. So 'water on the brain' is not so bad. We *should* have water on the brain, otherwise we're in trouble. It's just a question of how much.

I remember reading, some years back, about an experiment carried out in a home for older people. Brain maps were done, and some of the residents were shown to have shrunken brains. These were also those who appeared to have the most trouble with their 'marbles'. The experiment was to see if drinking water would improve brain function. Every hour a trolley came around and all were encouraged to drink a glass of water, except for two hours after meals. In a few months many had improved in several ways, and brain mapping showed comparative brain expansion. A salutary lesson for us all. (Unfortunately, elderly people tend to live on tea and toast. Tea is dehydrating, as is coffee.)

So, apart from the air, water is the single most important substance we can consume. It circulates through 60,000 miles of veins and arteries. Every function in the body needs water, and it becomes a part of every cell.[1]

Apparently one of the causes of pain is insufficient water, which causes dehydration of both brain and body. The brain will then express its desperate need for water by signalling us with pain. For **we cannot rely on our thirst alone to tell us when we need water**, especially as we grow older. People have found that drinking several glasses of good water will actually ease pain.[2] No! As noted, tea and coffee *will not do!* They are both *dehydrating*. We must drink plain water or suffer the consequences in both body and brain.

The problem today is, given that we no longer have fresh running streams to drink from and few of us have uncontaminated deep wells, it is now up to local governments to deliver us safe and drinkable water, conducive to human health.

But Colin Ingram, in *The Drinking Water Book*,[3] argues that there is hardly a drop of water left in the world safe to drink. And generally you cannot tell by the look of it, the taste of it or the smell of it.

For one thing it is necessary to chlorinate water to kill bacteria, but we need to be concerned about the effects on our health of long-term ingestion of chlorine. For there is no question that chlorine creates toxicity when it bonds with some of the organic chemicals ever-present in water. It forms compounds known as THMs (Trihalomethanes), which are known to be carcinogenic, that is they can cause cancer in vulnerable people. Chloroform is only one of these chlorine compounds. Most public water supplies will have measurable levels of THMs. In Europe the EU has set a maximum level of 1 ppb (parts per billion) of THMs as safe, meanwhile the US safe level is considered to be 100 ppb.[4]

With such 'wide-apart' differing standards, it seems likely that nobody really knows what is or isn't a 'safe' level, and that these are just guesses, like the original 'safe' levels of radiation exposure, which had to be frequently revised downwards as the years went by and people exposed to supposedly 'safe' levels developed cancer. And anyway, given our biochemical uniqueness, what is safe for one may not be safe for another.

A US Environmental Protection Agency study comparing women who drank chlorinated water with those who did not found among the chlorinated water drinkers a 44% higher rate of death due to intestinal and urinary tract cancers than in those not drinking chlorinated water.[5] Others believe that THMs can also contribute to heart disease.[6]

Beyond the danger from THMs, we also know that it is possible for certain viruses and parasites immune to chlorine such as the protozoan parasites giardia and cryptosporidium to creep into the water. In April 1993 cryptosporidium got into the water supply in the city of Milwaukee, killing at least 40 people and causing severe illness in over 370,000 residents.[7] Those with strong immune systems can survive such an onslaught, but as we must by now be aware there are a host of other things working against our immune systems.

In most Western countries there has been such widespread use of pesticides that they have leached into almost every water source. For example, in New Zealand, although 245T is now belatedly banned, there is almost no water anywhere without its minute traces of 245T. People who have in the past been accidentally 'sprayed' with 245T and subsequently develop severe sensitivities to it and to water, are simply 'out of luck'. In really bad cases there is no solution known to us.

Jeff Breakey claims that every year more and more of the 700,000 tons of toxic hazardous waste flung into the American environment gets into the water supply.[8] The evidence lies in the thousands of what used to be pure water wells now shut down from chemical contamination.

As Rachel Carson said over 35 years ago, 'It is not possible to add pesticides to water **anywhere** without threatening the purity of water **everywhere**.'[9]

Linda Weiss[10] says that there may be contamination in our water supplies from heavy metals such as mercury, lead, cadmium and nickel; asbestos, radon, road salt, leaking gasoline storage tanks or industrial wastes that seep into the water table. Again, for most of these there is no indication when they are in the water. For example, dissolved lead cannot be seen, tasted or smelled.

Another 'silent' toxic metal deliberately added to our water is aluminium, there to reduce 'that cloudy look'. According to Dr Morton Walker, DPM, aluminium is one of the toxic metals on the list of substances implicated in Alzheimer's Disease.[11] This relationship was truly established in a huge UK survey of 88 counties (reported in the *Lancet*) wherein there was found a direct relationship between the level of aluminium in the water supply and the level of Alzheimer's Disease. Scientists found a 50% increase in the risk with the higher concentrations of aluminium in the water, particularly true in Wales.[12] These findings have also been corroborated by other such studies in Australia, France, Norway and the US.[13]

Aluminium is not just in our drinking water. It is also to be found in numerous products we use: tea, coffee, baking soda; deodorants, beer cans, aluminium foil, cow's milk, soya milk, prescription and over-the-counter drugs; and particularly from aluminium cookware.[14]

The very worst I have come across is this:

aluminium concentration in infant formulas increases considerably during their preparation. The permeability of the gastrointestinal tract is greatest in the first days after birth, enhancing the potential for absorption of substances from the diet that normally get excluded.[15]

Consequently, the seeds of Alzheimer's Disease may be planted during the first days of life.

PHARMACEUTICAL WASTE IN WATER

A recent report from Janet Raloff in *Science News* concerns the addition to our water of pharmaceutical drugs coming from human body wastes.[16] As much as

50–90% of a medicine still in its original form can find its way from the body into the water supply. And now and then a chemical reaction with other substances in the water can turn partly degraded drugs back into an active form. Also, antibiotics in the water supply can contribute to antibiotic resistance, a question we will look at in more detail in Chapter 31.

Jules Klotter, commenting on this in the *Townsend Letter*, was struck by the irony of the situation:

How often have we heard disparaging comments about supplement-takers with 'expensive' urine? No one points out that the body also excretes pharmaceuticals, which are a heck of a lot more expensive than supplements and, being foreign to the environment, have unknown effects.[17]

These effects of drugs in our water are beginning to worry European officials responsible for the safety of water supplies. As for me, it is annoying to think that I've faithfully avoided taking drugs, only to have them forced on me in the water supply.

BREASTFEEDING, BREASTFEEDING!

Whatever we do as a community to treat water, the expense stems from the fact that only .5% of it actually goes for drinking and cooking in the home. The rest goes to industry or down the drains. That is perhaps why most people who study the problem of water end up believing that the most economical way to treat water is at the point of use. This makes sense because even if we had extra clean water from a treatment plant it can be contaminated by the time it gets to us. The delivery system includes piping systems of cast iron, cement-asbestos and PVC, all of which can pollute the water. Where there is a site of repair and alteration there will be further contamination from the asbestos fibres. Even changes in water pressure within the pipes can cause high levels of asbestos to enter the water. And finally, just before the water enters our homes, Ingram says that 'lead, cadmium and other toxic metals leach out of the valves and couplings of the pipes'.[18] It is particularly inadvisable to drink water from the hot water cylinder instead of from the cold tap, because hot water leaches out lead.

Nor is bottled water the answer. In most countries bottled water does not have to be more pure than tap water. 'Bacteria and chemicals have been found in all bottled water that has been tested.'[19] This finding was made by US government water experts analysing numerous well-known bottled-water products. Also there is a 42-page document put out by the California State Assembly as a result of an extensive study of bottled water which comes to similar conclusions. In fact, bottled water is often found to be less safe than our tap water. But then again, 93 out of 140 community water systems failed to meet the American Federal Government's minimum testing standards.[20]

The different ways of purifying one's own water at 'the point of use' involve lengthy and complex explanations beyond the scope of this book. I will say though, **please** avoid water distillers with plastic inside the lid, or those that catch distilled water in plastic, because those very hungry molecules coming up in the steam will bind with any of the highly mobile plastic molecules they encounter. The distiller should be of glass or the best stainless steel. (That is, one that will cause a fridge magnet to 'stick'.) Neither the steam nor the newly processed water should come into contact with plastic. I regard this as a serious danger. (See Chapter 16 on plastic.)

Another danger with water distillers is that they deprive you of the good minerals found in water. One must take supplementary minerals if one drinks distilled water.

Above all, it is essential to retain a country's water supply in public ownership, because people who 'buy' it to make a profit are not going to waste that profit by upgrading when possible and as new knowledge comes along. The owners are in there solely to make money and that should never be forgotten. The British have seen quite clearly that when water is privatized, the price goes up and the quality goes down.

When our health, our very lives are at stake, it is essential to see beyond ideology and into reality.

And then there is the fluoride in our water, which deserves a chapter all on its own.

⚠

10: FLUORIDE

'And then there's that wonderful fluoride.
It's safe and it protects us from tooth decay.'

Many years ago we were told that fluoride would improve our teeth, and at the same time that it was harmless to human health. To date there is not a single honest study to establish either that it works or that it is safe. Early Soviet writings reveal that fluorides had customarily been used to calm intractable prize bulls, making them easier to handle. Similarly, in the 1940s sodium fluoride was added to the water given to prisoners of war to make them stupid and docile. Apparently the Germans also made use of fluoride in this manner.[1] For similar purposes the former Soviet Union administered increasing dosages of fluoride to their prison populations in that huge empire, the Gulag Archipelago, 'the largest network of concentration camps in the world'.[2]

In the West we use high levels of fluoride components in most of the major tranquillizers given to our mentally ill. These are used to keep patients quiet and submissive, just as they were used in the former Soviet Union and Germany to keep prisoners quiet. The most widely used anti-depressive drug today is Prozac, or fluoxetine hydrochloride, a fluoride compound. And then there is the fluoride used in rat poison.

Clearly all these brain-controlling uses of fluoride involve significantly larger doses than we have in our water, but perhaps had we known of them we might have been less gullible. Moreover, there *are* people who speak of the 'dumbing down' of our society and wonder if fluoride has been among the causes.

Another of the more sensational aspects of fluoride concerns its use in the production of atomic bombs. Government documents recently declassified at the 50-year mark reveal that fluoride was the key chemical in atomic and nuclear bomb production, necessitating millions of tons of the stuff. And it was not radiation that was considered to be the leading health hazard of the bomb research programme, both for workers and for nearby communities. It was fluoride. In fact, apparently the first lawsuits against the American A-bomb programme were not over radiation, but over damage caused by fluoride.[3] But evidence for the adverse health effects of fluoride was censored by the US Atomic Energy Commission 'for reasons of national security'. This knowledge is more or less censored still, but for other reasons now.

Fluoride today is an industrial chemical of major proportions. It is used in the production of numerous items, from aluminium to pesticides, and is an ubiquitous part of most modern environments. From all these uses there are huge amounts of waste fluoride produced.

As early as 1937 the Danish scientist, Kaj Roholm, had warned the world of the dangers of fluoride ingestion.[4] Many others have done so since and we will be looking at some of them.

The first person to promote fluoridation as a means of preventing tooth decay was an American, Dr Trendley Dean. He was subsequently taken to court twice (1955 and 1960) and forced to admit that the statistics from the early studies he used to promote fluoridation were invalid – that is, fraudulent.[5]

And even as fluoridation was spreading around the globe, reports on the toxic effects of fluoride were beginning to surface: Tumour formation in mice (1952 and 1956); genetic damage to plants (1966) and fruit flies (1970, 1971). By 1972 the hypothesis (that fluoride prevents tooth decay, and is safe) was in doubt, and there were widespread concerns about some of the 'scientific evidence' for the benefits claimed for fluoridation.

A former Special Consultant to the Minister of Health, British Columbia, Dr Richard G Foulkes BA, MD, was originally the one who recommended that fluoride be added to the water supply in British Columbia. Dr Foulkes has since emphatically changed his mind, and says of that early recommendation that 'a powerful lobby' misled him into believing that the practice was safe and prevented tooth decay. One wonders if this was not the same 'powerful lobby' that originally persuaded Dr Trendley Dean. 'Huge financial concerns lie behind the promotion of this industrial waste product as a health benefit.'[6]

Of his complete reversal Dr Foulkes now says:

In the light of what is currently found in reputable journals with peer review mechanisms and in various Government documents and correspondence, I now hold a different view. That is that the fluoridation of community water supplies can no longer be held to be either safe or effective in the reduction of dental caries. Therefore, the practice should be abandoned or 'put on hold' until all available information is evaluated by persons who are competent in the principles of research and who have no vested interest in those institutions or professional organizations that are currently involved.

In fact Dr Foulkes, now actively campaigning to get it out of the water, believes that fluoride causes brittle bones in the elderly and may be a factor in certain forms of cancer.[7]

Most of us believe, or want to believe, that high level decisions affecting our health, our very lives, are made with the utmost care and based on 'scientific knowledge'. But this is not necessarily so. To illustrate the vagueness of the decision-making process in the area of fluoridation, we need to look at the *Townsend Letter for Doctors*,[8] which in 1989 reproduced a transcript of a meeting held in Washington DC in 1983. (This had been obtained under the Freedom of Information Act by Martha Bevis of Houston, Texas, with the aid of her Congressman.)

The transcript is a record of a discussion among the nine top American world-class 'experts on fluoride', doctors and scientists, who deliberated on the question of the maximum safe dose of fluoride to be put in the water. This was, of course, nearly 40 years after the initial fluoridation of US water supplies. In 1975 it was declared that no undesirable effects of fluoride could occur in water using 10 ppm (parts per million) at a time when the level used was 2 ppm.

The following discussion was to decide on a 'safe' level for that time, in the light of then-current findings on adverse effects of fluoridation. The meeting and its recommendations were requested by the US Environmental Protection Agency.

The transcript reveals a group of people who don't know what they're doing, feeling their way to a consensus. Here are a few excerpts, sentences selected from the discussion:

Dr W: 'I realize that we have few facts and many unknowns.'

Dr S: 'We could cut it that close. I just don't know where the truth is. That is what I don't know.'

Dr W: 'Let me go ahead on what we don't know. First of all, any problem with a low latency isn't going to show up by anything available to us at the present time.'

Dr S: 'I am saying that I accept that we do not have the numbers from what it is in the literature.'

Dr M: 'Just as dental fluorosis is a manifestation of moderately low levels of fluoride excess, osteosclerosis is the next stage, and crippling fluorosis is a much more severe stage.'

Dr K: 'What is the level of fluoride in the drinking water in those communities that get ... crippling endemic bone fluorosis?'

Dr S (1): 'You don't know what the level is, but certainly you're talking 8–10 ppm [parts per million] and above.'

Dr S (2): 'The problem with that literature is that they tell you the ... waters contain 1.6 to 15 or 18 or 23 ppm, and you never know what well the guy is using that shows this.'

Dr S (1) 'I think that you have to conclude that we haven't looked for it and we really don't know.'

Dr S (2) 'Let's just say, because we really don't have the information to come off of this, that osteosclerosis occurs and we really don't know whether it is positive or not. We don't have the data.'

Dr M: 'But we can still vote on it. That's what we're here for.'

Dr K: 'From all the available data, we can't state that there is no apparent adverse health effect on a water fluoride level of 2 ppm or below.'

Dr W: 'You would have to have rocks in your head, in my opinion, to allow your child much more than 2 ppm.'

Dr R: 'I think we all agree on that.'

Despite these expressed misgivings on the part of some of the safety of even 2 ppm, a majority of the committee eventually voted unequivocally for the safety of fluoride levels at 4 ppm. And when it came time to the question of age and toxicity:

Dr K: 'If you're talking about potential toxicity, we have no idea whether it is 18 or puberty. We have no idea.'

When it came to vote on the question, the chairman said: 'All right. How many people feel that 18, picking that one out of the air, is a more appropriate age to run the 12 ppm up to than nine?' ... 'I know I mentioned every age under the sun. I guess I will settle with a recommendation for 18.' But split down the middle, the committee voted 5–4 for age nine.

Thus this committee's 'deliberations' reveal an astonishing lack of safety data about a dubious chemical then being added to more than half the water supplies in the US, and throughout this discussion it apparently did not occur to any of them simply to recommend that fluoridation be stopped.

Fluoride is dangerous. And those countries with intelligent leadership have simply stopped fluoridation, or never started it. Among these countries are: Norway, Sweden, the Netherlands, Denmark, West Germany, Belgium, Finland, Russia, Japan, Greece, India, Sri Lanka, China, Burma much of the Middle East and Northern Africa. In addition, 500 cities elsewhere in the world have stopped it or never had it. The European Commission has definitely ruled against it.

Very few governments actively promote it apart from those of New Zealand, Australia and the US.[9] South Africa was free of fluoride thanks to the opposition of Douw G Steyne, Professor of Pharmacology at the University of Pretoria, now deceased. But unfortunately now that he has gone, recent Western aid to that country seems to have a fluoridated string attached to it.

Studies have revealed numerous health problems occurring as a result of fluoridation. The first concerns were to do with mottled teeth (endemic dental fluorosis). The late, very great, Dr John Colquhoun PhD, BDS of New Zealand, for one, did considerable research in this area.[10] Several different studies by professional researchers found a range of 20 to 50% of children with dental mottling in fluoridated areas. And this at 1 ppm in New Zealand. In non-fluoridated areas it was approximately 4.25%. This mottling is called dental fluorosis, but it often describes more than simple mottling. There may also be pitting, even crumbling of teeth. And as our teeth are the hardest part of the body, if they are in trouble the chances are the bones are also. And in fact overgrowth and weakening of bone *have* been found in association with dental fluorosis in both boys and in male rats.[11]

One of the problems is that today fluoride can be found in so many things beyond the drinking water: foods, soft drinks, toothpaste, mouth rinses and topical application gels. No one knows who is actually getting how much. (It has been estimated that children will swallow about one-third of the toothpaste they use.) Moreover, you can get as much as 5 mg per day from a combination of tea and the water with it. You get more in boiled water than in unboiled, and you get it sometimes in high amounts in bottled water. Even if the countries who artificially fluoridate the drinking water were to stop tomorrow, the environment is already overflowing with it.

Even infants, or perhaps especially infants, can be at risk from too much fluoride. According to a recent *Journal of the American Dental Association* article, some modern commercially-prepared baby foods contain such high levels of fluoride that babies who consume them are at risk of dental fluorosis (the white flecks, or irreversibly brown- or yellow-stained permanent teeth).[12]

Then there is also cow's milk, containing increasing amounts of fluoride despite the fact that Nature attempts to filter it out. As we noted in Chapter 3 on homogenized milk, there is an imbalance of calcium and magnesium in cow's milk, that is for humans, because it is not a milk that was designed for us; it is designed for calves. And this imbalance can contribute to osteoporosis, or bone deficiency disease. But unfortunately fluoride also is antagonistic to magnesium, and negates it. So that we have the normal imbalance of calcium to magnesium in the milk plus the fluoride, which makes it worse.[13] Additionally, the usual inappropriate agricultural techniques now in use and the toxins used will also deplete magnesium.[14]

You can certainly increase bone **mass** with calcium and fluoride, but without the magnesium, which is the mineral which provides the elasticity in bone, and other minerals, it is a seriously defective bone which may simply crack, fracture and shatter under strain.[15]

Recently an animal study has demonstrated that with increasing fluoride levels in the diet the quality of bone decreases. The scientists' conclusions: 'Ultrastructural disorientation of bone tissue and articular cartilage is a toxic effect of fluoride.'[16]

Thus, as another antagonist to magnesium, fluoride contributes to faulty bone structure. And yet we have today a situation where people are actually advised to take both fluoride supplements and calcium supplements 'for the good of your bones'. And it affects far more than bones. Fluoride actually *increases the requirements* for calcium as well as magnesium, which can result in a general state of deficiency with secondary hormonal problems as mentioned in Chapter 3.[17]

Indeed a Mad Hatter's tea party.

It is no wonder that we have an epidemic of osteoporosis with this kind of advice being given to so many women. There are now seven studies which show an association between fluoridated water and hip fractures.[18] And hip fractures from osteoporosis are serious matters. Today they cause more deaths in women than cancers of the breast, cervix and uterus combined. And those who manage to survive the fracture will be extremely debilitated.[19]

Moreover, for the first time researchers are beginning to see fluorosis and hip fractures in those fluoridated parts of the world where it has never been seen before. Senegal and India are both seeing dental and skeletal fluorosis.[20] One study also demonstrated significant increase in hip fractures in fluoridated areas.[21]

On the other side of the problem, selenium tends to protect the skeleton from the effects of fluoride.[22] The populations of countries with low selenium in the soil such as Finland and New Zealand will therefore experience more bone problems from fluoride than those with good levels of selenium in the soil.

It is also not in the least surprising that the incidence of heart attacks among women is also increasing every year, whereas a few years ago it was negligible. The Framingham study has revealed that heart disease is now the most frequent cause of death in women over 67 in the US;[23] in fact women have caught up with men and surpassed them. This has possibly been caused by the Xanthine Oxidase in homogenized milk and the magnesium deficiency caused by milk, as well as from the fluoride-induced magnesium deficiency. For as we have noted (Chapter 4), it is magnesium that guards our hearts as well as our bones.

There is also a problem with fluoride in combination with aluminium, as we have noted, added to our water to reduce cloudiness. For the most minute amounts of aluminium will potentiate (increase) the effects of fluoride.[24] Aluminium is also not only in our water supply but also in numerous products we use, as well as in aluminium cookware (see Chapter 9). Thus when you cook in aluminium you are adding more of a toxic metal. You are also depleting your magnesium and calcium.

(As noted, aluminium is on the list of substances long-established as implicated in Alzheimer's Disease. And we put it in our water supply!)

The good news is that once we get the fluoride out of our water, our bones will gradually normalize provided we have enough magnesium and selenium in the diet. The living skeleton is constantly being mineralized (or demineralized, as the case may be), so that we get a completely new one about every 8 to 10 years.

But there are numerous other studies to warn us of the dangers of fluoride. To cite only a few: In 1967, Dr M A Roshal of Canada pointed out that even at the so-called 'safe' levels of 1 ppm, blood sugar metabolism is adversely affected. People with diabetes or hypoglycaemia should not take in fluoride.[25] Rosetta Schuman, veteran health researcher, cites a prominent US allergist, Dr Jonathan Forman, who wrote

In our practice we have run down cases of hives in several patients with behaviour problems and others who have been labelled neurotic, and have found the cause to be fluoride contamination. When these people were put on distilled water and when fluoride-containing foods were removed from their diets, they recovered. When fluorides were re-introduced into their diets, the symptoms returned.[26]

Since 1994 it has been known that fluoride can accumulate in brain tissues and affect behaviour, IQ and/or learning abilities, depending on the age at exposure, and moreover that it has the potential to cause motor dysfunction.[27] That is, fluoridation can affect the CNS (Central Nervous System). Dr Phyllis Mullenix et al. have shown this by demonstrating hyperactivity in rats after prenatal exposure to fluoride. 'Experience with other developmental neurotoxicants teaches us that changes in behavioural function will be comparable across species, especially humans and rats ... also indications of a potential for motor dysfunction, IQ deficits and/or learning disabilities in humans.'[28]

Chinese investigations into the effects on humans taking in high levels of fluoride in the drinking water also report that the Central Nervous System is affected, and this would also suggest that children with dental fluorosis are at greater risk of decreased mental activity and increased risk of disturbed behaviour.[29] In fact, children living in areas with a high fluoride level were of lower intelligence than those children with the lowest levels of fluoride in their water. This was attributed to exposure as an embryo when the differentiation of brain cells occurs. Both the human research in China and the animal research in the US point to the neurotoxicity of fluoride in drinking water. That is, it can cause brain damage.

Meanwhile, American National Cancer Institute surveys found that, since 1973, in fluoridated areas around the country there was a 53% increase of bone cancer (osteosarcoma, a rare form of cancer) in males under the age of 20.[30] There were similar findings from a state study: in 1992, Dr P D Cohn studied bone cancer (osteosarcoma) in three counties of New Jersey and established that the ratio of osteosarcoma in males under 20 years was 5:1 in fluoridated vs non-fluoridated areas.[31] This means, of course, that fluoride may not just damage bones and cause hip fractures in older women, but it can cause cancer in the bones of others also.

Perhaps most damning of all, fluoride also reduces the mobility of white cells, which thus depresses the immune system, our defence against infections and cancer.[32] Altogether, about 10,000 excess deaths a year in the US have been attributed to the fluoridation of water.[33] And finally, it has been noticed that airborne fluoride can cause surface deterioration in both marble and Portland cement.[34] **Pretty powerful stuff!**

However, as most people are unaware of these serious side-effects of fluoride, the most basic issue for many may be, 'Does fluoride do the job? We are concerned about our children's teeth. Surely it has reduced dental decay?' When we try to find evidence as to what has caused the reduction in the incidence of tooth decay, however, we come up against a blank wall. When all published studies were examined by Dr D Ziegelbecker in 1981,[35] no correlation was found between the level of fluoride in water and numbers of decayed teeth. This, along with other studies reported previously (e.g. Japan, 1972) actually destroyed the basic hypothesis that supports the case for artificial fluoridation of community water supplies.

Professor Mark Diesendorf PhD, of Sydney University, Australia,[36] studied the incidence of decay in both fluoridated and non-fluoridated areas in eight developed countries over 30 years, and found large reductions in tooth decay in both the fluoridated and non-fluoridated areas. So the reduction in tooth decay cannot be attributed to fluoride.

The courageous and highly principled ex-chief dental officer for Auckland, Dr John Colquhoun PhD BDS,[37] reported that studies in New Zealand based on official government data, collected over 50 years, indicate that reductions in tooth decay were taking place *before* the fluoridation of water supplies and the introduction of topical fluorides and fluoride toothpaste.

Even the studies done by *pro-fluoridation professionals* show that the difference between the two areas is, on average, a difference of one tooth, or one tooth surface only.[38] These studies do not, of course, discuss the risks involved.

There is also evidence that data have been manipulated, for example in New Zealand and in Scotland, where fluoridation has since been discontinued.[39]

But if it's true that tooth decay has declined in our world, the question must then arise, 'Why has tooth decay been significantly reduced at all? If not the fluoride, then what?'

The fact is that nobody really knows. Tooth decay is caused by a bacterium and as such is a microbial disease. We in fact have to ask the same question about why many other microbial invaders such as diphtheria, scarlet fever and tuberculosis have declined. Most infectious diseases were in decline long before the advent of antibiotics, mass vaccinations and fluoridation, all of which have had miracles attributed to them. (See page 129 in Chapter 17.) Since the beginning of time there has been a constant state of flux between people and microbes – for centuries there were those occasional pandemic plagues which killed enormous numbers of people in a short period. But we have not had one of those since 1920.

Some claim that the cleaner environment (the improved sanitation and improved diet in the early part of the 20th century) generally strengthened the immune system, which meant the gradual decline of many of those infective agents. And it is an ominous sign that some of them, such as tuberculosis, are returning.

It is without doubt extremely ironic that around the time that tooth decay was undoubtedly in decline, much of the world decided to contaminate its water with something to reduce tooth decay. Now *there's* something to amuse those observers from the future. But it is not terribly amusing to us, for it seems there is always a price to pay when we try to take a short-cut to health. We pay the price personally in reduced health and more expense, and the environment pays a most terrible price.

Dr Foulkes says this:

It has long been recognized that fluorides, in their various forms, are toxic to plants, insects and animals, including humans. Fluorides are an industrial pollutant as they are byproducts of numerous industrial processes. These include the manufacture of fertilizer, the smelting of aluminium, the generating of power from coal and high octane gasoline.

We do not perhaps think about what happens to the water when we've done with it. However, the damage to our environment from simply dumping tons and tons of this waste product into our waterways is incalculable. We have flooded our environment with fluoride. It is into everything that uses water. If we were to stop adding it to the water supply right now, we would still have it around for millennia to come.

And there is a cash cost involved. Despite the fact that fluoride is a waste product, a side-effect of producing something else, it costs us all, everyone of us, plenty. In fact it has been a most expensive experiment, not just in terms of the environment and human health, but also in monetary terms. From the University of North Wales, Geoffrey Dobbs: 'Children have been reported to drink about 0.04% of the public water supply, so that the remaining 99.96% of the fluoride added is pure pollution with nothing to recommend or justify it...' In fact, for every $1,000 spent by the rate/taxpayer for fluoride chemicals, less than 50 cents goes towards the purchase of fluoride for children.[40]

In Tacoma, Washington, out of a total annual expenditure of $125,000 for chemicals, only $10 of this is consumed by children, except for a very small amount ingested by other age groups. The excess fluoridated water is used for all other purposes and is put into the environment mostly through the sewer system ... for example, Seattle, Washington puts an estimated 225 tons of fluoride (hydrofluosilicic acid) into its water supply each year.

Another example:

The current estimated annual costs of water fluoridation in Calgary are $230,000 a year just for the chemicals, and 99.9% of this will not be drunk, but will be flushed straight down the city sewers. The effect will be to deposit roughly 150 tonnes of fluoride into the Bow River and environment each year. Under pollution control regulations the Reynolds Aluminium Company of Canada Ltd, is legally permitted to discharge only 36.5 tonnes of fluoride into the St Lawrence each year.[41]

It is clear that were these huge industries unable to sell their waste fluoride to local governments, they would be up for considerable cost. As it is, they are actually earning money for their waste. A double win for them! A double cost for us! And the rest.

And what is this enormous dumping of a toxic substance into our waterways doing to the fish and other sea life? It is probably not just overfishing by the greedy that is depleting our fish resources. Fluoride is also playing its part. Dredging brings up the fluoride from the bottom where it falls and accumulates. Immature fish are the most sensitive to it. If exposed to fluoride they will make unproductive eggs and develop bone abnormalities.[42]

Dr Foulkes believes that if children must have fluoride it would be significantly more cost-effective, as well as more health-effective, to give them fluoride tablets. Moreover, these would then be *pharmaceutical grade fluoride rather than industrial waste.*

But in truth only topically-applied fluoride (that is, fluoride applied to the actual teeth) seems to make a difference.

Foulkes also declares that decisions on such matters as fluoridation should be made by elected officials and the general public, rather than the 'health authorities'.[43] This would be because once the latter have made a commitment to a certain position it is very hard to budge them, because that may imply an admission of past wrong-doing. But there is nothing wrong with responding and acting upon new knowledge as it comes along. That is the admirable path to take.

The journal *Fluoride*[44] (edited for many years by Dr John Colquhoun) features editorially an apt quotation from Leo Tolstoy, which is applicable not just for the fluoride question, but for most of the issues we have been discussing in this book:

I know that most men ... can seldom accept even the simplest and most obvious truth if it be such as would oblige them to admit the falsity of conclusions which they have delighted in explaining to colleagues, which they have proudly taught to others, and which they have woven, thread by thread, into the fabric of their lives.

One can only hope that these are threads which will soon become unravelled, along with many others. There are indeed signs that this is happening. The UK's *Guardian Weekend* recently featured a huge article on fluoride, 'Clear and Present Danger':[45]

Since childhood we have been told that fluoride is good for our teeth ... but fluoride toxicity has now been linked to bone disease, infant mortality, and brain damage. And the line between safety and danger, purity and poison, is a thin one.

Moreover, as there is a class action (500 people suing because of teeth mottling and crumbling) in process against the makers of fluoride toothpastes, the British Dental Association has urged such companies to give clear information as to the fluoride content of toothpaste. Professor John Murray, Dean of Newcastle University's School of Dentistry, said such precise information was necessary to enable consumers to make 'informed choices'. This follows in the wake of 'a series of academic studies suggesting that its long-term use can damage bones, the immune system and the central nervous system'.[46]

And finally, the conservative American Food and Drug Administration is now requiring warning labels on all fluoride toothpaste as follows:

WARNING: Keep out of the reach of children under six years of age. If you accidentally swallow more than used for brushing, seek professional help or contact a poison control centre immediately.

If that is not an admission that fluoride is a poison, what can be?

Once one becomes 'water conscious' the feeling of 'water, water, everywhere, but not a drop to drink' becomes overwhelming at times, especially if one is striving for optimum health.

Fortunately there is a better way to purify most water. Today over 3,300 cities in the world treat their water with ozone. Most of these can be found in Europe, but in the US in 1985, Los Angeles California installed the largest ozone water treatment plant in the country, perhaps because this city with its vast freeway system had become pollution-conscious.[47] Ozone treatment not only purifies the water in terms of bacteria, but also it *oxidizes* out heavy metals like mercury, lead and cadmium.[48] (However, as we noted in Chapter 9, this does not take care of the problem of water gathering toxicity en route to us.)

As we have noted, since we evolved the oxygen in our air has declined drastically, from 30% down to about 19%, which in cities can be reduced to 12% or less.[49] Ozone water treatment not only purifies the water but it actually adds an extra molecule of oxygen to the water. This extra oxygen, readily absorbed by the body, brings renewed energy, health and vitality to those consuming it.

It is essential in our oxygen-poor world that we do what we can for the health of our children and ourselves with this most vital of natural resources. The steps we need to take are as crystal clear as ozone-treated water.

1. As mentioned in Chapter 9, *we must retain in public hands anything to do with the number one natural source, our country's water supply.* We will never get any improvements put in by people buying our precious natural resource with the aim of making money from it. The evidence from the UK shows that water quality deteriorates after privatization, while prices increase.

2. We must insist on our water being ozone-treated, and of course, without the addition of fluoride. When it is a question of our health, our children's welfare and a little money, there should be no question about it. And of course we will put those enormous sums we used to pay for a waste product, fluoride, into the ozone plants.

It is long past time to get rid of what the late Philip Sutton, dentist, called *The Greatest Fraud: Fluoridation.*[50]

11: SUGAR

'A little sugar can't hurt!'

Many years ago I read John Yudkin's book, *Pure, White and Deadly*, and ever since have looked at sugar with a jaundiced eye.

US government statistics indicate that over half the calories of the average American diet consists of processed or 'dismembered' foods that have been stripped of their balanced nutrients; foods such as white sugar, white flour and hydrogenated fats and oils.[1]

The intake of sugar around the turn of the century was around 10 lb a year per person. At the present it is closer to 120 lb; the average diet is about a quarter sugar, and this average person consumes about 12 teaspoons a day. It isn't difficult to get to that level if you drink soft drinks, for each bottle contains at least 10 teaspoons of sugar.[2]

Even the American Food and Drug Administration in 1986 put out a report claiming that when 25–50% of the diet calories are sugar, one is at risk of: diabetes, glucose intolerance, heart attack, behavioural changes, excess calcium in the urine, gallstones and mineral deficiencies.[3] When the normally complacent FDA says something like that, we'd better listen. In fact here is the hard statistic on diabetes, which was a rare disease in 1935: Between that year and 1978 it increased 600%.

But there are other less immediately obvious problems in connection with sugar. For one, the question often on our minds whenever we get a cold or a flu: 'Why me? Why do some get 'em and some not?' Well, we know it is the immune system which is supposed to defend us from these foreign invaders. So why is it that the immune system fails us?

We have already looked at some of the reasons: the fact that margarine and hydrogenated vegetable oils in clear glass bottles will depress the immune system.

But these are not the only things. There are other foods and non-foods that do it. From the *American Journal of Clinical Nutrition*: 'Any form of concentrated sugar, when taken in more than small amounts, can greatly impair the ability of white cells to kill bacteria.'[4] That is, sugar will impair immune function even when derived from fruit juice or honey.

Dr Nancy Appleton PhD, a self-confessed ex-sugarholic and probably the world's foremost expert on the role of sugar in the diet, nutritional consultant, researcher, lecturer and author of *Lick the Sugar Habit*, *Healthy Bones*, and *Balanced Body Secret*, has this explanation:

Every time we eat as little as two teaspoons of sugar, we change the delicate balance in the biochemistry of our bodies, and throw them out of homeostasis [from an ideal balance into an imbalance]. After we take in sugar, blood tests would show that some of the mineral levels have increased while others have declined. Usually it is the calcium which increases and the phosphorus which decreases. Minerals work only in relation to each other and when there is too much of an imbalance a mineral can become toxic (or poisonous) to the body. Toxic calcium can cause kidney stones, arthritis, and hardening of the arteries, among other things.[5]

(We have also looked at this in connection with dairy foods which are top-heavy with calcium. And see the chapter on fluoride for its effect on calcium metabolism.)

For it is our minerals which make it possible for the enzymes to work, and it is these enzymes that help us to digest our foods, among other tasks. Thus the two teaspoonfuls of sugar will also make it difficult for us to digest our food, and that partially-digested food may thus go on to putrefy in the gut, to cause all sorts of havoc further down the track.

The immune system does its valiant best for us, but when we overuse it, it will get exhausted just as we do in a marathon. And unfortunately it is not just sugar that causes the body to go out of homeostasis. It is also an excess of alcohol or coffee, fried foods, foods to which we are allergic, overeating, corticosteroid drugs, antibiotics and many other over-the-counter drugs, prescription drugs and recreational drugs.

Wearing out the immune system is not a safe thing to do, because it is that system which we have in place to protect us from cancer as well as the mild respiratory illnesses of short duration. One can perhaps see why there is an epidemic of cancer today, considering the average diet, even without all the other environmental hazards. A statistical study done by Drs Seely and Horrobin, published in the July 1993 *Medical Hypotheses*, established that breast cancer rates in various countries are proportional to sugar consumption. The theory as to why this is so is that sugar makes insulin, which, like oestrogen, is believed to increase the incidence of breast cancer.[6] Of course the chances are there will be several contributing causes to most cancers.

But there is more, much more! Dr Appleton summarizes 'the whole catastrophe' in a list of 49 reasons why sugar can contribute to the ruination of our health. After all, it is not a true food. It is not something our bodies were designed to handle:[7]

1   Sugar can suppress the immune system.
2   Sugar upsets the minerals in the body.
3   Sugar causes hyperactivity in children.
4   Sugar produces a significant rise in triglycerides [fats].
5   Sugar contributes to the reduction in defence against bacterial infection.
6   Sugar can cause kidney damage.
7   Sugar reduces high density lipoproteins [desirable fats].
8   Sugar leads to chromium deficiency.
9   Sugar leads to cancer of the breast, ovaries, intestines, prostate and rectum.
10 Sugar increases fasting levels of glucose and insulin.
11 Sugar causes copper deficiency.
12 Sugar interferes with the absorption of calcium and magnesium.
13 Sugar weakens eyesight.
14 Sugar raises the level of neurotransmitters called serotonin.
15 Sugar can cause hypoglycaemia.
16 Sugar can contribute to eczema in children.
17 Sugar can raise adrenalin levels in children.
18 Sugar can lead to anxiety, difficulty concentrating and crankiness in children.
19 Sugar can cause ageing.
20 Sugar can lead to alcoholism.
21 Sugar causes tooth decay.
22 Sugar contributes to obesity.
23 Sugar can cause acidity in the stomach.
24 Sugar can cause changes frequently found in persons with gastric or duodenal ulcers.
25 Sugar can cause arthritis.
26 Sugar can cause asthma.
27 Sugar can cause Candida albicans (yeast infections).
28 Sugar can cause gallstones.
29 Sugar can cause heart disease.
30 Sugar can cause appendicitis.
31 Sugar can contribute to multiple sclerosis.
32 Sugar can cause haemorrhoids.
33 Sugar can cause varicose veins.

34 Sugar can elevate glucose and insulin responses in oral contraceptive users.

35 Sugar can lead to periodontal disease.

36 Sugar can contribute to osteoporosis.

37 Sugar contributes to saliva acidity.

38 Sugar can cause a decrease in insulin sensitivity.

39 Sugar leads to decreased glucose tolerance.

40 Sugar can decrease growth hormone.

41 Sugar can increase cholesterol.

42 Sugar can increase the systolic blood pressure.

43 Sugar can cause drowsiness and decrease activity in children.

44 Sugar can cause migraine headaches.

45 Sugar can interfere with the absorption of protein.

46 Sugar causes food allergies.

47 Sugar can contribute to diabetes.

48 Sugar can cause toxaemia during pregnancy.

49 Sugar can contribute to eczema in children.[8]

Other researchers also have attributed a whole host of illnesses to sugar. They all compile their own lists:

The mass indictment of refined carbohydrates as the cause of many of the ills of Western countries today was advanced by Surgeon-Captain T.L. Cleave, MRCP, formerly Director of Medical Research of the Institute of Naval Medicine, Great Britain. In 1956 he designated 'the saccharine disease' as the master disease, incorporating diabetes, coronary disease, obesity, peptic ulcer, constipation, haemorrhoids, varicose veins; *E. coli* infections ... appendicitis, cholecystitis, pyelitis, and diverticulitis; renal calculus, many skin conditions and dental caries.[9]

Moreover, Dr Cleave and his associates noted **one factor common to all healthful traditional diets: the absence of sugar and all simple carbohydrates.**[10]

Others see the high intake of sugar as an addictive problem:

Refined sugar is particularly insidious as it produces addiction as severe as any drug addiction. The only difference between heroin addiction and sugar addiction is that sugar doesn't need injection, is readily consumable because of its availability, and isn't considered a social evil. However the strength of sugar addiction is just as strong as heroin addiction.[11]

The most recent ploy to enable manufacturers to deceive us as to how much sugar we are taking in, is in labelling techniques. If the word SUGAR were to appear first, then we would be aware that there is more sugar in the product **than any-thing else**. So some manufacturers now employ the following device: one popular breakfast cereal has labelling as follows –

OATS, SUGAR, BROWN SUGAR, CORN SYRUP, MALTED BARLEY, MALT SUGAR, HONEY.[12]

Also, under the current gross misconceptions about the role of fats in health, many products are marketed as 'low fat', 'reduced fat' or 'fat free'. But to compensate for the loss in palatability, sugar is increased as fat is decreased. This excess sugar is, of course (oh loathsome fate!) converted to fat in the body when it gets there.[13]

There is, however, a solution to our sugar craving. It's just that those who produce sugar and those who produce sugar substitutes, which appear to be almost as dangerous (only with the emphasis on the brain and nervous system; see chapters on MSG and synthetic sweeteners, to come), do not like the idea. And apparently they carry enough clout to keep it from us; never mind the avalanche of diseases these may cause, diseases which could possibly be avoided.

There is a herb in the Chrysanthemum family, *Stevia Rebaudiana*, used by the Guarani Indians of Paraguay for centuries to sweeten their foods.[14] Stevia is today cultivated in Paraguay, Brazil, Japan, China, South Ontario, Mexico, California and even in the south of England. It can be grown in a hothouse just about anywhere.

Stevia is the sweetest, most naturally sweet plant on earth, and in tiny amounts it will sweeten just about anything without any of the negative effects of sugar and artificial sweeteners. It may even, it is claimed, inhibit dental decay. Apparently it has virtually no calories. Sounds like the answer to all our sweetest dreams? Yes. I use it very occasionally. Occasionally because I have virtually lost my taste for sweet things, except for chocolate. What I dream of now, is a wholesome chocolate bar made with Stevia instead of sugar. I could probably get it in Japan. One day!

Since 1931, studies have been done to look for any toxic effects of Stevia, and none has been found. More recently numerous toxicity studies have been done in Asia, and that is why we will find there a famous sugar-free cola-flavoured drink sweetened with Stevia, and sugar-free gum made with Stevia. Stevia can be found, sold as a sugar in most countries, except for the US and its satellites, for the reasons mentioned above. In fact, the FDA permits Stevia to be imported and sold in the US, but it must be sold not as a food but as a food supplement. This situation is testimony both to its safety and to its threat to conventional sweeteners. (However, late in 1998 in the US the FDA conducted a huge book-burning enterprise – the burning of books on the subject of Stevia. Do we have even a semblance of democracy in this primitive stage in human development?)

This entire grotesque charade makes me long for a decent honest concern for the health of people on the part of governments, a concern that goes way beyond the need for a few to make millions out of us, so that we may all live as well and as long as we are entitled to. The sugar we eat today, with its implication in numerous degenerative diseases is, of course, only one small part of that infinite carelessness with our lives.

We will give the expert, Dr Appleton, the last word on this:

We create our own sicknesses by upsetting our body chemistry, but we can also actually create health. Stop doing to the body what you did to make it sick and the body will heal itself. It is a fact that the average person who lives to be over the age of one hundred, does not die of a disease. These people simply die, peacefully, of old age. And we can too.[15]

Dr Appleton's address is PO Box 3083, Santa Monica, California, 90403, US.

⚠

12: JUNK FOOD

'Junk food is no big deal.
A little of what you fancy ...'

Have you ever dreamed of having purple hair? Or perhaps bright green or cherry red? Apparently you can do it easily at home with *Kool-Aid*, the drink of choice for millions of young people and children in the United States. The kids just add water and dye their hair with it. They say the unsweetened version works best. The dye is more concentrated in that. But one must be sure to rinse well so you won't 'run in the rain'.

But *if this stuff will actually dye hair*, just what does it do to people's insides? We can't be certain. When one day they are autopsied, will these kids end up with a purple liver, a cherry red heart and green kidneys?

What can one say about junk food that hasn't already been said many times? The problem is that, considering the vast array of plastic and depleted foods we have to choose from, it is somewhat difficult to get a decent diet these days.

In 1740 James Lind observed that sailors went berserk when deprived of fresh vegetables, that is when they had to live on a diet of vitamin-deficient food. People are going berserk today on dry land for the same reason, in fact on deficiencies seldom observed except in countries where starvation exists. (Incidentally, it was to be another 60 years and thousands more deaths before Lind was listened to. Sound familiar?)

Dr Marion Stewart, visiting New Zealand in 1997 to promote her *Every-woman's Health Guide*, told the story of how she and her husband drew straws to see who would be the one to go on a junk food diet for six weeks to see what it would do to them. Her husband drew the short straw and after extensive tests launched himself into the project with gusto.

Gradually he became lethargic. The libido disappeared. He began sleeping on the job. He was grouchy. By the end of the six weeks his blood tests showed that his health was definitely declining. They were relieved to get him off this junk food diet. It took another six weeks to get him back to where he had been. What some people will do for science! Anyway, a diet of solid junk food *will* eventually kill you, one way or another, if you give it a chance.

Some years back, there was an American doctor by the name of Weston Price who was interested in the effects of food on health. He travelled extensively, observing the effects of different diets in different parts of the world at different times. Over and over again he found the same story in all parts of the world. On their traditional diets the indigenous peoples of the world had strong healthy bodies free from cancer, heart disease and immune system weakness. And surprisingly, tooth decay and cavities were almost nonexistent, despite the fact that these people usually had no dentists or fluoride toothpaste. But when they switched from their traditional diets to modern Western foods, there was a noticeable, significant and continual degeneration in health.[1]

The same story comes through in many walks of life. Take Merino sheep, for example. Recently the world of sheep and wool was astounded by the fact that New Zealand's High Country Marino wool was selling for 15 times the price of other Marino wool. The secret as to how this feat was accomplished was eventually told. These sheep are reared organically with the best of food, without 'drenches' and other medication; and they are fitted out with raincoats in the winter! So if we want to be healthy we must eat the best of food, avoid drugs and always wear a raincoat in winter!

Beyond that, I will just pass on to you this fairly hilarious/sad piece by an American humorist of the wise variety, Howard Belkamp. It is my personal belief that if you can eat well and prudently six days a week, you're allowed to go a bit mad on the seventh, given that we're surrounded by the stuff. It's what you eat six days a week that counts. Of course after a while you won't even want to go mad once a week. I go mad only about once every six weeks.

AMERICA EATS AND GETS SICK[2]

by Howard Belkamp

Dog Food and Videos

A friend and I went to the video store the other night. I wanted to get a 'food' movie. I like food movies – *Babette's Feast, My Dinner with Andre, Like Water for Chocolate*, etc. We rented one called *Eating*, about a bunch of women who get together and eat out and talk, or so I thought, and another, French-Vietnamese film called *The Scent of Green Papaya*. OK. Two movies. At the counter, the woman tells me it's a 'special' night and I can get two more movies for free and keep them all for four days. This is a dilemma of sorts because I can go nuts trying to find a video when I haven't got something specific in mind. But back into the bowels of the store we go. Five minutes go by and not a clue. Nothing looks good. Finally I find something called *Delicatessen* – a food movie, right – so I pick it up.

Suddenly, I *smell* something. Something unpleasant. For a minute I can't identify it, but then it hits me: Dog food. It smells like someone has come into the store, opened ten cans of Kennel-Ration, and dumped them on the heater.

I ask my friend, 'Do you smell dog food?' She replies, 'Is *that* what it is?' I'm close to gagging on this odour. I think of another movie they might have – *Shirley Valentine* – about an Englishwoman who goes to Greece and has an affair because her life is a dull routine and her husband is an inconsiderate bore. And there's food in the plot. I approach the counter and ask for it. They have it. Now we can get out of here, away from the dog food smell. While I'm paying for the video my friend comes up and says, 'I found the smell. Look over there. Over there is a woman eating a McDonald's hamburger and fries.'

The movie *Eating* was awful. Couldn't stand more than ten minutes of it. Boring, badly acted, badly directed. But the big surprise was the movie, *Delicatessen*. It was not, strictly speaking, a food movie, but it was extremely bizarre and very funny. I recommend it.

Watching America Eat

The dog food incident reminded me of going to McDonald's in Willits, California, ten years ago with Jim Gibbons, the outstanding runner and health fanatic, my old friend with the 50-year-old face on a 25-year-old body, who is not exactly a friend of the overweight. We were in town on some errands, decided that we were hungry, and had a mutual inspiration to do something disgusting and perverted: eat a McDonald's burger. Both of us knew better, but as I told him on the way, 'I've got a terrible craving for a dose of grease and salt.'

This may have been a seminal moment in the formation of my runner friend's war on the obese, because as we sat there chomping on our gut bombs, two grossly overweight women, with their pitifully fat children at their sides, waddled up to the counter and ordered Big Macs, fries, 'apple pies' (deep-fried sugar and fat) and *diet Cokes*. (The TV tells them that diet pop will make everything all right, will somehow cancel out the fattening, nutritionless food). Far from being the insensitive lout that some in the Overweight Community make him out to be, Gibbons is actually hypersensitive to the health and well-being of others. So sensitive that he nearly threw up at the spectacle we were witnessing. It was his last McDonald's burger, and mine too.

But you can't escape the brutal reality of the mainstream American diet by wiping McDonald's off your list. All you have to do is be reasonably conscious of your surroundings at the supermarket checkout counter. It never fails: the sickest and unhappiest-looking, pale, squishy, blotchy, mostly overweight people all have the same stuff in their carts – hot dogs, Wonder bread, marshmallows, Kraft macaroni and cheese 'dinner'-in-a-box, Pop Tarts, big jars of mayonnaise, baloney, six-packs of Diet Coke and Pepsi, Captain Crush and Fruit Loops-types cereals, cake mixes and canned frosting made with nothing but sugar and lard. Twinkies, Ding-Dongs, Ho-Hos and other such unperishable chemical concoctions that one observant friend puts under the general category of 'shit-pie doodles'; Cool-Whip, fake cheese in individually-wrapped slices (better suited to patching the roof than eating), and quite often sausages – not just any sausages, but those large variety, shrink-wrapped, grease-and-salt bombs with wholesome-sounding names like Grandma's Favorite, Friendly Farms or Paradise Valley.

All this amounts to media-fed abuse of the public, a continuing and successfully-orchestrated corporate campaign to maintain huge profits on relentlessly advertised crap, promoting and maintaining feeble physical and mental health in large portions of the public. As the late jazz musician and writer John Stephens said 25 years ago, 'The plan is to have the entire population ill or mediocre by the year 2000, and they're already way ahead of schedule.'

PS A confession: I am also one of those terrible people who sneak a look in other peoples' trolley carts at the market. And then suffer agonies because I want to explain to them why they shouldn't be eating some of that stuff. Then suffer more agonies because I don't dare say it. (I tried it only once and got HELL!)

⚠️

13: NICOTINE

'Lower-nicotine cigarettes are better for your health
than the older higher-nicotine cigarettes.'

Two internal reports put out by the Brown and Williamson Tobacco Corporation, and not intended for general distribution, reveal that today's lower-nicotine cigarettes actually carry more of a clout than yesterday's higher-nicotine varieties. This is because the tobacco industry, while lowering the nicotine levels, began using ammonia to 'retain the flavour'. Ammoniated nicotine actually enters the smoker's bloodstream more quickly and has a stronger effect than non-ammoniated nicotine. But industry officials will not admit they add ammonia to the nicotine for any reason other than to improve the taste.[1] The report does not say what else the inhalation of ammonia does.

An excellent book, *Smoking: The Artificial Passion*[2] details the tragedy that is nicotine addiction. Smoking kills far more people each year than does AIDS, heroin, cocaine, alcohol, car accidents, fire and murder combined. In the US alone, smoking causes 2 million preventable deaths every year. These are the cancers of the lung, mouth, larynx, oesophagus, bladder, cervix and kidneys. But smoking also contributes to heart attacks, vascular disease and emphysema. Moreover, recent findings indicate that people who live with smokers, but do not smoke themselves, have twice the rates of heart disease as do other non-smokers who do not live with smokers.[3]

More interesting, the 'War on Drugs' propounded by several Western countries does not include tobacco. Is it because of the tax revenue, the influence of the tobacco companies, or both? If it is the revenue, then the figures have not been done, because the health costs of dealing with the aftermath of tobacco are incalculably higher than any revenue collected from selling cigarettes.

In the US and elsewhere, the medical profession has a poor record in this area. For many years the financial mainstay of the *Journal of the American Medical Association* was cigarette advertising. Some of this advertising even boasted that prominent doctors smoked their brand rather than one of the others. And if we go back much further to the heyday of smoking, there is one advertisement that appeared almost everywhere in the thirties and forties. It featured a doctor sporting a monocle and a stiff wing collar, declaring, 'As a doctor I cannot recommend any particular brand. But personally, I always smoke Craven-A.'

Well, that was an age of innocence, comparatively speaking, was it not? But long after that innocence was sullied, both medicine and the cancer institutes were very late in getting behind the drive to reduce smoking deaths. Today as always, it is a case of 'he who pays the piper calls the tune.'

And just as smoking kills other people as well as oneself, wearing perfume is another lesser-known hazard to both oneself and others. Because almost all perfumes are based on petrochemicals; you might as well be breathing in exhaust fumes all the time you're wearing perfume. It depletes one's stores of vitamin C. There are many of us who hope that one day perfume-wearing will become as anti-social as is smoking.

EMERGENCY ADVICE

Get the book *Smoking: The Artificial Passion*!
Many like me look forward to the day when people will wear perfume and after-shave only in the privacy of their own homes, with consenting adults.

14: MSG

'Perfectly safe. The American Food and
Drug Administration says so.'

MSG, or Monosodium Glutamate, is a food additive found in many processed foods today. 'MSG is safe for almost everyone. Only significant amounts will cause mild and temporary reactions in a few.' Thus spake the American Food and Drug Administration (FDA).

But only days after the above announcement, David Livingston, 42, almost died after eating MSG in a restaurant. Apparently he knew he was highly sensitive to MSG. So when he ordered his meal he was most emphatic about his problem and was assured that the meal he was ordering would not contain MSG.

However, on finishing this meal Livingston felt so unwell that he went to his doctor where he went into respiratory arrest (stopped breathing). He was revived and transferred to the local hospital where he went into cardiac arrest (stopped heart). In the hospital it was found that the food he had ingested contained MSG. Clearly, had he not gone straight to his doctor he would have died.

Livingston is now suing the restaurant owners who nearly caused his death for $100 million, such is the level of suing in the US. And moreover, in the absence of easier ways, suing for large sums has been one way to focus attention on a problem, to initiate legislation, to effect change.

The problem with much health information today is that there is a scarcity of disinterested (in the sense of impartial), accurate and fair knowledge and research. Because of the expense involved in undertaking research, modern governments tend to leave much of the work they used to do to business interests. And research funded by companies into their own products can hardly be impartial. The funding can also go to an 'outside' laboratory which acts as a 'front' for the company endeavouring to get a favourable outcome (*he who pays the piper calls the tune*).

As we will note in the chapter on the FDA, this has been apparent over and over again with drugs which, as a result of research, are 'found to be safe'. On this basis, these drugs are then placed on the market, only to be withdrawn within a year owing to the horrific side-effects and deaths which consumption of the drug is causing. The drug Thalidomide was only one, and one which received a great deal of publicity. But there have been numerous other similar situations.

Nowhere is this kind of questionable research more apparent than in the multibillion-dollar food industry. As a result, of course, groups of concerned consumers, some of whom have been affected by supposedly 'safe' foods, or who perhaps have lost a loved one, will form a group to oppose the sale of unsafe foods and merchandise. They have scant resources to oppose the 'big boys', but they fight valiantly on.

One such group in the US is the Chicago-based **Truth in Labeling Campaign**, with its leaders Dr Adrienne and Jack Samuels; they have recently filed suit against the American Food and Drug Administration over the necessity to label all foods containing MSG.[1] They are also backing David Livingston in his court case.

They claim that the FDA's position on MSG, that this additive is essentially safe and may cause only mild adverse reactions in very few people, is 'an inaccurate reflection of the results of a report on the food additive MSG ...' This refers to a safety report conducted by the Federation of American Societies for Experimental Biology (FASEB) under the auspices of the FDA. The **Truth in Labeling Campaign** (TLC) claims that FDA ensured the results it wanted 'by posing narrow and limited questions for FASEB to answer'. The resulting findings, according to the TLC, 'ignored volumes of data that prove that MSG causes brain damage, learning disorders, obesity, stunted growth, infertility, and other endocrine problems in laboratory animals'. Also the report 'minimized the number of people affected by MSG and the severity of their reactions'.[2]

If it is true that 'the FDA asked FASEB to answer 18 specific questions, designed to guarantee that the report would conclude that MSG is safe,' then we can see how the FDA could claim that there was no need to exclude MSG from the safe list and/or to label all those foods containing MSG. It also gives us an idea of how the FDA functions in this world. And that ordinary people like thee and me haven't got a dog's chance of protecting ourselves unless we have other kinds of knowledge. That goes for the UK and most of the Commonwealth countries too, of course, because our health authorities tend to function as satellites of their US counterparts.

Another group with a similar purpose is **NOMSG**, the American **National Organization Mobilized to Stop Glutamate**,[3] a group which works hard to circulate information on the subject.

MSG has no nutritional value whatsoever, which is not unusual these days. But beyond that is the fact that it does not work on our food. MSG works to change *us*. Classified as an excitotoxin, it is designed to 'excite', to stimulate our tastebuds. But the problem is, it is also a neurotoxin. That is, in addition to exciting our tastebuds, it also excites the neurones in the brain. Once the excitotoxin is consumed, these neurones then begin to fire off rapidly, till, like the young woman forced by the magic red shoes to dance on and on, they may become exhausted and die.[4]

In 1968 came the first report of a serious adverse reaction to MSG. And in 1969 research on excitotoxins using laboratory animals established that MSG can damage the brain and nervous system through the induction of brain lesions. Pregnant monkeys who were fed MSG gave birth to brain-damaged offspring. This was also found with pregnant rats.[5]

Two years later the baby food manufacturers took the MSG out of baby food, but what they did was to remove the 'pure' MSG and substitute hydrolysed protein, which apparently is almost as bad. It was not until 1978 that infant food was completely free of it. In the meantime, who warned pregnant women not to eat it? And not to use the baby food? Who was looking after our children, our health?

Perhaps worst of all, a child today consuming a cup of soup containing MSG (almost all of the processed soup contains it) and a soft drink with an artificial sweetener (aspartic acid, *another excitotoxin*) in it, will be taking in *six times* the comparative level that destroys the neurones in the hypothalamus of baby mice. In other words, the consumption of quantities of both MSG and the artificial sweetener can damage the developing brain in both foetus and child. The hypothalamus is immature at birth. And the damage to this 'master' gland by these products can lead to severe endocrine problems later in life. Among these problems: decreased thyroid hormone production, increased tendency towards diabetes and higher cortisone levels than normal.

After these findings were published, the FDA remained silent on the issue. Gynaecologists and paediatricians were not told to warn their patients of this danger.

Unfortunately, according to **NOMSG**, MSG is today back in some baby foods and in some infant formulas.

MSG (monosodium glutamate) is all-pervasive, ubiquitous these days. **NOMSG** warns that MSG is *always* found in autolysed yeast; calcium caseinate; hydrolysed oat flour; hydrolysed protein; sodium caseinate; textured protein; yeast extract; yeast food and yeast nutrient.

It is *often* found in barley malt; bouillon; broth; flavourings; malt extract; malt flavouring; 'natural' flavourings; 'natural' beef flavouring; 'natural' chicken flavouring; 'natural' pork flavouring and seasonings.

Clearly 'natural' does not always mean what it says. The substance may once have come from nature, but it often bears little resemblance to its original self by the time we see it on the grocery shelf, or in the refrigerator and freezer sections.

There are also substances which actually *create* MSG: fungal protease, protease and protease enzymes. In addition, the **NOMSG** is suspicious of: carrageenan; enzymes; smoke flavouring; soy protein concentrate; soy protein isolate; torula yeast; vegetable gum; whey protein and whey protein concentrate.

MSG can be found in almost all processed food, including soups, crisps, fast and frozen foods, prepared TV dinners, salad dressings, meats, most canned foods, some crackers and breads, 'low-fat' foods; canned fish, frozen entrees, ice cream and frozen yoghurt. If the manufacturers are required to list it on the label they often get around it by calling it 'hydrolysed vegetable protein', 'natural flavouring' or even 'spices.'[6] Drinks, candy and chewing gum are also potential sources of hidden MSG and it may also be found in substances other than food. It may be in soaps, shampoos, hair conditioners and cosmetics (why I cannot tell; so that they smell better? So that they cause our brains temporarily to 'feel better'?). The most obvious are those that contain 'hydrolysed protein' or simply 'amino acids'.

Worst of all, perhaps, MSG may be present in tablet binders for medication, both prescription and non-prescription, including enteral feeding materials and materials administered through IVs in hospitals.

The other possible menace, the artificial sweetener aspartame, is found in over 900 products worldwide. There was controversy over its initial entrance into the world. Beatrice Trum Hunter, author of many books on environmental health, in a letter to the *New England Journal of Medicine*[7], deplored the fact that aspartame had been approved for public consumption before appropriate studies had been conducted, and the inadequacy of those studies when they did appear:

Having had numerous contacts with consumers, I can attest to the fact that many people are adversely affected by aspartame. When they avoid the substance, symptoms disappear, when they challenge themselves, symptoms reappear. By now the files of the FDA bulge with reports, from both consumers and health professionals, describing adverse reactions...

When the scientific studies did come, giving aspartame a 'clean bill of health', they caused an angry scepticism among those who have worked among patients with problems caused by artificial sweeteners. Dr Derrick Lonsdale MD, for one:

...we physicians 'in the trenches' have overwhelming evidence that sugar and various chemical sweeteners have a drastic effect on many of our patients of all ages. In my view ... they are probably the major cause of the pandemic of hyperactivity and learning disability syndromes which plague our society. Who amongst us has not seen a dramatic difference in behaviour and health patterns both physical and mental when these substances are withdrawn from the diet?[8]

Dr Lonsdale made the point that just giving a dose of these substances and observing behaviour does not work in testing. The harm comes with use over time, when a sensitivity or maladaptation is built up. And he found numerous other inadequacies in connection with the studies done.

Dr H J Roberts MD of West Palm Beach, Florida, a diabetes specialist, is one 'in the trenches' who has written extensively on the subject of aspartame and health from a database of over 1,000 victims whose symptoms improved after the withdrawal of aspartame from the diet.[9] He has also written books on the subject[10], including *Aspartame: Is It Safe?*, *Sweet'ner Dearest: Bittersweet Vignettes about Aspartame*, and *Defense against Alzheimer's Disease*.

Dr Roberts points out that aspartame is 50% phenylalanine, compared to 4% to be found in meat and other proteins. But it is the 10% methyl alcohol that is the most risky part. At a recent World Environmental Conference, information was brought forward about an American 'epidemic of multiple sclerosis and systemic lupus', serious illnesses attributed to aspartame, or methanol toxicity. Apparently the symptoms of these illnesses resolve after withdrawal of the aspartame from the diet.

Dr Roberts claims that it is unsafe to subject aspartame to heat because it frees the methanol which can cause damage to humans. And he speculates that the fact that diet drinks sent to the Gulf War were left out on pallets in the 120°F (49°C) Arabian sun for weeks at a time, and drunk all day long by the servicewomen and -men, is a possible reason or component of Gulf War Syndrome.

The Ada Parker newsletter records that Dr Louis Elsas, Professor of Pediatrics and Genetics at Emory University in the US, recently gave evidence on aspartame before a US Congressional hearing claiming that the ingested phenylalanine from aspartame concentrates in the placenta, and can cause mental retardation. In laboratory tests, 'Animals developed brain tumours: phenylalanine breaks down into DXP, a brain tumour agent.'[11]

Aspartame and MSG are both potent neurotropic drugs, that is they are substances that affect the brain and nervous system. When we realize that Valium and Lithium, which are neurotropic drugs, may produce any number of side-effects, then the same may hold true for MSG and aspartame. People sensitive to these substances have reported as many responses as one can imagine, from migraine headaches, racing heart, vomiting, diarrhoea and fatigue to depression, mood swings, mouth lesions and hyperactivity in children. Of course other things may cause these symptoms, but apparently they *can* be caused by MSG or some artificial sweeteners.

Both MSG and aspartame can bring mild discomfort or just gradually lower one's overall level of health. Or, in the case of MSG, it can bring very serious reactions and even death, as in the case of David Livingstone, had he not gone immediately to his doctor.

In excitotoxin-sensitive people the amount they can tolerate varies, from one molecule to many grams, before there is a reaction. It is estimated that between 25 and 30% of the population will be sensitive to MSG and aspartame in varying degrees, only we are often unaware of it because one can either react immediately or within up to 48 hours. Or there may just be an ongoing lower level of health. The only way to tell for sure is to eliminate all MSG and aspartame (that is every single molecule) from the diet for two weeks and see if one does not feel better overall.[12] To be certain of truly eliminating it one has to stick to all whole natural foods which have not been altered in any way; that is, eliminate anything with a label on it! Not a bad policy for most of the time, anyway.

The US Air Force has warned all pilots off aspartame because a pilot drinking a sugar-free soft drink containing aspartame is more susceptible to dizziness, memory loss and irritability.[13] Two pilots, Charles King and Michael Collins, had seizures after drinking soft drinks with aspartame in them, and lost their jobs. They regained their health by eliminating the sweeteners, but could not get their jobs back.[14]

What follows was reported to the *Townsend Letter* for June 1998 [page 116] by Betty Martini, founder of Mission Possible International, the American anti-aspartame information group:

Pilots continue to report grand mal seizures and blackouts while the FAA [Federal Aeronautics Association] has done nothing to warn pilots off this neurotoxin. Joe Neill, a co-pilot ... has just died in-flight. The other pilot landed the plane. When his widow was contacted she reported that he drank diet drinks ... The wood alcohol in aspartame and the altitude appear to affect pilots faster. Another pilot about a year ago, also hooked on aspartame, also died, but at least he had landed the plane. It has been reported that there have been other deaths.

Dr John Olney MD has established a link between aspartame and brain tumours.[15] Dr H J Roberts has found an association between joint pain and aspartame consumption. He suggests that doctors try asking patients with these pains to try aspartame avoidance before getting involved in tests, consultations and drugs.[16]

Concerning the nervous system, MSG and aspartame more readily affect the most vulnerable, our young children and the elderly. These additives can intensify or even initiate such neurodegenerative diseases as Parkinson's Disease, Alzheimer's Disease, Huntington's chorea and other nervous system diseases.[17]

It is of course the glutamate part in both MSG and aspartame that can cause problems; in addition there is the methyl alcohol in aspartame. Dr Richard C Henneberry PhD says on the subject:

I consider it ironic, that the pharmaceutical industry is investing vast resources in the development of glutamate receptor blockers to protect neurones against glutamate neurotoxicity in common neurological disorders, while at the same time the food industry with the blessing of the FDA, continues to add great quantities of glutamate to the food supply.[18]

Dr Russell Blaylock MD, in discussing the treatment of children suffering from Hyper-activity, Attention Deficit Disorder and so on, said this:

Special emphasis is placed on the avoidance of chemical additives, especially MSG, the artificial sweetener aspartame, and artificial food colourings and flavourings. Numerous animal experiments have shown that MSG and aspartame are capable of causing brain and retinal damage.[19]

The law suits against the manufacturers of aspartame are beginning to blossom, as for MSG. Four writs have been filed in Oklahoma against one manufacturer of the artificial sweetener. The plaintiffs in these cases claim in their submissions to the court that aspartame has caused several different health disasters in the US.[20]

I myself was taken in the last time I had my six-weekly treat: a new small chocolate bar. It tasted OK, but when I looked at the list of ingredients on the wrapping I was amazed to discover I had eaten aspartame. (I should have checked *before* I purchased, but was not expecting it. How can good chocolate need such an addition? Chocolate has done fine without it for decades!)

The question must always be why has the public not been informed as to the dangers of these substances? Who is in charge of our health? Why is it allowed in our foods?

PS They are now adding excitotoxins to cigarettes to 'enhance the flavour'. So now you get the ammonia, and the cadmium and the excitotoxins, all of which may cause brain damage. Just who is looking after the health of smokers? And the rest of us?

15: GENETICALLY-ENGINEERED FOOD

'Genetically-altered "Frankenfood"
is fun! Fun! Fun!'

One of the most recent entrants in this pantheon of modern horrors is genetically-modified food. Margo White puts it this way:

We're talking about a revolution – of an entire food chain, seeping across the borders of the world, before governments, regulators, consumers and ethicists are able to understand it fully, a revolution that could change the nature, production, ownership and the very DNA of our most basic commodity, possibly forever.[1]

Dr Morton Walker DPM, long-time health researcher and author of numerous books on health, has drawn up a menu of tasty treats to tempt us. All these are foods now being sold to unknowing consumers all over the world.

Appetizer

spiced potatoes with wax moth genes
juice of tomatoes with flounder gene

Entree

blackened catfish with trout gene
pork chops with human genes
scalloped potatoes with chicken gene
cornbread with firefly gene

Dessert

rice pudding with pea gene

Beverages

milk with genetically-engineered bovine growth hormone (BGH)[2]

(Perhaps he could have done better with the dessert. What about a pesticide-drenched soy-based pudding, spliced with walrus gene, flavoured with vanilla and Scotch Thistle?[3])

Dr Walker describes genetically-altered food as 'food which has been changed by biotechnology through the splicing of genes from one organism to another, to incorporate a particularly desired trait'. And he is concerned about the risks of eating such genetically-engineered foods, as possible 'precursors to an even greater incidence of cancer, atherosclerosis, allergies, immune suppression, and other physical and mental degeneration for all who consume them.'[4]

Beware if you have a severe food allergy problem. For the food you've spent your whole life avoiding might just pop up in an entirely different food. For example, a small percentage of the population will die if they eat fish. Naturally they avoid fish like the plague. But what if some other food harbours a fish gene, like a sort of modern Trojan horse?

That is exactly what has happened. The latest crop of juicy tomatoes contains flounder genes. These new fish-tomatoes are known as 'Flavour Savrs' and can now be found in supermarkets in most of the Western world. They look just like ordinary tomatoes, but they last and last. In fact they can last for a month and look exactly as they did when you first bought them. I do not find this reassuring. Nor would those fatally allergic to fish.

Another hazard is the insertion of nut genes into soybeans. Another small percentage of the population is hypersensitive to nuts and must avoid them at all costs. In Australia there has already been one death from a severe reaction to soybeans spliced with a walnut gene, and unlabelled as such.[5] How can one be certain to avoid such things when today soybeans are used in numerous foods?

Beyond these unfortunates there is also a much larger percentage of the population who are restricted in their choice of foods due to food intolerances or sensitivities. Some of the reactions can be mild; others can be severe and incapacitating. How are they going to cope when they do not know if the foods they are allergic to are lurking in other foods?

But the American Food and Drug Administration, which hounds doctors who prescribe vitamins and other supplements – in fact is wont to raid their surgeries with sheriffs waving drawn guns – has given the green light for any of our foods to be genetically altered and sold to unsuspecting populations without warning labelling required.

One of the worst possibilities of genetically-engineered food was voiced by Dr Walter Dorfler of the University of Cologne speaking at the International Congress on Cell Biology in San Francisco, December 1996. He made the claim, before all those experts in the field, that based on his research, DNA fed to a mouse could ultimately make its way into the cells of the mouse body. It was a finding to make the blood run cold. For if true, this means that the genes from genetically-engineered foods may not be destroyed in the stomach but could pass into our genetic coding.[6]

During the process of this genetic engineering, 'artificially constructed parasitic genetic elements, including viruses, are used to carry genes of one species into the genes of another and "smuggle" them into cells. Once inside, these vectors insert themselves into the host genome.'

By transferring genes across species barriers which have existed for aeons, we risk changing the blueprint of each organism's biological processes – and according to Dr Peter Will, biologist at Auckland University in New Zealand, 'Cellular proteins replicated in other species can give rise to infectious neurological disease. Other researchers say that there are virtually unlimited health risks.'[7]

Meanwhile, the American National Wildlife Foundation compiled the following list of possible risks involved:

1 New toxicants – Apparently the American Food and Drug Administration which holds sway over us all will not be requiring testing of genetically-altered food, and therefore any new toxicants (dangerous substances) may not be recognized. Because they are alive, these organisms are inherently more unpredictable than chemical products. They may reproduce, mutate and migrate. 'Once released, it is virtually impossible to recall these living Frankenstein-like products back to the laboratory.'[8] Genetically-engineered foods reproduce themselves and can never be recalled from the environment, nor can they be kept apart from their wild and non-altered relatives. One field test of genetically altered potatoes indicated that, over distances of 1,100 metres, 72% of the non-modified potatoes contained the transmuted gene.[9]

2 Diminished nutritional quality – Consumers may be unaware that the juicy-looking tomatoes they are eating may not have the nutritional value of ordinary tomatoes.

3 New allergens – warnings are supposed to be placed on the food package if allergenic effects have been noted. This is rather useless, as the substances we react to, and in what combinations, may be biochemically unique to us and us alone or to a small percentage of the population. And as this is left up to the manufacturers it is not a reliable form of labelling – they are not about to slit their own throats.

4   Unexpected effects – The genetic stability of engineered plants is supposed to be tested, but because of that personal biochemical uniqueness the results of eating these things cannot be predicted.

Many of the recent experiments on genetically altered foods are out of science fiction. US Department of Agriculture researchers last year produced a 'transgenetic' pig with human growth hormone gene. But rather than the hoped-for larger pig, it became lame, arthritic, sterile, skinny and excessively hairy. [10]

5   Harmful side-effects from deleted genes –

Even worse than leaving out a food's gene is the introduction of a complementary gene for suppression of an 'undesirable' gene. Such suppression may diminish the immune ability of the consumer to take that complementary gene into the body.

6   Counterfeit freshness – They can remain 'fresh' for weeks, but are they? They are more likely 'dead' from the start.

7   Hazards to domestic animals – Same as for humans, only they would get more of it.

8   Harmful effects on wildlife and habitats – Developers are supposed to detect adverse environmental effects, as well as harmful effects on humans and animals, and report them. But given the fact that they could lose billions by doing so, does anyone these days believe in Santa Claus?

9   Unchanged genetic material combined with gene products – there are genes which are designated as matching other genes, but what happens when there is an error? 'A true Frankenstein monster could be created that grows out of control.'

Dr Walker rightly points out that the American FDA is not doing the job it is supposed to be doing, that is protecting people's health. Moreover, if there is absolutely no warning about the fact that one is eating altered foods it could transgress religious dietary restrictions as well as health restrictions. For example, if there are pig genes hidden in the broccoli, where does that leave those pledged not to eat pork? And then there are those pledged to eat fish on Fridays. What happens when there are meat genes hidden in their vegetables? And how can vegetarians be sure they are not eating meat?

Apparently hundreds of billions of tax-payers' money have been spent on these genetically-altered plants and animals. Dr Walker rightly maintains that, had this money been redirected to sustainable, ecological farming methods, the US would have taken a giant stride towards a safe organic food supply for its people. Instead a fortune has been spent on developing this risky, depleted food of dubious nutrient capacity. And the rest of the world is rapidly being exposed to it.

There is already a strong precedent for concern in the fiasco surrounding tryptophan, but the story on this useful amino acid is interesting for more than its G-M aspect:

L-Tryptophan is a nutritional supplement found in many protein foods in small amounts. For some years it was prescribed by the best of doctors and naturopaths as a safe, effective and inexpensive aid for depression and sleep difficulties. However, because of its ever-increasing success it became a target for those enterprising people who wish to make money out of something popular. Also, it was not difficult to predict that sleeping pills were headed for the 'endangered' category. So L-Tryptophan gradually came under the scrutiny of both drug companies and those engaged in the business of genetic engineering.

The full story on this, and all the legal, ethical and political issues involved, occupies three lengthy articles by Dr Morton Walker DPM, in the *Townsend Letter* published in 1994 (under the title 'Shocking Truths Behind the Tragedy of Tryptophan'). Numerous others have lectured and written about it over the years, including Dean Wolfe Manders, Senior Lecturer in Humanities and Sciences, California College, Oakland/San Francisco.[11]

How can one do justice to this lengthy and complex story in a few sentences? But to attempt the impossible: First, in late 1989 one manufacturing company produced and flooded the US market with a cheap genetically-altered version of tryptophan. Following this, among those who took it some 10,000 became seriously ill with EMS (Eosinophilia-Myalgia Syndrome), and 39 died. (Dr Walker is of the opinion that 'Genetically-altered Strain Five ... turned out to be stressful to human cells. It was incompatible with the immunology of recipients.') Naturally the US FDA recalled it immediately. Then the lawsuits began. Cummins and White of Newport, California, went into battle for numerous applicants. After the usual slow turning of the legal wheels, the firm paid up over $500 million in penalties and over $650 million in legal fees. But that, of course, is an extremely over-simplified version of the legal repercussions.

The reaction from the FDA to this horror story was to ban all sales of this 'dangerous tryptophan' permanently from the market. This meant a ban on *all* tryptophan, not just the genetically-engineered variety. But the sickness and death following on from people taking the altered version was *not* an example of the dangers of tryptophan. It was an example of the potential dangers in genetically altering anything.

This ban on tryptophan occurred on 22nd March 1990. On 26th March, a leading article in the journal *Newsweek* launched the new drug, Prozac. Not only did *Newsweek* devote many pages to the wonders of this new drug, but a huge Prozac was depicted on the front cover, floating ethereally and enticingly. Some are inclined to note a possible connection between the two events – the banning of the natural form and the promotion of an expensive drug, five times the price of the natural product.

The fact is that L-Tryptophan and Prozac act in a similar way, to enhance the use of the brain neurotransmitter, serotonin. However, only L-Tryptophan can actually *produce* serotonin, so that individuals who do not produce enough will not be helped by Prozac-type drugs, but may be helped by tryptophan. This could go some way towards explaining the differing successes among those who take this drug. (Also see the chapter on Prozac.) Dr Manders concludes:

The story of L-Tryptophan illustrates a sad and perverse picture of the politics and priorities of public health in America: A safe dietary supplement, a serotonin producer, is publicly unavailable to people, while daily fed to animals by corporate agribusiness ... And, while publicly exclaiming that L-Tryptophan is a dangerous and untested drug, the FDA quietly allows human-use L-Tryptophan to be imported, and then marketed and sold by the pharmaceutical industry. To allow the FDA ban on L-Tryptophan to continue unreviewed and uninvestigated condemns millions of Americans to unnecessary financial expenditures and needless suffering.

So, those who could benefit from the true and natural form of tryptophan are now deprived of it. And it is well to remember (see the chapter on prescription drugs) that no safety assessment methods are fully reliable. In the case of new drugs, over 10% of serious 'side-effects' at first go undetected. How much worse could it be in the technologized food industry?

(Actually, the natural L-Tryptophan is now available as 5-HTP. But who knows how long before the FDA gets wind of it and bans it?)

Naturally it is cheaper to have foods that will last indefinitely. All the problems of delivery before perishing can be resolved. And the same company known for its experimental genetically-engineered bovine growth hormone (BGH) which forces cows to produce more milk, is also, as we noted, doing wonders with soya beans. They have engineered them to survive even greater doses of the company's herbicide, and thus you may get more herbicides, or biocides (as Rachel Carson would have it) than ever if you eat soyabeans, today present in hundreds of foods, sometimes where one would least expect them if not an avid reader of the fine print on the label. The New Zealand Green Party Co-leader, Jeanette Fitzsimons, claims that soy is used in 60% of processed foods. 'It's hard to imagine a New Zealand diet which would not include something genetically engineered.'[12]

Most of all,

One of the biggest problems with engineered food, is that it presents our digestive and immune systems with never-before-seen combinations of amino acids and chemical compounds, because they are not always broken down prior to crossing the gut wall into the body's general circulation.[13]

In other words, they are constructs like the TFAs (see Chapter 2) which we may not be evolutionarily designed to process and cope with. Since the TFAs came in we have seen an epidemic of heart disease all over the Western world.

There is a global network of physicians and scientists, PRAST (Physicians and Scientists for Responsible Application of Science and Technology) which has circulated the following concerns on the subject of the genetic engineering of our food, as published in a factsheet produced by PRAST:

1   Genetic Engineering is Fundamentally Different From Breeding: The artificial insertion of foreign genes represents a traumatic disturbance of the close genetic control in normal cells. It is completely different in nature from the combination of maternal and paternal chromosomes brought about by natural mating mechanisms.

2   Genetic Engineering of Today is Technically Primitive as it is impossible to guide the insertion of a new gene: Therefore it is impossible to foresee the effects of an inserted gene. But even if the position of the gene can be localized afterwards, the knowledge of DNA is far too incomplete to make it possible to predict the result.

3   Hazardous Substances May Be Generated Unpredictably: Because of the artificial insertion of a foreign gene. These may, in the worst case, be toxic, allergenic or otherwise damaging to health.

4   No Safety Assessment Methods Are Fully Reliable: Over 10% of serious side-effects are undetectable in the case of new drugs in spite of rigorous safety assessments. The risk of not detecting a hazardous property of a new GM food is probably considerably greater than in the case of drugs.

5   The Present Rules for Safety Assessment Are Seriously Inadequate: They have been explicitly designed so as to simplify approval procedures. They accept very insensitive safety testing. Therefore there is a considerable risk that foods harmful to health may pass undetected.

6   The GM Foods So Far Developed Are of No Significant Value for Mankind: The products mainly satisfy purely commercial interests.

7   The Knowledge Is Very Incomplete about the Ecological Effects of Releasing Genetically-modified Organisms: It has not been positively proven that GM organisms may not cause environmental harm. Various potential ecological complications have been anticipated by ecological experts. For example, there are many routes for uncontrolled spread of engineered and potentially hazardous genes, including gene transfer by bacteria and viruses. Environmental complications will probably mostly be impossible to repair as the released genes cannot be retrieved.

8   New and Potentially Dangerous Viruses May Emerge: It has been experimentally demonstrated that inserted virus genes may unite with genes from infecting viruses (so-called recombinations). Such new viruses may be more aggressive than the

original virus. Viruses may also become less species-specific. For example, a plant virus might become harmful to valuable insects, animals and to man.

9　The Knowledge of the Hereditary Substance DNA Is Very Limited: Only the function of about 3% of the DNA is known. It is risky to manipulate complicated systems that are incompletely known. Extensive experience from biology, ecology and medicine shows that this may cause serious unexpected problems and disturbances.

10　Genetic Engineering Will Not Help Solve the World Hunger Problem: The claim that genetic engineering may contribute importantly to reduced world hunger is a scientifically unsubstantiated myth.

Billions have been spent with the view to making even more billions in the future. And they will be made at our expense, if we let it happen.

William E Swartz, Director of Technology for Rhone-Poulenc Food Ingredients in Cranbury, New Jersey, likens the inter-splicing of genes in food to 'inserting a few seconds of rap into a Beethoven symphony'. But with food, when you have no idea what you're eating it could actually turn out to be a major rape of our health. Nature doesn't 'get it right' all the time, but she gets it right most of the time. We evolved to be a living part of Nature, and we evolved to get our foods from Nature, not from the laboratory.

The irradiation of food is another problem area and it is worth noting that these alien foods are generally permitted to be sold without any identifying labelling required, meanwhile there are ongoing efforts from vested interests to discredit and restrict people's access to centuries-old herbal remedies which are derived from **real** plants. It would seem that much is dependent on the amounts of money at stake and who is making it. Again, check Chapter 27 on prescription drugs. In my opinion we should eat only the food we have evolved with, for that is what we are designed to metabolize.

Needless to say, governments which permit genetically-engineered and other 'tampered-with' products to be sold without the appropriate warning labels are ignorant, uncaring and possibly in the pockets of the multinationals who make the stuff. The **most fundamental right of any free people should be a choice in the matter of what we do and do not eat**. Moreover, the failure to label can threaten those who *do make real food*, and hence a country's trading capacity. In the case of New Zealand, it could ultimately threaten a very dismal and not exactly thriving economy.

The salient point in this argument over labelling was made by consumer rights activist, the American Jeremy Rifkin, who said,

'If food producers are so proud of these "Brave New World" products, why are they so afraid to label them?'[14]

Perhaps the greatest worry of all in connection with genetically-altered food is that now there are crops which contain the genetic instructions not to reproduce themselves – a kind of built-in self-destruction at the end of the season. It has been speculated that this has been done so that farmers will have to buy new seeds each year.[15]

From the *New Scientist* (30th January 1999) we learn that these self-destruct seeds may actually be partially transferred into us through the process of digestion of the crop from these seeds. Does that mean we may not be able to reproduce ourselves?

But even without that possibility, life on our planet is at risk. The biggest threat is that seeds from these crops will be carried by wind, water and other means (as so many have already) to other crops, until we lose the older seeds. In fact the world could be held to ransom by the loss of them. It is even possible to foresee a time when the earth is bare from the loss of plant reproduction, and the human race could then perish from lack of the oxygen usually provided by the plant world. For it is plants and plants alone which enable us to inhabit this planet.

A GLIMMER OF HOPE?

The good news in the UK is that several of Britain's largest supermarket chains have determined that they will not sell genetically-modified foods.

Iceland's founder, Malcolm Walker, has said on radio: 'Consumers are being conned. Genetically modified ingredients in food are probably the most significant and potentially dangerous development in food production this century.'[16]

Iceland, Tesco and the others stand to and deserve to do well over this stand, as market research shows that 81% of food consumers are concerned about buying genetically-modified foods and would avoid them if possible.

When I contemplate the rows upon rows of smoothly identical tomatoes in the supermarket there is something unnatural, almost sinister, about their rank perfection. They are all exactly the same size, shape and colour, like Christmas-tree decorations. They last and last. They do not squish when pressed. They taste like tomato-flavoured cardboard.

I prefer to buy the Italian acid-free variety, each one unique in size, shape and colouration. They squish; they die; they taste like tomatoes 'orter'.

And I remember that when a human being dies, an extraordinary thing happens. One moment there is life. A few seconds later there is death. Something has flown. That spark, which is the essence of a unique biological entity, has flown, just disappeared.

What is this 'spark of life', this indescribable wonder? This spark that is found in every living thing?

When we tamper with the very life-force of a plant, its DNA, do we cause that spark to die? Do we risk eating something essentially strange and dead, but somehow artificially 'embalmed' to look alive?

But let us give the last word on the subject to Dr Paul Butler, medical chairman for Physicians and Scientists for Responsible Genetics in New Zealand:

The public must be protected from being unwitting subjects of uncontrolled experimentation with their food supply and environment. An immediate moratorium should be placed on the release into the environment of genetically engineered organisms and on the use of genetically engineered foods.

16: PLASTIC

'Plastic is such loverly stuff!'

In our century plastic is just about everywhere in our everyday lives. It is also used in the building industry, the electronics industry, the health care system, in transport and just about everything else. The problem is that although we use plastic in so many ways, until recently there has been no research into any possible associated problems, either in the short or the long term.

Barry Densley of Melbourne, Australia, has been taking a look at it and finds that plastics and PVC (polyvinyl chloride) are actually toxic byproducts of the petroleum industry. And they are not inert materials at all. In fact, the mixture of dangerous molecules emanating therefrom, known as phthalates, seems to creep into just about everything it comes in contact with.[1]

Densley calls this chemical mixture 'a deadly cocktail' partly because the stabilizers used are known to be carcinogenic and also because the phthalates act as **xeno-oestrogens** – that is, false or pseudo-oestrogens (sex hormones). We have in the plant kingdom substances known as phyto-oestrogens with which we have been associated for millions of years. They do not harm us. But these xeno-oestrogens we have been consuming inadvertently for only the last 50 years are actually poisonous to the human body, and **can** harm us because they disrupt our hormonal systems which in turn influence every aspect of our bodies and our lives.

It has been shown that fish will change sex under long-term exposure to such synthetically oestrogenic compounds. Meanwhile among humans, sperm counts have fallen by up to 50% over the last 50 years in many countries, with testicular cancer rates increasing dramatically in the same period. Moreover, several kinds of phthalates are **known** to be 'testicular toxicants'. Perhaps worst of all, a recent study on aborted male foetuses found that they were already developing testicular cancer in the uterus, while figures obtained by Densley from the Australian

Bureau of Statistics indicate that the main cause of infant deaths in the first year are related to endocrine (hormonal) disorders, congenital defects, diseases of the nervous system and complications immediately before and after birth.

Another finding which may be related to the plastics in our world: males are declining in numbers, and have been for the last 20 years, because fewer are being born. Although the statistics don't look bad, that is a percentage of 0.515 of the births down to 0.513 or 2, in terms of actual numbers it can truly add up. In Canada during the last 20 years approximately 8,600 fewer males than usual have been born; in the US 38,000 baby boys; the numbers of baby girls increased proportionately.[2] While some may be inclined to applaud this, it is not good news for the future of the human race, nor are the reasons why it is happening anything to cheer about.

Phthalates are suspect in this world of horrors because they migrate from everything plastic. They enter the body and become a part of our body fluids, which in a pregnant women will cross the placenta to affect the future child. They are also there in breastmilk.[3]

There are phthalates in the plastic packaging or wrapping materials surrounding just about everything. In other words, phthalates will migrate from the wrapping around the cheese into the cheese we eat and hence into us. Extremely worrying, they can also migrate from the plastic containers for blood used in the blood banks, into the life-bringing blood they contain. They are also there in the plastic mattresses, bumpers and toys for infants. And it is the toxic fumes from these and/or the fungus which grows on them, that are suspect as one of the possible causes for SIDS, or Sudden Infant Death Syndrome.

One of the worst likelihood's is that xeno-oestrogens from plastics as well as pesticides and other things are part of the cause of the ever-increasing breast cancer rates in women.

We should be aware that the United Kingdom Ministry of Agriculture, Fisheries and Food, conducting numerous experiments, has found phthalates present in every food sample taken since 1993, including meat, fish, eggs, milk and milk products. Every infant formula tested contained phthalates.

Thus it is on the cards that phthalates can affect reproductive ability and the developing foetus, and can cause spontaneous abortions, stillbirths, toxaemia, low birthweight, congenital defects and childhood cancer, as well as breast, testicular and other cancers.

A recent book, *Our Stolen Future*[4], has comprehensively reviewed the potential impact of synthetic chemicals such as phthalates on human health, and has stirred up the powerful plastics and chemicals industries. But as always they will use their wealth and influence to stall and deny so that it will be difficult to get anything done for perhaps generations. Witness the decades-long debacle of the cigarette industry resisting any attempts to contain its billion-dollar empire, aided and abetted by various others.

There is a vast array of studies and references for all of the statements made in this brief look at the problem.

In the meantime, perhaps we should go back to using the more inert cellophane for wrappings. And now we know why it is so often used in health food stores.

PS People using water distillers should ensure that those 'hungry molecules' in the steam do *not* encounter plastics, either in the collecting vessel or on the way to it. Your health, even your life, may depend upon such avoidance.

⚠

17: IMMUNIZATION

'Vaccinations are effective and safe.'

To rational human beings, the ultimate test of both the safety and efficacy of vaccinations would be: prolonged use over a period of time, with vigilant reporting of 'side-effects' and deaths. But for some extraordinary reason, doctors are not routinely required to report either deaths following vaccination, complications following vaccination or even if and when people contract the illness against which they have been vaccinated. And it has always been this way.

As such, those health officials who trot out the old chestnut, 'The benefits of immunization far, far outweigh any adverse reactions'[1] are speaking not from knowledge but from ideological positions – that is, for propaganda reasons. And inasmuch as such pro-vaccination propaganda is so widespread, the wise, the cautious will look at what evidence to the contrary *is* available.

The idea behind immunization is 'scientific' and seems quite sound. We are told that if we give a healthy human a tiny dose of something we are trying to avoid, then the body will make antibodies against it, and thus win out when the actual disease arrives in all its strength.

This is, of course, one of the principles of homoeopathy as well. However, there is a big difference between the extremely dilute substances used in homoeopathy and the much larger amounts of known biotoxins used in vaccinations.

And there are enormous 'selling jobs' and 'propaganda' to convince health officials and the general public that the immunization procedure is sound and a good idea, even for tiny infants or especially for tiny infants. But the most serious charge against the process of immunization is that it is a risky business injecting foreign biological products into infants barely born and just getting their bearings in this world, just beginning to develop that all-important but tricky immune system. The US Taskforce for Safer Childhood Vaccines went so far as to report that, 'Safety is only relative and cannot be absolutely guaranteed.'[2]

But if we truly want to look at possible infant deaths in relation to immunization procedures, in the absence of the appropriate reporting procedures we have to look at overall country-wide statistics. For example, when Japan stopped injecting infants with the DPT (Diphtheria-Pertussis-Tetanus vaccine) and moved up the age of immunization to two years, cot deaths (Sudden Infant Death Syndrome or SIDS) virtually disappeared in Japan. There was also a decline in spinal meningitis. Japan went on to have the lowest infant mortality rates in the world, followed by Sweden where the use of the pertussis immunization was dropped in 1979. (Italy does not use the DPT either.)

Similarly, when the Australian government made DPT immunizations a voluntary choice, half the country opted not to vaccinate and dropped out of the programme. The incidence of SIDS then dropped by 50%. In the UK, deaths also decreased when immunization became voluntary. In the light of these statistics it would seem that the immunization of infants *may* be a risky business.

Very few of us in the English-speaking countries are aware that in some Western European countries the pertussis vaccine is no longer used at all because 'they have decided the risk of vaccine damage is greater than the risk of catching the milder form of whooping cough prevalent in developing nations today.'[3]

One wonders why it has taken so long to 'find out' a significant possible cause of SIDS when it should have been obvious now for many years; moreover, those countries which continue to vaccinate most infants have the highest rates of SIDS in the world. For example, in the US there are nearly 10,000 baby deaths every year from SIDS, a tremendous increase in the last two decades, an increase which may reflect increased immunizations of infants.[4]

New Zealand has one of the highest rates of SIDS in the world, a rate of 2 per 1,000 live births (approximately 100 deaths per year); we also have high rates of immunizations, 91% in 1996; 87% in 1997. The DTPH3 (diphtheria-tetanus-pertussis-haemophilus influenza, referred to as 'The Quad') is given at 6 weeks after birth, and then again at 12 weeks after birth, among the earliest exposures to the needle in the world. That NZ cot deaths tend to cluster around the 8- to 16-week mark is proof of nothing; the timing is, however, suggestive.

One possible explanation is that cot death can follow breathing difficulties from damage to cerebral (brain) nerves occasioned by immunization.[5] Of course immunizations will not be the whole story in SIDS. There are other likely causes. For example, incorrect infant feeding.[6] We noted in Chapter 2 that for the best health and brain development infants require Essential Fatty Acids not found in hydrogenated fats and oils. Also, that in these 'technologized' fats and oils will be found Trans Fatty Acids or molecules the body was not designed to process.

In Chapter 3 we looked at problems which may be associated with homogenized milk and the dried milk solids. Most mass-produced infant formulas contain both TFAs and homogenized milk, and sometimes also dried milk solids.

As far back as 1974 Dr Robert Riesinger expressed the belief that one of the reasons breastfed babies fare better is that there is far less *E coli* in their gut and that it is this bacteria in the gut which, in combination with the DPT vaccine, causes endotoxic shock, heart and breathing failures.[7] He has been ignored.

There are also mattresses designed for babies containing fire-retardant substances which give off potentially damaging fumes. This theory has of course been disputed, as has the fungal growth on plastic theory, but ask the chemically sensitive how they react to such fumes. Everything that is close to an infant, particularly petrochemical substances, particularly in a space where the air is close, as in the depths of some Moses baskets, should be suspect.

It is also claimed that the position an infant lies in has a lot to do with SIDS and that the placing of infants on their backs has decreased the death rate in NZ. It has. But infants have been found dead in every possible position. Infants have even died in their mothers' arms. It is wise to put an infant on its back or side, but position is possibly a final factor; it cannot be the main cause.

But to look at the question of infant immunization from the point of view of individual medical researchers, as early as the 1930s in the US, 'researchers reported that some children reacted with fevers, convulsions and collapse'. In the same period, Thorald Madsen of Copenhagen reported the death of two infants within a few minutes of the injection.[8]

In 1982, Dr William Torch of the Nevada School of Medicine submitted a report to the 34th Annual Meeting of the American Academy of Neurology, showing that two-thirds of 103 children who died of SIDS had been immunized with DPT vaccine up to three weeks before their deaths, most dying within a day of the immunization. Dr Torch believes in a causal relationship.[9]

In 1983, there was a report in *Pediatric Infectious Diseases* from a combined UCLA School of Medicine Department of Pediatrics and a Los Angeles County Health Department study of 145 SIDS victims, 53 of whom had received DPT immunizations in close proximity to their deaths. The researchers concluded that these findings 'further substantiate a possible association between DPT shots and SIDS'.[10]

Most recently, *Pediatrics* carried an article, 'Interleukin 6, C-Reactive Protein, and Abnormal Cardio-respiratory Responses to Immunization in Premature Infants.'[11]

In 1994 the US Institute of Medicine, looking at the up to 10,000 cases of SIDS per year in that country, admitted that the evidence is consistent for a causal relation between DPT vaccine and acute encephalopathy, encephalitis or encephalomyelitis and 'unusual shock-like state'. This was reported in the *Journal of the American Medical Association*.[12] In fact it has also been demonstrated in laboratory animals.

Meanwhile Dr Archie Kalokerinos MBBS, PhD, of Australia, was serving as Medical Superintendent of Collarenebri Hospital when he noted that after immunizations were carried out in the Aboriginal community, up to half of the children went into endotoxic shock and died. He was able to rescue a few near-deaths by administering large doses of vitamin C (a detoxifier) into the muscle or veins. He realized that these poor infants were so malnourished that they could not cope with the impact of the vaccines. So before the procedure he built them up with vitamins, especially vitamin C, in doses proportionate to their age, and most of them thereafter survived the immunizations. He also wrote a book on this subject, *Every Second Child*.[13]

But the deaths were not just among Aboriginal children. For Dr Kalokerinos also found a high infant death rate following immunizations in Caucasian (white) infants. 'Infants who were apparently well or who had a trivial illness, became suddenly shocked or unconscious, often preceded by an irritable or apprehensive state, and died. Autopsies failed to explain why.'

Unfortunately, what Dr Kalokerinos had to tell the world was not welcome to officialdom. He says 'When I sought assistance from other general practitioners, specialists and government departments I was told:

1 That nobody else had such a problem.
2 That I was obviously doing something wrong.
3 That I was not suited to practise medicine in such an area.
4 That I should see a psychiatrist because I was "over concerned".'

Dr Kalokerinos claims that all doctors had (and have) this problem. But they keep quiet about it. Colleagues and contemporaries of Dr Kalokerinos, as well as the authorities he sought to influence on behalf of helpless infants, not only ignored his work but became extremely hostile, even when he was able to get to infants with the vitamin C in time. 'Several times I was able to demonstrate to colleagues the dramatic reversal of the shock or unconscious state. They remained hostile.'[14]

But there are numerous other accounts of studies recorded in medical journals and elsewhere which give hints as to the correctness of the above-mentioned doctors' conclusions. And all these accounts should have alerted concerned authorities as to the dangers of vaccines to infants, but they have not. For the official policy all over the world is to deny that vaccines have anything to do with SIDS.

No matter what carnage lies in the wake of immunizations, the basic but unsubstantiated belief of the pro-vaccinators is that, as noted, 'the benefits to millions always massively outweigh the risk to the very few.'

Apart from the devastation that has been wrought on those individuals whose children have died, it is not only the deaths which should concern us. There are also numerous reported adverse reactions to vaccines. In fact the US Department of Health and Human Services early in 1997 reported that an estimate of 60,000 children per year receiving the DPT vaccine experienced convulsions, shock, colic etc.[15]

In 1988 a case brought before the High Court in London revealed 2,081 neurological (nervous system) problems in 80% of those inoculated with whooping cough vaccine,[16] while more than 90 cases of autism, or inability to talk, in the UK are considered due to the after-effects of immunization. The term 'autism' was first described in 1943 by the American child psychiatrist Kanner. It is doubtful that this handicap even existed in significant numbers before that period.

But cases of encephalitis (inflammation of the brain) mentioned as a part of the statistics cannot convey the terrible burdens of the parents whose children sustain this assault.

Here is an excerpt from a letter to the editor from a mother in New Zealand caring full-time for her brain-damaged child:

My son was brain damaged by the state's mass-medication vaccination programme as an infant. Now in his thirties, autistic, epileptic, mentally retarded with no speech, no writing ability or communication, he needs full care with every aspect of his life ... 24 hours a day.[17]

She could not see how she was going to manage, as the NZ government was clearly planning further inroads into the assistance given to such people.

The New Zealand *Listener* reported another mother's experience with her 15-month-old healthy child:

About an hour after he'd had the vaccine, he became sleepy, and wasn't able to be woken for 19 hours. He slept for 19 hours solid. The next morning he woke with a high-pitched scream, back arched, body all rigid, and screamed for five and a half hours.

This formerly healthy child then went on to develop autistic tendencies, allergies, swollen joints, seizures and bizarre behaviour problems that took years to bring under control. His mother sums it up:

I believed in vaccinations and that's why we did it ... I didn't want a child brain-damaged or dead, which is what they told us if you don't vaccinate – and unfortunately I got a child brain-damaged anyway.[18]

In the UK after a massive immunization campaign in 1994, it was reported that

26% of cases experienced swollen arthritis or painful joints after the first dose and that children's lives were thereafter disrupted by swollen joints, severe allergic reactions, swollen glands, violent headaches, inflammation of the brain, brain damage, autism, coma, epilepsy, ME, speech and behaviour problems, inflammatory bowel disease, difficulties with sight and hearing – all of which may contribute to evidence that challenges the very foundation of immunization policy: the notion that the benefits to millions always massively outweigh the risk to the very few.[19]

In fact the aftermath in Britain following that particular campaign was so severe that Dawbarns, a firm of solicitors with a long heritage, put out a 39-page fact-sheet on the dangers of vaccines.[20]

But as we noted at the outset, extraordinarily, in most countries **doctors are not required to report adverse reactions and deaths suspected to be due to immunizations**. We can therefore never have a true picture of the situation. But the following figures of adverse reactions were *volunteered* by some doctors to the US Vaccine Adverse Event Reporting System, a division of the US Food and Drug Administration, during an 18-month period:

COUNTS OF EVENTS BY VACCINE TYPE[21]

Reports	Serious	Life-threatening	Hospitalized	Disabled	Died
DTP 246	7,327	1,269	133	975	72
Oral Polio 229	5,633	1,015	114	759	49
Haem B Conj 225	5,060	1,027	121	781	36
Hepatitis B 17	4,227	383	57	241	108
Measles MR 26	3,502	434	50	372	43

That is, after immunization, over 3% of the subjects reported on as having had DPT immunizations died; 4% after Polio. But one has to go on to ask the question: Of what possible use is a voluntary system which results in no follow-up, no relevant study or conclusions as to safety?

Also in the US, since 1988 $724.4 million has been awarded to the families of children injured or killed by immunizations. And we should perhaps be asking the question as to why American insurance companies generally refuse to cover problems ensuing from immunizations.[22] But no matter what the outcome, as with almost all medical interventions those who manufacture vaccines are not called to account when disaster occurs.

The record of immediate severe illness and death in a small percentage of children following immunizations is inescapable; moreover we cannot know of the true **long-term effects** of individual immunizations, for these show up only when broad statistical data are studied. In 1994 the *Journal of the American Medical Association* published the result of a survey which found that British children receiving the whooping cough (pertussis) vaccine were nearly six times more likely to develop asthma than those who had not received the vaccine.[23] In fact, a 1989 US study at the Bronx Municipal Hospital indicated that asthma is increasing both in frequency and severity, with more than a fourfold increase in hospitalizations between the years 1960 to 1987.[24]

In New Zealand, a highly vaccinated country, according to the Asthma Foundation over one-sixth of the country suffers either from asthma or a similar respiratory condition. While in the UK, between 1958 and 1970 the incidence of allergic eczema more than doubled.[25]

A study conducted by the Inflammatory Bowel Disease Study Group of the Royal Free Hospital and reported in the *Lancet* in 1995, found that people who had received the measles immunization were three times more likely to develop Crohn's Disease, and more than twice as likely to develop ulcerative colitis (both are chronic gut diseases) than people who did not receive the vaccine.[26] Autism was another aftermath noted.

Then in 1996 a US science researcher, J Barthelow Classen, using a Christchurch, New Zealand register, suggested that Hepatitis B vaccines given since 1988 are linked to a 60% increase in diabetes in those vaccinated in New Zealand.[27] Strangely enough, it has also been linked to the rare disease alopecia (complete baldness in either sex, but predominantly in women), which jumped from 11.2 cases per 100,000 to 18.2 cases per 100,000 after the immunization programmes.[28]

Dr Russell Jaffe MD, PhD, a prominent US scientist, researcher and physician, has declared that overall the incidence of autoimmune disease has increased more than tenfold in the past two generations.[29] Autoimmune disease is a derangement of the immune system whereby the body attacks itself. Many diseases formerly not understood are now known to be autoimmune in nature, such as juvenile diabetes, pernicious anaemia, rheumatoid arthritis, multiple sclerosis and many others. As one example, in the US the incidence of juvenile diabetes per capita has nearly trebled in the past 30 years.[30] One explanation for autoimmune disease as a possible aftermath of immunization is that 'the body, unused to doing its own detection work, can no longer distinguish between foreign invaders and ordinary tissue and begins to destroy itself.'

Most modern illnesses (AIDS, asthma, cervical cancer and other '20th-century illnesses') are related to immune system problems.[31] Something is causing the immune system to 'do the unthinkable' – to turn on its own body, the one it is there to guard.

Dr Harold E Buttram would add,

Perhaps most ominous of all is the rise in childhood behavioural disorders, hyperactivity, and learning dysfunctions, with approximately one out of five children now being classified as learning-disabled. Some experts believe that such mental and emotional impairments are, in many instances, a direct result of immunological derangements.[32]

Dr Kris Gaublomme MD, Dip Hom of Belgium has summed up:

The potential advantages of vaccination are presented using falsified statistics. In certain cases, the results are not nearly as good as we are led to believe. There are scientifically verified cases of serious illness and deaths linked to vaccination: Problems of meningitis, encephalitis, mental retardation, paralysis, autism, diabetes, asthma, pneumonia, bronchitis, depression, sterility, chronic fatigues, eczema, allergies, aggression, learning difficulties, and deficiencies in the immune system have all been linked to vaccination.[33]

However, despite all such empirical evidence that vaccines *do kill and damage*, the courts invariably rule that vaccine manufacturers are not responsible. There is also denial and misinformation in the selling of vaccines, with very limited testing for safety. Nor do the recipients see the long lists of potential adverse reactions, now legally required to be listed on the manufacturer's information enclosed with the vaccines. Meanwhile, billions and billions have been made, and are being made from the sale of vaccines.

But is it not worth all this carnage to be rid of some deadly infectious diseases? Not so, apparently. We noted in the chapter on fluoride that tooth decay was dramatically declining before the introduction of fluoride to our water supplies. Similarly, there is plenty of evidence that the infectious diseases which used to decimate populations in Europe 100 years ago were already in decline by up to 90% long before immunizations came into use in large populations. On this,

Dr R Mendelsohn has gone on record as saying: 'We cannot credit the mass immunizations in the US for the decline of some childhood diseases, for they declined simultaneously in Europe where the mass immunizations *did not take place*'.[34] Ivan Illich, author of *Limits to Medicine: Medical Nemesis: The Expropriation of Health*, has also commented, 'Higher host resistance due to better nutrition, sanitation and housing is the cause of the decline of infectious diseases.'[35] And he gives as evidence:

The combined death rate from scarlet fever, diphtheria, whooping cough, and measles among children up to 15 shows that nearly 90% of the total decline in mortality between 1860 and 1965 had occurred before the introduction of antibiotics and widespread immunization.[36]

What these doctors have noted has been fully authenticated by the story on diphtheria. By 1940, the annual death rate from diphtheria in Germany was less than 300 per million. But after the mass immunization for diphtheria there followed 'unprecedented diphtheria epidemics' in fully vaccinated subjects, and the death rate far outweighed the pre-1940 death rate.

A graph based on statistics from the Government Bureau of Statistics in Wiesbaden, Germany, indicates that the incidence of diphtheria from 1920 to the 1990s actually increased each time there were immunization programmes. Yet

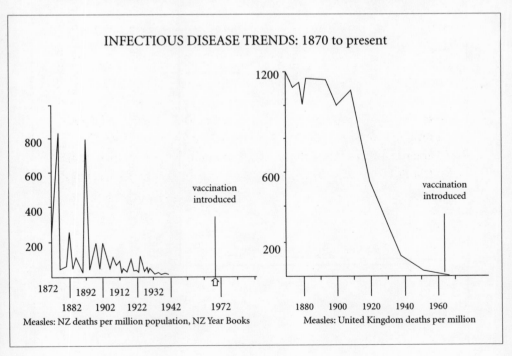

INFECTIOUS DISEASE TRENDS: 1870 to present

Measles: NZ deaths per million population, NZ Year Books

Measles: United Kingdom deaths per million

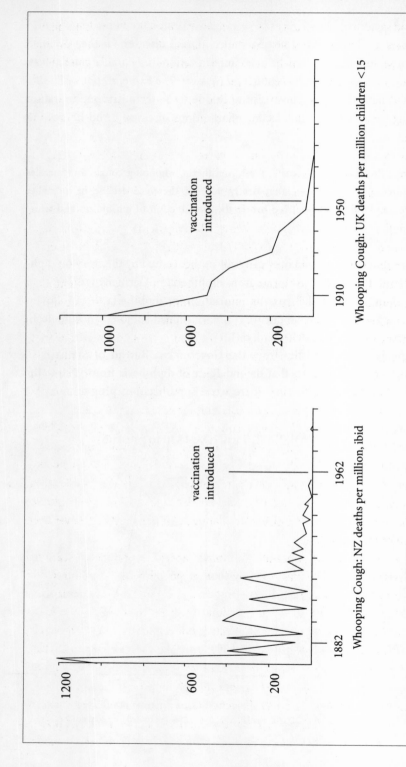

Whooping Cough: NZ deaths per million, ibid

Whooping Cough: UK deaths per million children <15

The graph clearly shows that death rates were declining rapidly, well before mass immunization programmes were introduced. These sharp declines are thought to be due to improvements in sanitation and nutrition in the previous 100 years.

the cases had steadily declined after the Second World War even though no immunizations were carried out for a few years after the war. They declined again after 1980 when immunization ceased, in a context of an overall decline, as for all infectious diseases in our century, immunizations or no.

Meanwhile figures from the UK reveal that between 1860 and 1948 measles declined 94.1%; scarlet fever 99.7%; and whooping cough declined 91%, all without vaccines.

Diphtheria's most obvious decline occurred between 1945 and 1949 in 4 million unvaccinated children.

Now, 50 years on, as smaller epidemics continue to appear in vaccinated children, we are told that the reason they still occur is because we are not using enough doses, and that 'more' will be better. Hence parents, who were assured from 1969–1990 that one dose of measles vaccine would protect for life, are being told that two doses, and sometimes three, will be necessary.

In 1994 the US Centers for Disease Control (CDC) reported that in an area of 100% immunization there had been a measles outbreak. It's conclusion, 'The apparent paradox is that as measles immunization rates rise to high levels in a population, measles becomes a disease of immunized persons.'[37] Not a statement to inspire confidence in either immunization or the CDC. A similar situation had been seen in 1987 when the CDC reported that measles outbreaks had occurred in schools with immunization levels greater than 98%. What is more, these measles epidemics occurred in areas formerly measles-free for years.

When it comes down to individual accounts, a New Zealand mother in a letter to the *Northern News* (7 November 1996), tells of her daughter who had been fully immunized for whooping cough but who soon after contracted whooping cough and was very ill for three months. Later her younger son received a measles shot. He soon became very ill with measles and did not fully recover for a year. Another mother who wrote in response to this letter claimed that her child had 'never been the same' since immunization.[38]

There is a monstrous amount of similar 'anecdotal evidence' scattered through newspapers and in the conversations of people when they meet, but as such it is evidence discounted by supporters of vaccination. Of course these accounts can be and are dismissed as 'anecdotal' by those who wish not to know the truth. But when the reporting of ill-effects is not required of medical people, how else are we going to know the worst that is possible? Moreover, as to efficacy, it is a fact that no vaccine has ever been used for scarlet fever or the bubonic plague, and yet they have both almost disappeared off the face of the earth.[39]

The effects of immunization over the generations are also a cause for concern. The history of measles is instructive. Formerly children acquired a natural immunity against measles after having the illness, an immunity for life, which was, in girls, later passed on to their babies and which provided these infants with protection for the first few years. Thus, before the 1980s only 3% of measles cases occurred under the age of one. But since the immunization process has compromised these immune processes, the protection lasts only 10 to 20 years, thus vaccinated women are no longer always able to provide protection for their babies in this manner.

Hence the increasing numbers of infants getting the measles. According to an Associated Press release,[40] 28%, or over one-fourth of children who now catch measles in the US are aged under one year. They are getting measles younger and younger, and at an age when they are least able to cope with it. Between one-quarter and one-third of these babies develop problems, some of them serious. Also, formerly vaccinated teenagers and adults are increasingly affected by 'atypical' – that is, a more serious kind of – measles.[41] We are advised to get 'boosters' and 'more boosters'.[42]

Another problem associated with the measles vaccine is that since immunization the risk of pneumonia and 'demonstrable liver abnormalities' has increased substantially to over 3% and 2% respectively among those vaccinated.[43] Before immunization for measles it was, for most, an unpleasant illness but not a serious matter for the majority who contracted it. As Dr David Ritchie, General Practitioner of Christchurch and anthroposophical physician says, 'with a normal child, there's no way you're going to die of measles.' Whereas after having interfered with the normal cycle of sickness and the acquisition of antibodies, the babies now contracting measles are at risk of dying from them.

Polio is another case where immunizations may make things worse. In 1954 the *Lancet* reviewed a half-century of research outlining the factors that either cause or increase the severity of polio (infantile paralysis). These included: '**Vaccination, especially pertussis vaccines**; trauma; tonsillectomies; and the injections of numerous substances such as cortisone, bismuth, buanine and penicillin.'[44]

Dr William F Koch MD, PhD has declared that

The injection of any serum, vaccination or even penicillin has shown a very marked increase in the incidence of polio, at least 400%. In Los Angeles, in 1949, after the largest smallpox vaccination campaign, an epidemic of polio broke out within two weeks. 26 deaths and 1,900 cases were reported. In 1933 in St Louis, Missouri, after a typhoid vaccination campaign, there was an outbreak of encephalitis (a form of polio) about 10 days after vaccinations, with over 100 deaths.[45]

Polio had already declined dramatically before the Salk vaccine came into use; moreover Neil Miller, author of *Vaccines: Are They Really Safe and Effective?*[46]

claims that doctors and scientists on the staff of the US National Institute of Health during the 1950s were aware that the Salk vaccine was both ineffective and dangerous. But there had been a large investment on the part of the American National Polio Foundation and the pharmaceutical companies, so they went ahead and used it.

Also, the New Zealand government of that time knew the reason they were getting the vaccine cheaply. It was known to be contaminated with at least one monkey virus (Simian Virus 40), from the monkey kidneys used in manufacture. However, NZ doctors and parents were told it was harmless. This crime against our children did not come to light until 1983, when it was exposed by the newspaper *Truth*, despite Health Department efforts to cover it up. And I have personally come up against some of the chronic and ruinous health effects in formerly healthy people of that criminal act, for which the officials involved in both countries should have been brought to trial.

On this use of contaminated vaccine, the journal *Science* commented in 1972 as follows:

There can be few graver opportunities for man-made disaster than the mass immunization campaigns that are now routine in many countries. Should the vaccine preparations become contaminated with an undetected agent ... such as a cancer-causing virus, a whole generation of vaccinated people could be put in jeopardy. This of course is no science fiction writer's horror story – it has already happened once; millions of people have been injected with a monkey virus ... which was found to be contaminating polio vaccines. The virus causes cancer in hamsters; no one yet knows what it may do in humans.[47]

They were referring to the SV40 used in New Zealand, a country which has among the highest rates of some cancers in the world. In 1962, according to records, over 2 million of the 2.5 million people living in New Zealand in that period had received either injectable or oral SV40-contaminated polio vaccine.

The polio vaccine is celebrated as the triumph of science over a dreadful disease, and yet as with the other diseases, polio declined equally in countries where the vaccine was not used. Also, **the data on polio has been grossly manipulated**. Before 1954, patients had to exhibit paralytic symptoms for only 24 hours (without lab confirmation) to be diagnosed as having paralytic polio. From 1954 onwards, after widespread use of the vaccine, the patient had to have symptoms for at least 60 days to qualify as a polio victim. Data manipulation is also accomplished by changing the name of the disease. Polio may have disappeared, but viral or aseptic meningitis has skyrocketed. In a California Report of Communicable Diseases, polio showed a zero count, while an accompanying asterisk explained 'All such cases now reported as meningitis.'[48]

However, before this salubrious solution,

Six New England states reported increases in polio one year after the Salk vaccine was introduced, ranging from a more than doubling in Vermont, to the Massachusetts increase of 642%. During the 1962 US Congressional hearings, Dr Bern Greenberg, head of the Dept of Biostatistics for the University of North Carolina School of Public Health, testified that not only did the cases of polio increase substantially after mandatory vaccinations (50% increase from 1957 to 1958, 80% increase from 1958 to 1969), but that the statistics were manipulated by the Public Health Service to give the opposite impression. However, by 1985, the CDC reported that 87% of the cases of polio in the US occurring between 1973 and 1983 were caused by the vaccine.[49]

It is a fact that Dr Jonas Salk himself, the creator of the Salk vaccine against polio, testified on the subject of live vs dead vaccines before the US Congressional Committee investigating outbreaks of polio, to the effect that **all polio cases occurring since 1970 were produced by live polio vaccine**.[50] He was once again advocating the use of dead viruses.

The strongest claims are made for the fact that immunizations 'wiped out smallpox'. But if we want to see the effectiveness of immunization in a fixed population we have only to look back at the history of smallpox immunization in the Philippines. Dr Guylaine Lancetot MD, writing in *The Medical Mafia*[51], points out that:

In 1905, the Philippines had a mortality rate of 10% due to smallpox. After a massive vaccination program, it reached epidemic proportions, killing 25% of the population, by now vaccinated. Despite this, the authorities stepped up the vaccinations. In 1918, the worst epidemic killed 54% of the people there, at a time when 95% of the population had been vaccinated. Manila, the capital, where everyone had been vaccinated or revaccinated, was the hardest hit with 65% dead. The Island of Mindanao, where the inhabitants had refused to be vaccinated, was the least hit. Only 11%. Despite this evidence, anti-smallpox vaccinations continued and, in 1966, the W.H.O. launched a world campaign which would last ten years, only to be abandoned because it proved to be ineffective.

The record of immediate severe illness and death in children following immunization should make plain the risks involved. And even more ominous, perhaps, we simply do not know the possible long-term negative effects of mass immunization. Both those who administer them and those who accept them are acting not on knowledge but on faith, blind faith.

Let us have a look at how these vaccines are made. In the case of vaccines against viruses, animal parts must be used in which to grow the cells. And these parts must come from a living creature. The cells could be from a monkey's kidneys, chicken embryos, rabbit kidneys or aborted foetal tissue, usually with the addition of foetal bovine serum. But obtaining materials from these sources is expensive, and in terms of the enormous numbers of vaccines made, monkeys and so on would soon be extinct. So the laboratory technicians have devised a way of *continuous cloning* to repeat these cells endlessly. One could say that they are therefore cancerous cells. But these cloned cells are thought to be safe until about the 38th usage, when they are supposed to be destroyed as they *then* become potentially carcinogenic. We have no guarantee, in the face of the costs of these procedures and the animals involved, that they *are* always destroyed at that stage or that it *is* at the 38th stage and not at, say, the 32nd stage that these cells become carcinogenic.

In addition, a growth factor must be used. Moreover, these are proteins foreign to the human body coming from an entirely different species. Since animal organs have been transplanted into humans, at least one new monkey virus has been detected. A virus from another species is particularly alarming because while that animal may be able to live with it, we may not, just as many native populations paid a heavy price with their lives from the 'new' diseases regarded as mere nuisances by the Europeans who brought them.

Perhaps the greatest concern of all is that in using live viruses in mass immunization campaigns we are practising biological engineering on an enormous scale,[52] for viral elements have a capacity to attach their own genetic material to that of the host cell. The host cell may then produce subtly abnormal proteins from the viral genetic code. On this subject, Dr Harold E Buttram MD, co-author with John Chriss Hoffman PhD of *Vaccinations and Immune Malfunctions*,[53] declares: 'From a large body of scientific literature, examples are readily available of the action of viruses in bringing about genetic changes in infected cells.'[54] 'Being made up of purely genetic material, they are highly susceptible to genetic change, a process referred to as 'jumping genes.'[55] 'Just as flies readily become carriers of disease, it would appear that viruses readily become agents for the transfer of genetic elements from one host to another. This foreign genetic material, in turn, may incite autoimmune disease, with the body's immune system attacking cells containing this foreign genetic material.' Dr Buttram concludes: 'Currently mandated childhood vaccine programs may be sewing the seeds of adverse genetic changes.'[56]

In the preparation of vaccines, in addition to the bacterial or viral mixture there are also adjuvants or diluents in which to culture bacteria and viruses. Some immunologists are concerned that these adjuvants may be toxic to the body, and possibly carcinogenic. These produce a generalized inflammatory reaction ranging from mild to severe. Among these adjuvants may be mercury, aluminium, thiomersal and formaldehyde.[57]

At immunization time this mixture of foreign material is injected directly into the body – that is, it bypasses the body's natural defence system: the mouth, the skin, the mucous membranes and the liver. (Except for the oral polio vaccine). On receiving this noxious mixture, the body, believing its defences have failed, is forced to produce blood antibodies.

Dr Trevor Gunn:

A vaccine tricks the body into thinking that the first lines of defence have been breached. Therefore the body no longer initiates a generalized inflammatory response, and is often forced to produce blood antibodies. But in addition, there is a drop in the immune system cells after the immunization. This can lead to an increased susceptibility to other diseases. There is no reason to believe this does not occur with all diseases.[58]

It has in fact been amply demonstrated that after immunization there is a significant if temporary drop in the immune system's T-lymphocytes. This is a direct blow to the immune system, our defence against all comers.[59]

Once one realizes what is actually in these vaccines there is something quite appalling about the idea of injecting a mixture of substances made up of bacteria or viruses foreign to the body, cultured on animal tissues with calf blood, possibly cancerous cells, and contained in a toxic and possibly carcinogenic solvent, into a helpless, unknowing infant whose brain, nervous system and immune systems are immature.

Also, in 'third world' countries where there is malnutrition and starvation, far from 'saving millions' the multi-billion dollar immunization industry contributes to the horrendous death rates in those places, just as it does among the Australian aboriginals. The donated money for these vaccines would be better spent on decent food and water; and/or self-reliance programmes designed by the people in the area for the benefit of their own.

Today we know a great deal more about the human immune system than we did when immunization was first so enthusiastically embraced, along with a rush to manufacture drugs, as the ideal ways to a nirvana of perfect health and multiple billions of profits. It is time that governments acted upon the newer knowledge.

It should be quite clear by now that the short-term effects of immunization, the adverse effects and the deaths; the medium-term effects of increased risk of autoimmune and other diseases, are quite worrying enough. Then, as mentioned, there is the longer-term possibility of immune suppression and even alterations to our genetic coding.

Neil Z Miller is another who has written on the subject. In his 1992 book *Vaccines: Are They Really Safe and Effective?* he says: 'There is an obvious effort to suppress negative findings, and as with fluoridation, children are the guinea pigs.

The long-term effects for our species are ominous.'

Julian Cribb of the Australian National Science Agency, author of *The White Death* (1996), another book on the subject of immunization, warned that the real danger in such vaccines as the polio vaccine lies in those diseases which take a while to emerge: AIDS, Creutzfeldt Jacob Disease and many others. For the worst possibility is that certain vaccines may set one up for AIDS or other immune system dysfunctions. The possible role of the polio vaccine (grown on media contaminated with Simian AIDS-like viruses) in the antecedents to AIDS is looked at in the chapter on AIDS. And the possible role of multiple vaccines in Gulf War Syndrome is looked at in the chapter on 20th-century illnesses.

I have long been of the opinion that the modern epidemic of immune system dysfunction as manifest in such diseases as AIDS, ME, CFIDS, EI, Total Allergy, MCS, etc. (diseases of a thousand names and millions of victims) are generally multi-factorial in causation, in susceptible people, mainly due to an overload of toxicity our immune systems were not designed to handle. And having looked at these writings and research on immunization, it looks as if immunization could play a part for some in the development of these diseases.

Even influenza vaccines have for some been disastrous. The US Government (that is, the tax payer) faces legal claims for billions of dollars because so far in the US there have been 1,100 cases of Guillain-Barre paralysis, and 58 deaths following swine flu vaccines.[60]

US Department of Justice files for August 1982, six years after the mass immunization campaign, indicated that 1,571 lawsuits had been filed by individuals claiming to have suffered serious side-effects from the Swine Flu Vaccine. Of those cases:

290 closed with a Federal Government payout of $57 million; 693 cases are still pending with amounts adding up to $1,027 billion involved; while 588 lawsuits were dismissed.[61]

The concept of immunization stems from an understandable desire to control natural processes and to save lives; also, on the part of the manufacturers, to make a pile of money. But it may prove to be a disaster for the human race. The great observer of humanity and health, René Dubos, warned us that if we tried too strenuously to control nature, nature would strike back. Or to put it grossly, 'There's no such thing as a free lunch.' Sometimes we get a short-term gain, only for a long-term loss. For example with malaria: the administration of quinine worked wonders for a time, but it also produced the drug-resistant, far more lethal form of malaria now sweeping the globe. (By 1975 the incidence of malaria worldwide had increased to 2.5 times what it had been in 1961.[62])

It is salutary to recall that we live in a microsoup of life, where the balance is crucial. And that the world of microbes can evolve a thousand times more rapidly than we can.

Erwin Alber of the Vaccination Information Network, New Zealand, says:

It is easy to forget that on the one hand, vaccines – stripped of their 'mystique' and the hype surrounding them – are simply a product someone wants to sell, much like soap, cigarettes ... while on the other, injecting the vaccines into a child is a medical intervention which carries considerable short- and long-term risks.

Hilary Butler, Researcher for the NZ Immunisation Awareness Society, insists that at the very least parents should demand the right to read the information from the manufacturer which comes with the vaccines, before they decide if they will accept the risks. As with the mercury amalgam tags, this is a 'truth-telling statement' which is required by law, also there to protect the vaccine manufacturer from any possible law suits. *(Well, we did warn you.)* The problem is that parents are not given these to read, and when they ask are often shamed for doing so with such phrases as, 'We wouldn't do anything that was unsafe.'

But here are the 'truth-telling' adverse reactions listed on a 1986 Connaught Laboratories vaccination product package insert:

Adverse reactions which may be local and include pain, erythema, heat, edema, and induration ... are common ... Some data suggest that febrile reactions are more likely to occur in those who have experienced such responses after prior doses ... Sterile abscesses at the site of injection have been reported ... Mild systemic reactions, such as fever, drowsiness, fretfulness, and anorexia occur quite frequently ... Rash, allergic reactions, and respiratory difficulties, including apnoea (breath holding), have been observed. Moderate to severe systemic events, such as fever of 40.5C (105F) or higher, persistent, inconsolable crying lasting three hours or more, unusual high-pitched screaming, collapse, or convulsions occur relatively infrequently. More severe neurologic complications, such as prolonged convulsions or an encephalopathy, occasionally fatal, have been reported ... Rarely, an anaphylactic reaction (i.e. hives, swelling of the mouth, difficulty breathing hypotension or shock) has been reported ... Sudden infant death syndrome (SIDS) has occurred in infants following administration of DPT ... Onset of infantile spasms has occurred in infants who have recently received DPT or DT.

Manufacturers thus have to 'tell the truth' in order to protect their millions in profits against possible lawsuits. But why is this truth so carefully hidden from us?

Immunization theory involves injecting disease into a hopefully healthy body. Many are beginning to question whether it is necessary 'to make ourselves sick in order to avoid sickness'.[63] It is my hope that before total health and environmental disaster strikes we will all become aware that the key to resisting disease is to strengthen the immune system.

Hilary Butler:

The medical profession maintains that immunizations 'strengthen' the immune system. I disagree. I hope that the strategy of the future, in determining a child's susceptibility to disease will not only involve resolving factors of nutrition, but also sanitation, housing, exposure to various environmental hazards, and possibly the level of tension in the family home.

I am totally in agreement with Hilary Butler on all points. For whereas in the past there was a link between poor sanitation and the dreaded diseases smallpox, typhoid and diphtheria, today the greater hazards appears to lie more nearly in the devitalized foods we eat and the many other environmental hazards we have looked at in this book.

And no child, constantly under severe stress, can grow up healthy.

Dr Robert Mendelsohn, in the *People's Doctor* (vol 4, no 5) said this:

I will continue to advise mothers ... to carefully study the known risks of immunization: arthritis from German Measles shots; encephalitis from measles shots; Sudden Infant Death following DPT immunizations, convulsions from whooping cough vaccine, and a host of others.

Mothers should also be aware of the documented failure over the past decade of diphtheria shots to protect children exposed to diphtheria epidemics, and they should know that Dr Jonas Salk has said that ⅔ of polio cases during this decade have been caused by the vaccine itself.

Daniel A Lander DC says this, 'The promotion of health is the only effective way to deal with any health problem.'

Irene Alleger, editor of the *Townsend Letter*:[64]

Our species will not long survive in an increasingly hostile environment, without an active immune system. Nor will we flourish as a nation producing neurologically damaged children. The proponents of vaccination consistently misrepresent the efficacy of vaccines, and the result of trials of vaccines, which show disastrous effects, especially in infants. One might wonder why there has been such a concerted effort in the past 10 years for mass inoculations of children now starting at two months of age and continuing through adolescence, when even a cursory reading of the literature indicates a lack of efficacy and such serious consequences.

Parents have been the victims of scare tactics and government bureaucrats who believe what they are told by the medical establishment.

Dr Kris Glaublomme, editor of *International Vaccination Newsletter*, calls for the following measures to be taken:

1 a guarantee of freedom of choice for parents
2 improvement in the information given to parents, complete and objective
3 a fair compensation in the event of vaccine damage
4 an ongoing compulsory monitoring system to examine the long-term effects
5 the exploration of alternatives to vaccinations
6 a system to deal with the secondary effects of vaccination.

Dr Edward Kasse MD, addressing the Convention of Vienna on Infectious Diseases in 1983, spoke as President of the Convention:

The goal of epidemiologists should not be the eradication of infectious diseases via the massive use of vaccines and antibiotics, but rather through the control and improvement of the quality of life. One must admit that there exists a certain number of cases of tuberculosis, polio or malaria and enter into a natural, ecological dynamic in making more effective the possibility of our body's defences, thanks to a health policy that is not contaminated by the interests of pharmaceutical multinationals.[65]

Jean Rostend: 'The obligation to endure gives us the right to know.'
    Perhaps we should give the penultimate word to Dr Robert Mendelsohn:

There has never been a single vaccine in this country that has ever been submitted to a controlled scientific study. They never took a group of 100 people who were candidates for a vaccine, gave 50 of them a vaccine and left the other 50 alone to measure the outcome. And since that has never been done, that means if you want to be kind, you will call vaccines an unproven remedy. If you want to be accurate, you'll call people who give vaccines quacks.

It seems to me that there is quite enough evidence for people to insist that the whole process of immunization be reviewed immediately. The enormous number of books published on the subject in the last decade, many mentioned in this chapter, provide ample support for this view.

    But at the very least, in the light of the foregoing experience and research cited it would seem that no country with any pretensions to 'freedom and democracy' should ride roughshod over their people's right to know the truth about immunization, and to make their own decisions as to whether their children, or they themselves, should be vaccinated. In fact even if it could be proved that vaccines were 'safe and effective' (it cannot), history should tell us that the right to dissent, particularly when lives are at stake, is among the most precious we have had, or have not had, down through the ages. Untold millions have died for that right. And it is as important today as it has ever been.

⚠

18: UNLEADED PETROL

'Unleaded petrol is better for us,
and for the environment.'

Yes indeed, leaded petrol was a menace. In 1974 Dr Henry Schroeder MD, Professor of Physics at Indiana University, wrote a trail-blazing book, *The Poisons Around Us*.[1] One of his main concerns was the effect of lead on the health of humans. In fact, he believed we were all suffering from lead poisoning, just as did the Roman aristocracy.

Professor Schroeder warned that lead was being extruded into the environment from the tailpipes of our motor vehicles at a yearly rate of about 2 kilograms (4.4 lb) per car. But the powerful petrochemical industry, the lead-based paint industries and others resisted any restrictions, and were able to do so, having strong representation on any boards or committees which could affect their freedom to pollute us all to death.[2]

From a combination of lead-based house paint, which tastes sweetish to children so they enjoy it and eat it, and leaded dust in the air (as high as 6.8% in some cities) settling on the streets and breathed in by children playing in the area, there were annually nearly 2,500 cases of lead poisoning in New York City alone. At the least it can cause mental retardation and cerebral palsy. Schroeder says this brain damage is permanent. At worst it can kill. And thus lead poisoning was declared a medical emergency.

And no wonder. Mice and rats fed lead for life in concentrations reproducing the levels in the tissues of humans showed a susceptibility to infections, loss of weight, hardening of the arteries, heart attacks, visible ageing and early mortality. When breeding rats were exposed to the same concentrations, the strain was dead in two generations, as were the Romans when they imbibed too much lead.[3] Only the Roman upper classes could afford the lead piping, lead plates and goblets, the lead wine storage containers and so on. (They even sprinkled lead in their wine to improve the taste.) The result was sterility, abortions, stillbirths and the end of the aristocracy. We may in part blame lead in our environment for the modern lowering of fertility and the flourishing of fertility clinics. But there are other candidates also, as we have noted.

When the results of all this research was out, Sweden began phasing out the lead from petrol. It took a little longer in the English-speaking countries.

So, all of us, especially our children, have, whether we realize it or not, been suffering from the effects of lead in our atmosphere. And now may we rejoice that it is at last out of the petrol?

Alas! I here reproduce a report by a Dr Maddock, just as I found it in the brilliant Seattle, Washington, *Well Mind Association Newsletter* for February 1997:

REPORT ON UNLEADED EXHAUST-PIPE EMISSIONS: LINKED TO LEUKEMIA

The aromatics spewed out by the exhaust pipe of a car with a catalytic converter burning unleaded fuel are far worse than the lead formerly emitted.

More than half of a litre of unleaded fuel is not petrol. It is actually a brew of aromatics and ... it could not be more evil. The aromatics that replace lead are dimethyl-benzine, mesitylene, toluene, xylene and benzine. All these are declared carcinogens and will cause leukemia and other cancer-related illnesses. Note that I have said will, not might.

'Not surprisingly,' Dr Maddock, our reporter, added, 'I have just read that in Sweden they have found unexpectedly high levels of leukemia in petrol station workers.' He cautions not to spill any of the fuel on your skin, as the aromatics absorb into your body through the pores of the skin.[4]

Anyone for an electric car?

And while on the subject of transport, the very least a 'civilized' country could do is to put in place a system of checking for polluting emissions when the car is inspected for safety. Sometimes it's just a question of fine-tuning the motor to correct spewing exhaust systems; at others the exhaust system or parts of it, must be replaced.

To ignore this question is to do neither personal health, nor the health of the planet any good.

19: ELECTROMAGNETIC FIELDS

'It's OK to graze around in those EM fields.'

When we drive along under high-tension power lines the radio will sometimes go mad with static, causing us to feel a minor annoyance at the break in our listening. But that isn't all that's happening. We ourselves are being exposed to the same influence as the radio. That is, we're being exposed to an electromagnetic field. And there are also the ones emanating from the car itself, from its own electrical systems.

Electromagnetic fields, known as EMFs for short, come into existence when electrical currents pass along wires and into appliances. As such we are surrounded by them.

All household appliances – computers, printers, cellphones, mobile phones, cordless phones, microwave ovens, electric clocks, electric blankets, water beds, lights, extension cords, plumbing currents, cell sites and so on – create fields. Some of them have these fields even when turned off. It is also important to remember that the wires we cannot see, such as those inside the walls of our houses, also create these fields.

This 'surrounding' by EMFs occurs both at home and in the workplace; and useful as they are, unfortunately there is a health price to pay. As we are electrical creatures as well as biochemical creatures, they may interfere with the electrical rhythms in our cells. Many of us have heard about the adverse relationship between heavy duty overhead power lines and people's health. But long-term exposure to household EMFs can also produce subtle changes in living cells.

EM Fields can cause headaches, insomnia, irritability and affect our mental stability because they may influence the production of our neurotransmitters (the electrical messengers in our brains). They can also weaken the immune system, and can cause an increase in miscarriages and birth defects.[1] Researchers believe that exposure to these fields can, over time lead to 'cellular proliferation' – that is, to cancer. Children are particularly susceptible.

It is extremely important to ensure that our bedrooms are as free as possible of EMFs, as we can spend one third of our lives in that room. Many of us know that children should not sit too close to a television set, but it is far worse to position a child's bed against a wall when there is the back of a television set on the other side of that wall. EMFs do not recognize walls (unless perhaps they are concrete blocks). Like ghosts, they just go right through them.

(Incidentally, we must not put our children to sleep in beds made of particle board and other dubious materials. For they are then breathing in all night the outgassing toxic glue or the formaldehyde used in cementing together these particles.)

These EM fields are measured in terms of milligauss of radiation. For example, a study conducted by the Karlinska Institute in Stockholm found that children exposed to 1 milligauss of radiation over long periods have twice the normal risk of developing cancer. Those exposed to 2 milligauss had three times the normal risk, and those exposed to 3 milligauss had four times the normal risk.[2]

'Of thirty-five international research studies on EMR (eletromagnetic radiation), thirty-three made a conclusive link between brain tumours, leukemia, and other forms of cancer, and electromagnetic radiation exposure.'[3]

But it isn't always cancer that is the first warning. To take one individual case: a New York couple lived high up in Manhattan's fashionable and very expensive Upper West Side. 'They began to feel ill when they spent time at home and felt better whenever they were out of the apartment.' Headaches, malaise, leg cramps and poor sleep caused them to have their apartment tested for EMR, after they'd seen a television programme on the subject.

One milligauss is the proposed standard set by the US Environmental Protection Agency; but Russian researchers (who have been testing these fields for many decades more than the rest of the world) have arrived at a much more stringent standard; $\frac{1}{1,000}$ of a milligauss is their safety standard. The New York couple made ill by their apartment found that it tested 6–22 milligauss. The reason was that the building's transformer was right next to their apartment. And so they moved, and presumably lived happily ever after.[4] (The article does not say what happened to the people who moved in next.)

Individual susceptibility will vary considerably. People with environmental illness, who are sensitive to chemicals in the environment, will also be more sensitive to these fields. Even weak electric fields can affect us. As for me, I'm saving up for one of those expensive new slim-line monitors with very little radiation. Then I'll be able to write books without all the anguish this one has cost me.

There are studies to establish that

pregnancies among couples exposed to the magnetic field generated by electric blankets and electrically heated water-beds appeared more likely to end in miscarriages, and foetuses conceived in electrically heated beds had a slightly slower growth rate than other foetuses. Other studies have found that frequent users of electric blankets had slightly increased risks of breast cancer.[5]

Then there is the worry about brain tumours. Apparently mobile phones tend to 'microwave' the nearby brain, which in fact could contribute to these. The *Medical Journal of Australia* recently featured a letter from a Dr Andrew Davidson concerned that the incidence of brain tumours has increased from 6.4 cases per 100,000 in males and 4.0 cases per 100,000 females in 1982 to 9.6 and 6.5 in the 1990s. He believes it could be 'related to the use of analogue mobile phones in the late 1980s'.[6]

Dr Neil Cherry, lecturer at Lincoln University, believes that EM radiation 'could well explain why cancer rates in New Zealand are rising, because this is one of the few potential carcinogens that we know is rising and everybody is exposed to it'.[7] In Europe one can now buy a low-radiation phone; while in the UK it is possible to buy covers which reduce radiation emissions.

Peter Sierck, another expert in this field, says that 'unfortunately wiring in compliance with national and local electrical codes does not necessarily mean low EMFs, sometimes quite the opposite.'[8] But the fields, and hence the risks, can be reduced with competent advice and treatment. The trick is to find it.

As Michael Riversong warns, 'Be very cautious of anyone who claims to be able to solve or neutralize all your electromagnetic problems. Since these fields are complex and invisible, there is plenty of opportunity for fraud.'[9]

EMERGENCY ADVICE

There is a device known as a Demand Switch that can be inserted in our electrical intake board which will contain the electricity there until we switch it on elsewhere in the house. There is then a four-second delay before the electricity reaches the point where we need it. This is in fact the only way we can sleep without a field around our heads, unless we position the bed against a wall where there is no wiring.

(There is one other thing one can do. We asked the electrician to give us a switch in the bedroom to turn off all the power in the house except for the refrigerator. This should not cost as much as a Demand Switch, but works like one.)

Electric clocks and so on should be placed on the opposite side of the room from the bed. Electric blankets should at the most be used only to warm the bed before we get into it, and should be switched off at the wall, not at the appliance. I use old-fashioned hot water bottles in preference.

⚠

20: MOBILE PHONES

'A cell phone can save your life.'

Sure it can. It's great to be able to dial up for help in an emergency.

But on the down side, recent studies in New Zealand indicate that cell phone in-car users have three times the injuries and twice the fatalities of those who do not use them.[1] In the US it's been found that people who talk on cell phones while driving have five times the risk of having a traffic accident than others: 'the more the phone is used in the car, the greater the risk of an accident.'[2]

The New Zealand studies found that it is even more risky to look for a missing object while driving; to reach to pick it up or to drop something and pick it up; or to alter the radio, cassette or stereo. Eating and drinking while driving may also be hazardous.[3]

For possible effects on the brain, see page 146 of Chapter 19.

The problem of cell phone danger while driving is somewhat lessened by the technology that does not involve holding an object to one's ear. But all the same it's a distraction at a time when one needs every ounce of concentration on the dangerous task at hand. Better pull over.

PS Are cell phones fattening? According to Dr Andrew Prentice of the Medical Research Council Dunn Clinical Nutrition Centre in Britain, they are. Because they can rob us of 16 kilometres worth of exercise per year. And when you add on all the other walking-saving devices like remote controls, Dr Prentice believes it can account for the increase in the numbers of overweight people.[4]

Yes, well, as we all know, just about everything we like used to be 'illegal, immoral or fattening'. Now we have to add the word 'dangerous'.

⚠

21: PESTICIDES

'A little spray won't hurt! Besides, we just
excrete all the "nasties", don't we?'

I like the story about the American couple who went to visit Oxford University. On encountering one of the gardeners, the husband asked, 'What d'you *use* on these lawns? How d'you get 'em looking like this? Never seen a lawn like it.'

Whereupon the Oxford gardener replied, touching his cap, 'Well sir. You just mow it every Tuesday morning for 400 years.'

He probably wasn't telling the whole truth, but it's likely their gardening methods haven't changed much since they began with that lawn. For centuries people grew their own foods, and often supplied others' food needs, by means of 'organic' methods. Moreover, there were no such things as 'sprays' until the second half of the 20th century. But people usually got fed, and fed much better. For the soils were used with care.

As Rachel Carson wrote in 1962,

Soil is in part a creation of life, born of a marvelous interaction of life and non-life long aeons ago ... life is not only formed in the soil, but other living things of incredible abundance and diversity now exist within it; if this were not so the soil would be a dead and sterile thing.[1]

It is the presence of those myriad organisms of the soil which creates and recreates it.

As Charles Darwin described for us over 100 years ago, it is the common earthworm which makes our soils possible, along with a few thousand other creatures. But when we fail to feed the soil with life-creating organic matter or we poison it, we starve or poison those inhabitants. And thus for centuries gardeners co-operated with that life in the soil. They returned nutrients to the earth and rotated the crops.

But in this second half of the 20th century was begun the practice of using manufactured 'fertilizers', which for the most part cannot truly fertilize because they are composed of highly-heated and 'dead' substances. Food grown on dead 'fertilized' soils compared with those grown on live, composted soils may look similar. But analyses reveal substantial differences in nutrients. There will also be differences that cannot as yet be measured, and all these differences will in the long run count in our overall health. For we cannot extract from our soils what is not there. Minerals, for one, are – like certain fatty acids – 'essential to life'. Without them our brains and nervous systems cannot function well. Without them we sicken and die 'before our time'.

And secondly in the 20th century, after the easy way out, the 'fertilization', began the bombing or blitzing with poisons of the unwanted wildlife and plants we called nuisances and weeds. This approach mirrored the war-like approach to life fostered by the war that had just been fought and the evolving faulty medical paradigm (the view of health and reality), the idea that a healthy body is 'invaded and becomes ill', which we will look at later.

It all seemed so 'modern' so 'scientific', so very clever, to create an array of poisons, one for every possible need. And when we consider that the discoverer of DDT (now banned in most places because it is so dangerous) was given a Nobel Prize, we get some idea of the stupendous arrogance and ignorance of the time. And we still live in that time. The idea that one can simply blitz nature into submission, that we do not have to work with her, is an arrogance peculiar to the 20th century, and is a 'side-effect' of our expertise in devising ever more effective ways both of killing and controlling each other.

For all these poisons had to do at the start was pass the test of, 'Does it kill well? Does it do the job?' None of them had to pass the test of 'Is it safe for people and other forms of life? The forms that we *do* want?' or 'What happens if it gets into the water supply?' These things were not worried about except by the occasional genius like Rachel Carson.[2] This was a gigantic oversight because we are all of us, the plants, the birds, the animals, linked in a 'great chain of being'. And if we poison one part of the chain, that poison will affect the entire rest of the chain. The Minamata disease, or mercury poisoning that we saw in Chapter 6 on amalgam fillings, was discovered when humans ate fish that had earlier eaten the mercury. The mercury stayed stored in the fish and accumulated over time. The bigger the fish, the more toxic it was. It is still the case.

By the time Rachel Carson wrote her shattering defence on behalf of the planet in 1962 there were already pesticide residues found in everything from the fish in the remotest mountain lakes to the earth worms burrowing deep in our soils, to mothers' milk. Because as she said, 'It is not possible to add pesticides to water *anywhere* without threatening the purity of water *everywhere*,'[3] a statement which has been echoed in our time by Professor W William Hughes: 'We may unknowingly breathe air, drink water, or eat food that was polluted with toxicants hundreds or thousands of miles away.'[4]

If, as it is said, every single dollar note in the US contains traces of cocaine, is it unreasonable to wonder how many other toxins are permeating our lives through travelling vast distances?

And if we consider the effects of these poisons on humans: yes, there may be a few hardy souls who seem to be able to use these sprays over a lifetime without protective gear and stay fit. And they're likely to pour scorn on those who say they're made ill by them. But on the other hand, many who do it for a living are forced to give it up and retire to take care of their acquired inferior health for a remaining shortened life.

It all boils down to our uniqueness, our biochemical individuality. Most of us were not designed to cope with anything like the level of toxicity in our environment today; 10% of the population, according to some doctors.[5] Certainly, when 'the design' was made up a bout of spray was never envisaged, because nothing like it existed. So whether or not one copes with sprays and other poisons or not has to do with the state of one's liver, and the strength of the individual immune system. Surveys reveal that people working with herbicides suffer a ninefold excess of cancer.[6] Other studies reveal that there are significant levels of DDT in the breastmilk of most American nursing mothers, especially if they are meat-eaters.[7] This will be true in most of the West.

But the problem can occur even earlier. According to researchers from the US Environmental Protection Agency, and the University of Minnesota, there is a relationship between pesticide exposure and birth defects. The Minnesota birth registry for 1989 to 1992 was surveyed, and rates of birth defects among those people certified to apply restricted use of pesticides on their land were compared with those for the state's population as a whole. It was found that 'Pesticide appliers had significantly more children with birth anomalies than did nonappliers.' Further studies resulted in the conclusion that 'families residing in predominantly agricultural regions of Minnesota are more likely to have children with birth anomalies.'[8]

Other studies have found not only more birth defects, but also lower percentages of males born in groups exposed to pesticides.

In Sevesto, Italy, in 1976, a group of people were heavily exposed to dioxin after an explosion at a pesticide factory. Dioxin is a potent poison ... Between April 1977 and December 1984, 74 children were born to parents in the zone of greatest dioxin exposure. Of these,

48 were female and 26 male, for a male proportion of 0.351. After 1985, the male proportion of live births began to return to normal.[9]

We also looked at this phenomenon in Chapter 6 on plastic. The male of the species is apparently more fragile, at least in the early foetal stages.

And from the New Zealand Toxins Awareness Group,[10]

A study from the University of North Carolina found that children who played in gardens sprayed with pesticides were about four times more likely to contract certain types of cancer than those whose gardens were not sprayed. Children from homes that used insecticide strips were twice as much at risk of developing leukaemia, and three times as much if their mothers were exposed to them during the last three months of pregnancy.

In the latest *New Zealand Toxins Awareness Group Newsletter* is a report on findings from the US Environmental Research Foundation:

Neither government nor the chemical corporations have seen it as their job to discover whether chemicals are harming children. Nevertheless, several studies have shown a link between childhood cancers and pesticides. Childhood leukaemias, lymphomas, neuroblastomas and brain cancers have all been linked to pesticides in recent years.[11]

Another favourite story of mine is the one about the Professor of Medicine from a well-known New England university, who learned a great deal one summer. He started applying a tick powder daily to his male cat, which was apparently having trouble with ticks. Within 10 days after he began this, he noted large numbers of dead or injured mice and birds lying on his formerly pristine front lawn. In addition to these efforts, the cat also brought birds and mice into the house where he viciously attacked them, 'red in tooth and claw'. All this was quite bewildering to the good professor, because up till that period his pet had been quite well-behaved and docile. The doting professor even went so far as to say heart-brokenly, 'My cat has become a murderer.'

But even as he said this there were personality changes going on in himself, for although he wore gloves during applications of the tick powder he often breathed in the dust as it escaped into the air.

Soon the professor's partner became alarmed by his increasing aggressiveness and 'continual rage'. And soon she left, for fear of almost certain physical attack from him. And it was about then that 'the penny dropped' for both the professor and his partner. They realized that the tick powder might have been the cause of these personality changes and it was stopped. Within one week, aggressive behaviour ceased in both cat and professor.[12]

This is, happily, a brief and humorous story. But let us suppose that the people in this story were not a 'learned professor' and his companion. And that they did not guess what was going on. The cat owner may have got into a routine, and may have continued to use the tick powder as before. There is then the possibility of the aggressive behaviour continuing to the point where a relationship is ruined, a job is lost, lives are irretrievably changed for the worse. And so on.

And if the cat became murderous on tick powder, is it not within the bounds of reason that the cat *owner* could also eventually commit murder? That he might develop a resentment against his former lover? For the ingredient in tick powder which does the damage is a cholinesterase inhibitor, which leads to a powerful overstimulation of the nerve endings, and hence aggression.

The idea that one could possibly kill with something so dangerous, and remain unaffected oneself, will truly be one of the many horrors future generations, if there are to be any, will surely look back on with amazement.

Our brains are sensitive. Our brains are vulnerable. They need to be watched over. It is not just the sprays and the powders. It's a plethora of other poisons in our lives also. And when people become ill from them, for reasons we will be looking at later in the book, there is seldom any understanding in medicine as to the causes and treatments for the condition. When people's poisoned brains react like that of the professor's cat, they will be called 'crazy' or 'hysterical' because in fact they are. And they will then be turned over to the mental health system because it is not recognized by many that these mental symptoms can follow toxic exposure. And of course they will not get the appropriate treatment, which is to get rid of the toxicity which might restore the victim to normal. Nor is there sensible treatment for those who become physically ill from them. (See Chapter 33 on 20th-century illnesses.)

There are particularly dangerous chemicals used to get rid of head lice in children. Some allege that one in particular may be the cause of nerve damage, seizures, comas and convulsions.[13]

Today, there are numerous ways we are taking in poisons: According to the *Self Help Cancer Cure Book*,[14] of particular concern are pesticides widely used in New Zealand on food products: pirimiphos-methyl and fenitrothion, both of which show up strongly in wheat (that is, in flour), apples and celery. Bran flakes and whole-meal bread showed the highest residues: 1.4 parts per million (ppm) and 16 ppm respectively. After reading this I understand why I react so severely to the bread many of us consider 'the best' and one of the most expensive. On the basis of figures like these and extrapolating from US figures, the New Zealand journal *Soil and Health* estimates 3,176 cancers per year in New Zealand (in 3.9 million people) probably induced by such poisons in our diet, '... some solid reasons for New Zealand's record-holding status in bowel cancer, breast cancer and childhood leukaemias'.

Other creatures can be affected: Dr Victor Penzer MD, DMD, FASCD, warns that family pets have been permanently blinded when exposed to pesticides at ground level.[15] And it is not just agriculture that uses poisons. Chemicals in medicine and industry also have undoubtedly speeded up the process of the poisoning of our world.

There is difficulty finding honest studies attesting to the safety of the poisons now so widely used in our daily lives, simply because one cannot deliberately expose people to them. But we know from the results with people *inadvertently* exposed that they can in some cases cause a lifetime of ill-health. There are also the survivors of the Vietnam War exposed to Agent Orange, a powerful herbicide, some of whom have struggled for years for recognition and compensation for their ruined health, their ruined lives. More on this in Chapter 33.

The worst of it is that one can be exposed to a poisonous spray entirely without one's knowledge. Many of them are like electromagnetic fields in that you cannot see them, smell them, touch them or know they are there. Someone sprays in a field some distance away. Then a wind can pick up a handful of the molecules and fling them right at you. You don't even know 'what hit you', or even that you've been hit. You may just gradually develop signs of illness, of immune system failure, depending on the dose you received and the response your immune system is able to mount, the ability of your liver to get rid of it. All you may know is that you have become ill in a way you never have before.

Anyone can in this way assault you. Your neighbour quietly spraying his roses, with or without a protective mask on, through the agency of a slight breeze, may also be spraying right into your house, with neither of you being aware of it.

The number of reported poisonings from sprays in the US is about 67,000 per year, which is thought to be about 73% of the actual numbers.[16] Herbicides and pesticides can damage the nervous system and the endocrine systems. But there is emerging evidence that it is the immune system, our defence system against infections and cancer, which is most affected. In the US it is calculated there are about 10,000 cases of cancer per year caused by these poisons.[17] Then there are all the other illnesses. The total damage to our health is virtually incalculable.

Thus after nearly 50 years of use, there is now plenty of experience and evidence as to what poisonous sprays and other things can do to us.

The most recent book I have come across, *Pesticides and the Immune System: The Public Health Risks*[18], has an Advisory Panel of distinguished scientists in the field. I will list them, so that the reader will know from what level are the statements to come:

Dr Michael Lister PhD, Head, Environmental Immunology and Neurobiology Section, National Institute of Environmental Health Sciences; National Institutes of Health; and Chief, Toxicology and Molecular Biology Branch, National Institute for Occupational Safety and Health; National Institutes of Health.

Dr Donald Kennedy PhD, Bing Professor of Environmental Sciences; Institute for International Studies; Professor Emeritus, Stanford University.

Dr Edward M B Smith FFOM, RCP, Medical Officer Assessment of Risk and Methodologies; International Programme on Chemical Safety (IPCS); World Health Organization.

Dr Norbert Hirschorn MD, Director, Family Health Division, Minnesota Department of Health.

The following are a few of the statements emerging from this book:

Although many pesticides have been reviewed for a range of acute and chronic toxicities, including possible risks of cancer and birth defects, they have not been reviewed in regulatory proceedings for potential toxicity to the immune system.[19]

Hundreds of millions of people are exposed significantly to pesticides each year.[20]

Roughly 85–90% of pesticides applied agriculturally, never reach target organisms, but disperse through the air, soil and water.[21]

Many organic and metal-based pesticides can also pass from mother to unborn child through the placenta, potentially leading to birth defects, abnormal development of the immune system, and foetal death.[22]

Infants are at great risk from pesticides in breast milk because their intake relative to body weight is so high.[23]

The laboratory evidence of pesticide-induced immunotoxicity may underestimate actual risks precisely because the test animals used are typically healthy young male adults fed carefully selected and nutritious diets.[24] [That is, diets most of us do not eat.]

Studies have shown that pesticide exposure significantly reduces resistance to bacterial, viral, and parasitic infections and promotes tumour growth in many animal species.[25]

Farmers ... experience elevated risk for many of the same cancers that immuno-deficient patients develop.[26] [For example, farmers, although healthier than most on average, have significantly higher risks for Hodgkin's disease, melanoma, multiple myeloma, leukaemia (all of which are cancers of the immune system) and cancers of the lip, stomach and prostate. Against a background of lower overall health problems and cancer incidence, these elevated risks suggest the presence of an occupational risk factor.]

Epidemiologists in the former Soviet Union have long observed that T cell counts and functions are suppressed after pesticide exposure.[27]

Among occupationally exposed farmers in particular, researchers found elevated rates of infectious diseases of the following organ systems: gastrointestinal, urinary tract, the female genital tract, and respiratory tract.[28]

Worldwide, malnutrition is the most common cause of secondary immunodeficiency.[29]

Many opportunistic infections that typically appear among immunocompromised patients, such as AIDS sufferers, are also resurgent in broader populations among those who do not carry the HIV virus.[30] [This means that today many besides AIDS sufferers are getting infections that one would expect to find only in patients with severely compromised immune systems. These infections would be tuberculosis mycobacterium, streptococcus pneumonia, listeriosis, candidiasis, herpes simplex and many others. The implication is that there are factors causing it, such as the poisons in our environment, our depleted soils, and many other things.]

Multiple assaults on the immune system, spreading disease vectors, and a diminishing range of control options surely are causes for concern.[31] [In this book, in Chapter 31 on antibiotics, we will have a brief look at what is meant by that 'diminishing range of control options'.]

The authors and the Advisory Panel conclude their analysis of the dangers of pesticides and so on as follows:

The World Health Organization should take the lead in designing and organizing an appropriate program of epidemiological and other research to address this risk. The major pesticide companies also have a responsibility to ensure that the products they sell do not pose a threat to the human immune system[32] ... Regulatory agencies should substantially strengthen their surveillance and control over the use of potentially immunotoxic pesticides.[33]

The good news is that the Danish government, which has in the past banned numerous pesticides, is now considering a total pesticide ban. That is, that *all* food grown in Denmark in the future may be organically grown. Let us hope that this initiative goes through and will spread to other governments,[34] for one of the most compelling pieces of evidence that pesticides may take a killing toll on human beings stems from what has been called 'The Israeli Anomaly':

In the 1970s young women in Israel were twice as likely to die from breast cancer as women in other countries with similar diets, lifestyle and child bearing patterns. Researchers investigating this tragic anomaly concluded that the Israeli women's exposure to pesticides was the cause of the epidemic of this disease. Prior to 1978, dairy products produced in Israel contained high levels of DDT, and lindane. Tests on breastmilk showed Israeli women had many times the level of lindane in their milk than American women.

These pesticides were subsequently banned, and the breast cancer rate in young women in Israel began to fall. Between 1976 and 1986, the death rate from breast cancer among women who had not yet gone through menopause declined by 34%. Significantly, Israel is the only example of a nation experiencing a decline in the death rate from breast cancer in pre-menopausal women.[35]

The fact that pesticides can cause breast cancer was also noted in the US *Journal of the National Cancer Institute* (April, 1992), reporting on a study done by the American chemist Dr Mary Wolff of the Mount Sinai School of Medicine in New York. Her research team noted a rise in the incidence of breast cancer following increased use of DDT. Also that blood tests of women with and without breast cancer showed that those carrying the highest levels of DDT had four times the breast cancer risk of women in the lower levels; and that even though DDT has been banned in most places it is still stored in our bodies and can even be passed on in mother's milk.

In contrast to Israel and Denmark, the government of New Zealand exercises very little control over the use of pesticides. Under its 1998 Hazardous Substances and New Organisms Act, New Zealand's policies will actually be less stringent than those of many third-world countries. The NZ government guideline says this: 'The Acceptable Daily Intake (ADI) is a unique value and humans can be exposed to this level of a substance without a toxic effect occurring.' Just how can an *Acceptable Daily Intake* be determined, given the cumulative nature of these poisons? Although there is a slim chance one could establish a 'safe level' with laboratory rats, human beings vary so much in their individual abilities to detoxify and cope with poisons that it is criminal in today's context of multiple insults to the body to so legislate in favour of chemical pesticides. The effect of this new legislation will be to make it impossible for damaged individuals to sue no matter what the levels of exposure, simply because it is so difficult to establish what that level is or has been after severe illness occurs. In the light of the evidence from other countries, particularly the Israeli experience and New Zealand's extremely high level of breast cancer, it is irresponsible to allow further pesticide inroads on the people.

Above all, no one can begin to calculate the actual and total amounts of pesticides, herbicides, industrial wastes, toxic heavy metals, radioactive materials and other toxic substances simply flung into the air, water, sea and soils of this our earth in the last 50 years. As mentioned, none of these things were there when the human organism evolved.

What is surprising is not that so many are sick in new and more horrible ways and in so many greater numbers than ever before. What is surprising to me is that *anyone* can remain healthy in the environment in which we now are forced to live. According to Dr Alan Gaby, even the remaining giant turtles are dying of something very like AIDS. Less than 50% of them are left.[36]

Unfortunately, almost all of us are exposed to pesticides and other poisons in our air, food and water, and against which our bodies must struggle on a daily basis. More than 700 chemicals have been detected in American drinking water, 129 of which the US Environmental Protection Agency calls 'dangerous'. Among these are industrial solvents, metals and radioactive substances as well as pesticides.[37] We are poisoning ourselves, mentally and physically. And there is no doubt in my mind that these products are shortening our lives.

Instead of creating our own food supplies, at least of vegetables and fruits, we take the easy way, the lazy way out. Instead of getting fit by working in our gardens to produce life-bringing organically grown vegetables and fruits, we spend time in a gym expending cash and effort to 'get fit'. Our forefathers had their gardens for their gyms. We risk taking our life-bringing foods from the hands of strangers, many of them more concerned with quantity than quality, and some of whom care for nought but 'making a buck' out of us. A Tufts University study testing different foods found that those bought in supermarkets had one-quarter to one-third the nutrients of organically grown foods.

From the polluted oceans to the destruction of the rainforest (the lungs of the Earth), the megacities, the poverty and the ever-present wars, we have created such an imbalance in Nature that we may not survive the consequences. We live in a microsoup of life where the balance is critical. And it is getting more and more unbalanced.

Professor Michael Crawford, whose work we looked at in Chapter 2, also takes an interest in other aspects of our food. With David Marsh, an agriculturist with a particular interest in the history of evolution and degenerative diseases, he co-authored *The Driving Force: Food, Evolution, and the Future*. In this they said:

Food is of such a commonplace nature that it is taken for granted, and its qualitative relationship with long-term biological considerations is overlooked. The historical changes in disease patterns, the contrast in incidence from country to country, suggest that *we are witnessing a signal of the potential power of food as a dominant factor in evolution.* These findings pose serious questions as to the impact of present day food and agricultural policies on immediate and future generations.[38]

A monumental series of books on the topic 'Modern Environmental Toxicology', includes Volume 21, *Chemically-induced Alterations in Sexual and Functional Development*, which reports on the findings of a multi-disciplinary group of experts. One of the conclusions: 'Unless the environmental level of synthetic hormone disruption is abated and controlled, large-scale dysfunction of the human population level is possible'.[39]

It was 1962 when Rachel Carson first warned us about the fact that we were consuming chemical residues along with our foods, storing them in our livers and our fat. Nothing has changed since then. A few of the worst poisons have been banned. But there are still enormous quantities of many different kinds of poisons: airborne, in our water, our soils and our foods. It can take some years for this kind of poisoning to show up in people's health. But it surely does.

Rachel Carson said these poisons should not be called insecticides and pesticides but *biocides*.[40] She wrote:

Future historians may well be amazed by our distorted sense of proportion. How could intelligent beings seek to control a few unwanted species by a method that contaminated the entire environment and brought the threat of disease and death even to their own kind?

Tragically, all this was begun in the 1950s while the US taxpayer was paying *millions of dollars a year* to manage huge food surpluses held in giant silos all over the country. But perhaps the most appalling irony of the whole situation is that, whereas before the sprays were ever used farmers lost 3.5% of their crops to insects, today with the evolution of numerous pesticide-resistant strains it is now around 12%.[41]

One could in fact say that the chances are we have thus, as it says in the Book of Genesis, 'sold our birthright for a mess of pottage'.

⚠️

22: GOLF

'Golf is a great game and good for your health.'

Well actually, playing golf can give you cancer, nerve damage, heart disturbances, and your offspring birth defects. But cheer up, golfers, these threats are not from the game but from the poisons used on the greens.

A 1990 study done in Japan uncovered the fact that many golf caddies were suffering from itching eyes and skin, blurred vision, congestion, throat problems, ankle and leg rashes and headaches.

Greenkeepers also reported becoming ill during or after pesticide applications.

The report also revealed that an 18-hole golf course 'requires' three to four *tons* of pesticides annually (weed killers, insecticides and fungicides).

In Japan there have also been reports of enormous fish kills and bone deformities in the fish in rivers and streams polluted by runoff from golf courses. Bird kills have also been reported in the US. Surface and groundwater becomes toxic. In turn, wells become polluted.

So there's a price to pay for that billiard green look.

But take heart, golf players. It is possible to maintain a golf course without the use of these chemicals (after all, they must have done so for centuries). There are chemical-free golf courses in the US, including one in southern New Hampshire, the Sagamore-Hampton course. Apparently this is such a popular course that golfers have to make reservations well in advance in order to use it.

There is also one in the Squaw Valley resort area in California. And apparently there are others working towards it, such as the Pine Ridge Golf Course in Towson, Maryland, and Florida's John's Island Club. There will doubtless be many others.

If you are a golfer and object to the use of chemicals on your course, make your concerns known. And for information on how to run a pesticide-free golf course, write to HANS, #202, 5262 Rumble Street, Burnaby, British Columbia V5J 2B6, Canada, sending him US$3 plus postage to wherever you are.

(The above information reported by Arline Brecher, Alternative Medicine Connection, on the ARC website: **http://www.arxc.com**)

23: MENTAL HEALTH

'The best way to treat major mental illness
is with drugs and psychotherapy.'

The method of treating serious mental illness with powerful drugs (usually fluoride compounds) does actually bludgeon the brain into a state more acceptable to society, and sometimes even to those suffering from such illness. On the other hand, the drugs may bring such unendurable 'side-effects' or consequences, both short and long term, that some victims are unwilling to take them. They dull, but do not cure.

People on these drugs can rarely 'pass for normal'. Also, they have more than twice the mortality rates than those of the general population (although I'm told the very latest rates are better).

The largest single cause is suicide, which is 10 to 15 times higher than in the general population.[1] It is also likely that, in the long term, these powerful drugs may significantly shorten lives of themselves.

As for psychotherapy for lesser mental problems, the 'neurosis', the life-crisis, the talking therapy, one can pore over numerous studies in an attempt to find any proof of efficacy. What one does find is that people on a waiting list for such treatment usually do as well as those actually getting it.[2]

Dr Louis A Gottschalk of the University of California at Irvine has evaluated groups of applicants for crisis intervention. Half were treated, the others put on a waiting list. At the end of six weeks Gottschalk's staff re-evaluated both these groups and found improvement in the members of both groups. Moreover, those who only waited did essentially as well as those who actually received the psychotherapy. Dr Gottschalk explains this as follows: 'Most patients suffering from life crises recover spontaneously within six weeks regardless of the kind of care they receive.'[3]

Worse, there are studies which show that psychotherapy can actually be harmful, such as the valiantly well-meant Cambridge-Somerville Youth Study, an attempt to assist young 'troublemakers', 'juvenile delinquents' as they grew up. These youths were given intensive therapy for many years until they reached adulthood. At the end of the experiment, 'the statistical result unnerved the faithful'. For it was found that the group receiving the years of therapy presented with more trouble with the law, and in fact every other kind of trouble, than another similar group which had received no therapy at all. 'The unpsychologized, uncounselled boys proved to have fewer delinquent episodes than their treated peers.'[4]

And then there is Woody Allen, who seems to have required, or desired, over '33 years of continuous therapy, 21 with the same doctor'.[5] But after nearly a lifetime of psychotherapy, despite it all, Allen seems never to change. Well, he can afford it! His dog also gets therapy at US$140 per hour. So much for psychotherapy and 'neurosis'.

But to return to the question of serious mental illness: How did the current paradigm, the basic concept, ever arise? That is, that serious mental illness is like 'neurosis' only worse? The psychiatrist deals in what the 20th century quaintly calls 'the mind'. The mind is somehow 'what the brain does'. You cannot find it anywhere, even at autopsy. It somehow floats around in the brain, just as 'the soul' somehow floats around in the body, possibly in the region near the heart.

Unfortunately the concept of 'the mind' has been an almighty stumbling block in the understanding of what actually goes on in our brains, our most precious part. I believe it is better to speak more precisely of 'the brain' which is, after all, the only thing we can observe. To think of 'the brain' instead of 'the mind' is to unmuddy the waters of a very clouded issue.

We have looked at the failure on the part of dentistry to see that what happens in the mouth affects people's health all over, and caused one of the most poisonous substances on the planet to be used as a material for filling teeth, resulting in untold damage and human suffering. Similarly, the business of separating the function of the brain into a world of its own, 'the mind', has caused incalculable suffering over a century of brain-damaging electric shock treatment, lobotomy and heavy drugging; and, if patients are able to converse, the practice of incessant 'jawing' between doctor and patient.

The extraordinary thing is that this latter part of modern 'psychotherapy', the talking on the couch, goes back to a rather nondescript little man named Sigmund Freud. And the fact that this inadequate human being managed, quite unbelievably, even after death, to lay his malignant hand across the entire 20th century and to finger just about every aspect of our lives, will doubtless be a source of both amazement and amusement to the people in the future for aeons to come. The emergence of this man who afflicted every one of us in numerous ways for our entire lives is perhaps worth looking at.

Freud's beginnings were inauspicious, middle-class Viennese. He must have had a strange childhood because it left him with a peculiar obsession about his mother. He grew up to become a small-time doctor with ambition. In those days doctors did not enjoy the comparatively fabulous incomes they do today. Like most of us he longed to be rich and famous, only perhaps more so than most. His most pressing problem was that for years he could not afford to marry his fiancée Martha. And it is quite astounding to contemplate that it was that difficulty in one ambitious man which caused our entire century to go down a long and blind alleyway, a very blind alleyway indeed, which was to have tragic repercussions for millions.

From his correspondence with others written during his early period of obscurity, Freud saw himself as Moses, leading his people to some sort of promised land, only he had yet to work out how to do it and where it was. His confidence in a great future was there as early as 1885 when he was 36 and there were no signs of it. But in anticipation of ultimate fame and biography, Freud described in a letter to Martha how he had destroyed any papers that could detract from that Moses-like image he wished to project.[6]

However, by the time he was 40 he had failure staring him in the face. He was a physician in private practice specializing in 'neurosis'. And he had already failed at everything he'd tried, projects most peculiar by today's standards:

Between 1884 and 1886 Freud had experimented with cocaine. He gave it to friends, his sisters, his fiancée and took it himself. He advocated that it be used as an anaesthesia. He seemed not to realize how addictive it was. He used it for his migraine headaches, and to 'fortify' himself before social events. In a letter of June 12, 1895 he said, 'I need a lot of cocaine', being truly addicted by then.[7] We will never know how much his long-standing use of cocaine (at least 15 years, judging by his correspondence) contributed to his bizarre theories and his self-obsession. But he lost his enthusiasm for promoting it as a cure-all, if not for taking it personally, when one of his fellow doctors took his life under the influence of the cocaine Freud had pressed upon him.

Then for a time he collaborated with an imaginative ENT (Ear, Nose and Throat) specialist, who believed that 'masturbation, coitus interruptus and the use of condoms caused damage to the nervous system and also to the tissues in the nose.'[8] 'Neurosis' could be cured by operating on the nose. In a text book published in 1893 Fleiss described 131 cases of 'neurosis' treated with cocaine and cauterization in the nose.[9] Freud believed all this implicitly, and even had his own nose operated on. It was also a nose that needed frequent applications of cocaine. Apparently there were 'genital' spots in the nose, and by applying cocaine and cauterizing them electrically one could be cured of sexual neurosis. Freud for a time saw nose operations as a cure-all for mental illness.

However the disastrous results of some of these 'operations', as in the case of Emma Eckstein, who in 1895 was suffering with 'stomach ailments and menstrual problems' considered by Freud and Fleiss to be due to masturbation, and whose operation went so wrong that the nosebone caved in, ruining her looks and possibly her breathing, somewhat dampened Freud's enthusiasm for the operation. The operation was bungled in that Fleiss had inadvertently left half a metre of gauze in the nose. Eckstein's subsequent dangerous and near fatal haemorrhage from the nose was, however, attributed to her own 'neurosis': 'Haemorrhages were hysterical in nature, the result of sexual longing.'[10]

(At this point it is perhaps relevant to ask the question: What chance do/did sane people have of being taken seriously when ill, when even a haemorrhage following bungled surgery can be attributed to sexual repression and neurosis? And there are many who have not to this day strayed much from this ridiculous stance.)

But even the disaster with Emma Eckstein did not dim Freud's regard for Fleiss. After it, he wrote to him: 'You hold in your hands the reins of sexuality which governs all mankind: you could do anything and prevent anything.'[11] Moreover, Freud asked that Fleiss's imminent child be named after him. It was, however, a girl.

Thus with both the cocaine project and the nose-operation enterprise Freud had contributed to the death of or serious damage in others, but his belief in his own manifest destiny remained undimmed. Freud also believed in mental telepathy and imagined he heard his fiancée calling to him. He took part in seances, psychic research, consulted 'soothsayers' and was unbelievably superstitious about numbers. He considered 28 to be particularly important because it was the number for the female menstrual cycle. A second sacred number was 23, the male cycle, as he saw it. (Actually, men living with women will eventually cycle with them. That is, a rise in temperature will occur at the same time in both, over a 28-day period.) Also, Freud believed he would die at 62, therefore he regarded 62 and 31, the half-way mark, as sacred numbers. (He actually lived long past that age, until his late eighties.) He performed magic to avert disaster. In fact it was a shared interest in the occult between Freud and Jung which was their original bond.

Freud once confessed, 'If I had my life to live over again I should devote myself to psychical research rather than psychoanalysis.'[12] Many of us would wish that he had.

As noted, one of his problems was that in terms of the rules of his day he could not for some years afford to marry his fiancée, Martha, or have a sexual relationship with her. Moreover, he was brought up to believe that masturbation was 'the root of all evil', and possibly, so were prostitutes. Forced to live under those harsh rules, the ensuing sexual frustration must have afflicted his vision somewhat. All of life was to him sexually charged, sexually oriented.

But beyond perhaps an understandable obsession with sex, clearly Freud was for some years looking for a gimmick, something to set him apart from his fellows; something to make him famous, luminous. So in 1901, at 40, facing defeat and a life of just plain ordinariness, he went on holiday alone to Rome, seeking a last chance, something to give him inspiration.

In Rome he toured the art galleries, just as we all do when in Rome. We look at endless gilt-framed oils. And over and over again, there is Mary and her child Jesus. But only Freud saw in those paintings anything beyond that which the rest of us see. And what he saw was bizarre beyond words. What Freud saw was a child lusting after his mother. There's an apt term for this, straight out of Freudian psychology. We call it projection! Now who but Freud could look at the Madonna and Child and see such a thing?

Sensible people should have laughed at his subsequent nonsense. In fact he *was* for a time very much laughed at in Vienna among his contemporaries: '... when someone mentioned Freud's name in a Viennese gathering, everyone would begin to laugh as if someone had told a joke. Freud was the man who saw sex in everything.'[13] But unfortunately some of us are seldom sensible, as a glance back at history can readily establish, especially when confronted by a determined patriarchal male. And in our 20th century, despite a little progress in 'science' we have perhaps established a record of errors and foolishness of such a magnitude so as at least to equal that of any other century. It does not do to think that because we developed and use computers and have gone to the moon, that we are also wise.

That the entire 20th century, especially our second half, was strongly influenced by the irrational views of a man like Freud, is perhaps some indication that many of us are incurably attracted to the bizarre, the 'interesting', anything to get us beyond the humdrum of everyday life. Logic and ordinary 'common sense' are too dull for most. There is no other explanation for the powerful hold Freud has had on our century, or for the related phenomenon – the renewed burgeoning of superstition, in the retreat back to the mysteries of the medieval by many in the last quarter of our 20th century. The infinite gullibility and longing of humankind for the impossible is perhaps boundless.

So Freud returned from Rome to Vienna with his inspiration, which was that everything pertains to childhood and that children are sexual beings lusting after their opposite sex parents. Little boys want to 'possess' their mothers and kill their fathers, and it is the resulting lifetime of guilt and anguish stemming from this that causes neurosis, mental illness.

Most students of the life of Freud believe that the 'lusting after mother' had perhaps been true of Freud himself. The fact that it makes no sense in evolutionary terms, or in any common-sense terms, did not appear to worry him. Theories of 'the unconscious' had been around for most of the 19th century, and had become fashionable in Europe since 1880.

Freud took up this idea, the idea that there is a vast reservoir of unknown dimensions somewhere who knows where, where we store all such unresolved problems and from whence, as if from some great black lagoon, creatures from its depths will emerge to destroy our equilibrium at critical moments. With this goes the theory that dreams can give us glimpses into this black lagoon (again not original with Freud), as against the modern more prosaic theory that in dreams our brains are sorting out the events of our lives, riffling through the memory banks as it were.

H L Mencken, the great American philosopher, humanist and humourist, ridiculed Freud's outlandish 'interpretation of dreams' thus:

The true meaning of a dream about a murder, is not that the dreamer is soon to be married, or that his brother, Fred, in Texas, has been trampled to death by hippopotami, or that the Philadelphia Athletics will win the Pennant, but that deep down in the dreamer's innards, somewhere South of the tropic of cancer, the cartilages of last night's lobster are making a powerful resistance to digestion.[14]

Having thus seized upon the concept of the unconscious, Freud then looked around for a method to solve the problems involved in the inevitable guilt over that childhood lust. At that time, a Dr Joseph Breuer had come up with the business of the patient lying on a sofa talking to the wise therapist, who would, of course, tower over the patient, and who is often hidden behind her. I say her, because in the beginning it was generally her. Freud seized on this as the way to solve all mental problems. As we have noted, the idea of the unconscious was not his, nor the couch business. Only the preoccupation with sex was his.

And when he began, the highly restricted middle-class ladies of Vienna, bored to death with their circumscribed lives which could never satisfy, challenge or extend the more intelligent among them, simply leapt upon Freud's couch and the novelty of taking part in such experiments. I mean, there they were lying on a couch in broad daylight, talking about life and sex, a bearded man hovering near, and it was all perfectly respectable. It was *'Science!'*

This vast difference in the relative status of the therapist and the patient mirrored the great differences in power and knowledge between professional men and the women permitted scant education in that period. But theoretically, in the therapeutic situation the difference was designed to make the patient regard the therapist as a father figure, an authority figure and a guide. The patient would thereby be impressed with the power of the therapist, would be receptive to the suggestions coming therefrom, and thus relaxed, incumbent, would be healed of the 'neurosis'. Or so went the theory.

And none can deny that many of the ladies of Vienna in that time were slightly batty. Just take any sane intelligent male and require him to spend his days doing beautiful embroidery, weaving in bits of people's hair (most of it from the dead), crocheting hats for horses and so on, and see how long he lasts as a sane, intelligent male.[15]

So of course the bored and batty middle-class women Freud persuaded on to his couch would say anything Freud wanted them to say. He handed them loaded questions and the ladies obligingly picked them up and fired them off. Yes of course they'd felt sexy about Daddy. Well, anyway hadn't Daddy felt sexy about them as children? Or was it Uncle Charlie? Really I forget!

Freud wrote screeds about these sessions he called 'analysis', which of course went to prove his basic theses. But I wonder if it left any of those early patients any happier with their lot? Because psychoanalysis can do little to solve the basically socio-economic and political problems, and does nothing for the biochemical ones.

As for the talk therapists, it works well for them. Also in some cases it is also that patients are sexually compliant as well as compliant in other ways. None can know the extent of the incidence of sexual encounters between therapists and patients. But when therapists end up in court they can always say it was for the good of the patient, and they have been saying that all this century. What the whole business of psychotherapy actually does for the patients may be something else. There is scant evidence that it does any good. I have talked to numerous people who have experienced it, and none of them was truly enthusiastic about the results of their 'analysis'. For example, I once talked to an extremely intelligent older woman who had been sent by her family for psychotherapy because she had insisted she was physically ill but the family doctor said it was not so. He had decided. And so this dear lady spent two years of her life going on a train some distance away to talk (at considerable expense) to a strange man about her childhood. There was no question of impropriety in this case, but she told me that at the end of the two years she felt worse, both physically and mentally, than she had at the beginning.

Freud was not the least interested in the major mental illnesses, schizophrenia and the others. He did not deign to treat any such people. It was 'neurosis' he was interested in. And unlike his fellow doctors, he did not accept 'charity patients'. His patients had to be financially well off both to be acceptable to him and to be able to afford him. Hence the medical fraternity in Vienna regarded him as unethical. He was not respected in his own city.

There is plenty of evidence that he was sexist, racist, elitist and avaricious: also very anti-American in numerous ways, which is ironic considering that it was to be the US that embraced his Freudianism so whole-heartedly. Freud referred to America as 'a gigantic mistake', and that the discovery of tobacco was 'the only excuse for Columbus's misdeed. America is useful for nothing else but to supply money.' On his trip there he complained that America had caused his handwriting to deteriorate and his intestinal problems to worsen.[16]

Freud also 'hated American ideals of equality, and in particular egalitarianism between the sexes'.[17] Freud had not a shred of respect for women, despite or because of the fact that even before fame came he always surrounded himself with a bevy of women slaving over him. In fact his wife even put the toothpaste on his toothbrush for him. And despite his earlier obsession about his mother, he did not attend her funeral even though he was but two hours away.

Misogynistic and patronizing, he believed that women's whole existence was damned by lack of a penis and that having babies was a compensation for this lack. Altogether his dubious personality and even more dubious theories should have been 'laughed out of court'. The fact that they were eventually taken seriously should give us, every one of us, pause. Because it tells us just how gullible the human creature can be.

Those who disagreed with Freud were accused of 'sexual repression and neurosis'. Similarly, men wishing to seduce the women in their lives could taunt them with the charge of 'inhibition and neurosis' if they did not co-operate. Some are still doing it.

(The point that was lost on Freud, and lost to his followers and many today, is that if sex were just an itch that needs to be satisfied, masturbation would and will do. But sex is so much more than that. It is, above all else, the desire for union with another, in some the desire for domination over another. But at its best it is so much more than Freud allowed, because he would give no status to women.)

However, despite the many shortcomings of 'Freudianism', before long the whole thing 'took off like wildfire'. The doctors of Freud's day loved it once they got over their original shock. It fulfilled a need in them, at least.

As we will see in Chapter 32, Freud's theories enabled them to both explain and justify all their failures to understand or cure. For the purposes of this book **the most significant aspect of Freud's influence on medicine is that it permits doctors never to be wrong**. To be able to transfer any problems back to the patient. Instead of having to say the awful words, 'I don't understand your illness. I cannot deal with it. I have no way of curing it,' ever since Freud, doctors have been able to maintain a god-like stance, to say instead, 'There's nothing physically wrong with you. It's all in your head. Get thee to a psychiatrist.' Ridiculous though it was, doctors soon found it very useful, for Freudianism works very well for them, if not for patients.

And this is not just a minor thing. For that neat little 'way out' has hindered the progress of medicine in our century incalculably. That quick exit from rational thought, combined with one other faulty concept we will be looking at also, the Pasteurean fallacy, meant that doctors never had to worry about exploring the difficult, the hard to understand. With these 'blind alleys' they occupied, they had no reason to worry when confronted by the vast array of illnesses caused by the ruination of our soils, our foods, our air and our water. Medicine was able to pretend they did not exist! And most doctors are still doing it.

Although as we have noted Freud was not interested in serious mental illness, his concept of the causes of 'neurosis' affected people dealing with the entire field of mental illness. Eventually the major mental illnesses were considered to be roughly under the same rules as neuroses, only more so. A psychosis, or major mental illness, was an advanced neurosis. And thus the true causes of mental illness were not considered, even though eventually through the use of drugs it was clear that behaviour *could be modified* by changing the biochemistry of the body, even if it did not bring victims back to normal.

In the First World War most of the men in Freud's family had fought on the side of the Germans. As the Second World War approached, in inscribing his book for Benito Mussolini Freud referred to him as a 'cultural hero'. And it is difficult to know whether Freud was being funny or serious when, during that war, as a condition of his release from Germany to London he signed a paper testifying to the fact that he had been well treated by the Nazis. But he did more than that. He added: 'I can heartily recommend the Gestapo to anyone.' We hope it was a joke – or perhaps just a Freudian slip!

Whether he had a sense of humour or not, at the end of his life when dying of cancer of the mouth, throat and face (probably from smoking a pipe and/or taking cocaine), Freud saw clearly that his illness was affecting his brain. Whether he then saw the truth 'in a flash' or whether the realization that his 'jawing on the couch' methods had 'cured' few had come gradually upon him, we will never know.

Chances are he also knew by then that he had been ridiculous, that his whole life had been a fraud. And possibly so that he would not go down in history, and I mean the long-term history, as a complete and utter nincompoop, he wanted to say something sensible before he died, for the record. And verily he did.

There is a legend that, amazingly, in a flash of honesty he made an official pronouncement. He said that he thought that in the end all mental illness would one day be known to be occasioned by *physical* reasons. (That is, *through the biochemistry of the body*.)

Predictably, his followers didn't want to hear of it. They wouldn't have a bar of it. In fact very few have even heard of it. Which just goes to show that we hear what we want to hear, or what we are permitted to hear by the professionals. The practice of psychotherapy and all the other varieties of 'jawing therapy' went on apace, undaunted.

We must perhaps give Freud the credit for two things. First the realization of the importance of childhood in the long-term lives of people, although not in the way he insisted. And it is debatable whether going over and over one's childhood does much good. Second, he began the loosening up of the guilt-ridden late 19th century and early 20th century attitudes to sex and anything to do with it. Because in a roundabout way what he did have that effect. Although of course it might have happened anyway without him, considering pendulum swings, the revolt of each generation against the parent generation. We'll never know.

But Fuller Torrey, author of *Freudian Fraud* speculates:

One cannot help but wonder what would happen to many of the people in long-term psychotherapy if they spent the same hours working in community service or volunteering their time for the benefit of others, that they now spend in the eructation of childhood trivia.[18]

And, 'the focus of all psychotherapy systems ... is not some higher ideal, not one's fellow man, but merely oneself.'[19] And indeed we have seen the ultimate flowering of the preoccupation with self in this our late 20th century. More on this in Chapter 35.

But despite Freud and his all-round convenience, not everyone was sucked into his questionable vortex. In 1942 when Freudianism was slowly infiltrating the medical schools and from thence to the couches and consulting rooms of the US, an American, Dr Linus Pauling, twice a Nobel prizewinner, presented a different view. In a paper published in *Science* magazine he described a system of treating mental illness with high doses of specific nutrients. He called this system *Orthomolecular Psychiatry*, as against Freudian Psychiatry.

This Orthomolecular Psychiatry had its beginnings in the study of pellagra, a vitamin B_3-deficiency illness with severe mental manifestations. 'Pellagrologists' – that is, those who studied this illness (not uncommon in the American South before the Second World War) – had learned that to prevent pellegra in most people, less than 20 mg a day of B_3 is needed. That is, most reasonable diets will do it. But once the condition has become entrenched it can take 600 mg a day both to control it and to prevent a resurgence of the illness. It is as though some pathway gets damaged through the illness, and one has to take extra measures to keep it open.

And it seems that some purely mental illnesses are also in this category. It requires a constant experimentation with doses and nutrients to get it right, but major mental illnesses can usually be corrected. If not, the condition is too long-standing and imprinted on the brain. But for most, once the ill person's brain has become biochemically stabilized, it is then a question of adjusting the dose to find the optimum level.

From this knowledge a small group of exceptionally intelligent psychiatrists and doctors experimented with the principle with other mental illnesses. And to their great joy they found they were able to bring back to normal, people with schizophrenia and many other serious mental illnesses. By 1942, when Pauling wrote up the account of this, a group of 12 psychiatrists and doctors had been using these methods in their practices for some years. Specific regimes were worked out for different psychiatric and physical conditions. They work.

By the end of the first quarter of the next century, if not sooner, mental health will be a question of correcting the biochemistry of the whole body and hence the brain, to bring sufferers, in most cases, to completely normal health. It will be over a century too late to prevent the entirely unnecessary sufferings of millions in our century; millions treated inappropriately, primarily because of the baleful influence of that one ambitious man who could not marry his Martha.

To take the most severe problem, the one that Freud deigned not to consider: As early as 1884 the biochemical view of severe insanity, what we now know as 'schizophrenia', had been put forward by a Dr J W Thudichum, the founder of modern neurochemistry. His book, *A Treatise on the Chemical Constitution of the Brain*, went a long way to establish that what we think of as madness or mental illness was primarily biological and chemical in origin. Thudichum had in fact pointed the way out of the snake pit.

Even before then, Wilhelm Griesinger of the University of Berlin had become convinced that all mental illness was basically physical, and theorized that insanity involved anatomical brain changes. The British psychiatrist Henry Maudsley echoed Griesinger's organic theory, while another German physician, Emil Kraepelin, advocated science rather than philosophy in the analysis of mental illness. He completed the Kraepelinian system in 1899, in a compendium still invaluable today.

But any such brilliant advances of the late 19th century were brushed aside by the Freudians, to the sorrow of all of us. But the work of these early geniuses did not completely die. And the biochemical cause of the major mental illness, schizophrenia, was anticipated by Drs Abram Hoffer PhD, MD, and Humphrey Osmond MD in 1952.[20] They believed that there was 'an abnormal diversion of adrenaline into adrenochrome, an hallucinogen'.[21] This means that when under stress one's 'charging-up hormone' may, in susceptible people, turn into a nightmarish concoction like a very large dose of LSD, with predictable results. (In 1963 Hoffer and Osmond's findings were published in the *Lancet*, Britain's most prestigious medical journal.[22])

No one knows why this should happen in some people. We are now in the realm of speculation. But it would seem that every human being has a unique biochemistry with unique needs. Some of us have a greater need for certain nutrients than others. In addition there are accidents which can cause one person's brain to need more of a particular nutrient than others, for example unfavourable foetal influences (extreme malnutrition of the parents at conception, as happened during the Second World War,[23] occasioning higher incidences of schizophrenia in Holland, to mention only one effect); premature birth, cyanosis (lack of oxygen), the Rh factor and other problems at birth may also predispose one to schizophrenia.

Whatever the cause, based on a hypothesis that people with mental illness have nutrient deficiencies, those extremely brilliant and compassionate doctors, Hoffer and Osmond, have since that time been treating people with this serious problem with large doses of niacin (vitamin B_3) and ascorbic acid (vitamin C, preferably in the ascorbate form) with enormous success. (In fact, after 40 years of successful treatment, in 1989 came the proof of their hypothesis: a laboratory study which established that adrenochrome could indeed be present in the body in the form of adrenolutin.[24])

From 1951 to 1960, Dr Hoffer's group conducted four double-blind controlled studies taking in over 5,000 sufferers from schizophrenia, with 90% well after one year of treatment. Only 15% did as well on conventional treatments.[25]

Other nutrient systems will similarly relieve other mental illnesses. But this practice, though demonstrably successful, has of course been entirely ignored by mainstream psychiatry, with their ubiquitous backers the powerful pharmaceutical companies.

And when we consider how comparatively inexpensive these supplements are, as against the enormous costs of treating such an illness totally inadequately with drugs (plus all the costs of supervising, etc.) and the even more enormous and unending agonies endured by sufferers and their families, the shortening of their lives, the failure to cure, now *there* is a feeding frenzy for people looking back at us from the next century. But one can see also that with such a rational treatment the entire profession of psychiatry will, except for the care of the physically brain-damaged, be dispensed with. Disturbances of brain biochemistry could be treated by family doctors – well, at least the more enlightened ones.

Thus we can see why this is a treatment which the psychiatrists will fight to the bitter end, even, of course, if that treatment can, as it does, bring to an end the incalculable damage done to people, their families and their lives.

According to Dr Hoffer, 'The American Psychiatric Association bears major responsibility for preventing the introduction of a treatment which would have saved millions of patients from the ravages of chronic schizophrenia.'[26]

And a British psychiatrist, Dr Hugh Freeman said, **'America's enchantment with psychoanalytic psychotherapy has done more to retard psychiatry in America than any other factor.'**[27]

The question that will concern future critics will be, who is madder – those suffering from mental illness or those unwilling to even look at the real cures for such illnesses, cures that have been going on for over 40 years, because they are based on nutrients and not on drugs? I don't think there will be much doubt as to the answer when looked at objectively. But it is a most common form of madness in our century, a madness in all forms of 'health care', and of course successfully promoted by the pharmaceutical industries.

Dr Hoffer himself has posed the question,

What is it worth to save a human from the fate of the chronically tranquillized psychotic, barely able to get by ... I would urge all physicians to reward themselves and their patients by witnessing these recoveries. Do not wait for their psychiatrists ... do it yourself.[28]

Drs Hoffer, Osmond, Carl Pfeiffer (Pfeiffer degrees in medicine, chemistry and pharmacology) and many others, as noted, have been treating schizophrenic patients with large doses of vitamin B_3 (3–9 and more grams per day), and vitamin C (ascorbic acid 3–20 grams per day), a treatment which was, in 1963, accepted for publication in the *Lancet*.[29] Since 1986 when Carl Pfeiffer's Brain Biocenter was established, more than 5,000 people have been treated. Dr Pfeiffer has cured epilepsy, and bipolar illness, as well as schizophrenia. Some of the ex-patients keep in touch, and so long as they continue to take their megavitamins, most have led normal, sometimes highly successful lives. There are doctors, lawyers and teachers among these ex-patients. And you would never know if you met them that they once had a serious problem.[30] Meet any other victim of this illness, on conventional treatment, and you will know it immediately. For conventional treatment does not bring the sufferers to normalcy. As Dr Hoffer says, 'I have yet to see one patient on tranquillizers alone who is practicing medicine or law, or piloting a plane.'[31]

For many years now, 12 of the physicians using these methods have explored the possibilities in megavitamin therapy. Other nutrients have been added to the regime: pyridoxine (B_6), folic acid and thiamine (B_1). Specific regimes have been worked out for different psychiatric and physical conditions. It soon became apparent that a good diet and minerals in optimum doses were also helpful. Specifically: copper, zinc and manganese were helpful; also amino acids such as tryptophan and methionine.[32]

Dr Hoffer recently outlined in more detail his current protocols for the treatment of schizophrenia, the result of years of observation of his patients. He says: I no longer treat schizophrenia with just one vitamin. The complete treatment deals with optimum nutrition, with the correct supplements in optimum dosages, with drugs as they are needed and with the type of psychotherapy every physician owes every patient.[33]

He pays attention to food allergies, and the diet in general. He instructs his patients to remove all the simple sugar from the diet, which advice effectively removes approximately 90% of the junk food. Then he recommends a basic intake of:

B_3 (niacinamide): 1 gram three times daily
B_6 (pyridoxine): 250 mg daily
zinc sulphate: 220 mg daily
ascorbic acid (vitamin C): 1 gram three times daily
B-forte: 1 tablet three times daily
Halibut liver oil capsules: 1 capsule three times daily.[34]
The patient's regular medication must not be removed until there are strong signs of recovery, and then only gradually.

As mentioned earlier, to describe this treatment Dr Linus Pauling in 1942 coined the name *Orthomolecular Psychiatry*, in a classic paper on the subject published in *Science* magazine. The article described the practice of using nutrients in the treatment of mental illness.

Lest anyone think I am here talking purely from research, let me clear that up right away. For I have played a part in the complete recovery to normality of two severely disturbed mental patients, both conventionally diagnosed by specialist psychiatrists under extremely expensive and 'highly trained' care for many years, with no improvement. We'll call them Richard and Maria. I saw the entrenched terror, the pain and the anguish in their eyes. And I saw both of them return to complete normality within three weeks, just by changing the biochemistry of the body and brain.

Maria suffered from bipolar illness (formerly known as manic depression). She had endured this for nine years, with no relief from lithium, the standard treatment. When I saw her she was 'at the end of the line', having twice taken overdoses. However, we suggested she try anti-fungal treatment in large doses, and within three weeks there was no mania, no depression.

Upon this miraculous recovery, Maria paid big money to go back to see the five specialists in her disease, the professional psychiatrists who had not been able to help her.

'I want you to know how I recovered, so that you can help others,' she said.

Whereupon all of them said the same thing in different ways: 'There there, dear. You were about to get better anyway.'

Richard suffered from schizophrenia. He proved to me several times over that the supplements work. On them he is completely normal. He has a highly responsible job. He lives just like anyone else. But like most people with a chronic condition returned to normal, after a year or two you say, 'Well I'm over that horror. I'm OK now. I don't need these any more.' You discard the supplements. Only to find the 'schizophrenia' crunchingly back again. And it takes three weeks to become normal again on the supplements. It is a most difficult three weeks. There is no question that once this particular illness has become entrenched, one must stay on the supplements for life.

This happened to Richard three times, enough to make it quite plain to me that Hoffer, Pauling, Pfeiffer and the others are 100% correct. And after all, *did not the great Freud say it on his deathbed*?!

Strangely enough, it is alleged that Jung said about the same thing on *his* deathbed, again to 'resounding' deafness on the part of listeners.

There is so much evidence for the biochemical basis of severe mental illness, that it of course requires a whole book to deal with the question adequately.[35] We are here just briefly looking at the subject. For example, the March 1997 *Scientific American* reported on recent findings among suicides.[36] Neuroscientists have found that suicide is attempted when serotonin levels in the brain are low. That is, there is a biochemical abnormality.

Suicide is now the ninth leading cause of death among adults, and the third among adolescents.

New Zealand has the dubious distinction of leading the world in these statistics. Also of interest, psychiatrists have seven times the suicide rate of the general population.[37]

It was, of course, the tortured Freud who promoted the nonsensical idea of a 'death wish', but if we are to be consistent, in evolutionary terms we are bound to strive always to live, and it seems likely that in most cases, not all, it is primarily disturbances of brain chemistry which alter that. For whatever life events precede the fact of suicide, they are not *always* sufficient to cause suicide.

Alcoholics have the worst suicide rates: 18% of alcoholics take their lives, compared to 15% of depressed or manic-depressive people and 10% of schizophrenics. According to Dr Kristin Leutwyler, the reason alcoholics have such high levels of suicide is because they have *a dearth of serotonin receptors*. And there are other biochemical abnormalities in suicide victims: 'the phospho-inositide system was found to be impaired by 30 percent.' We do not, of course, yet know to what extent life events and situations contribute to the lowering of serotonin levels, etc.

There is much of this biochemical evidence constantly coming forward. There is possibly a combination of life events and biochemistry. And yet psychiatry remains stubbornly wedded to horrific drugs that dull but do not cure.

So our Freudian 20th century has staggered on, full of nonsense about mental illness, and curing nobody. In earlier centuries the mentally ill were kept in jails where the good people of the town would come out to watch them for an evening's entertainment.

In our enlightened century we've shot electricity through their sensitive brains so that they are never quite the same again; we've stuck sharp surgical knives into their delicate brains and turned them into passive morons; and we've used massive doses of fluoride compounds which dull their poor brains and further wipe out their nutrients. And any time they've been capable of speech they've been condemned to talk on and on about their childhoods.

I do not know who has mistreated the mentally ill most – those who in past ages just threw them in a jail and fed them slops, or those who did our horrific 20th-century 'high-tech' things and the jawing. In neither case have many been 'cured'.

It is appalling, *appalling*, that when all along, as of before the middle of this century, there were wiser and kinder people actually getting the mentally ill better, actually getting them back to normal living. And they are still doing so.

Looking at the evidence it seems quite clear that within a few years, mental health – in fact all health – will be a question of detoxifying and correcting the biochemistry of the body and brain. And all this nonsense about analysing one's childhood will simply disappear.

Not that one's childhood is unimportant. Quite the contrary. I suspect that possibly about 10% of us were unloved or abused, or both, in childhood. And we will never truly recover. We will 'make adjustments'. But we have to live with the knowledge that we will never have the lives we could have had, for they are ruined by low self-esteem and other faulty self-assessments most difficult to correct. And the memories are simply not erasable.

It may be that the opportunity to talk it over with someone wiser than oneself might help. There are groups which people enthuse over, rebirthing and numerous other gimmicks. But when one settles down again there is still that unhappy childhood carried for ever within the memory banks of the brain, and all that goes with it, and one must just get on with living.

In my city, our most successful businesswoman, who started off with 10 dollars in her hand, has in a few years made millions. But she has gone on record as saying, 'I would trade it all for a happy childhood.' And I would say exactly the same thing for myself. But we are both quite sane, or so they tell me.

One rarely 'goes mad' because of an unhappy childhood. Provided the bio-chemistry of the brain is not too far out, provided one's nutrients are in balance, one will at least cope, albeit with a colossal handicap. And conversely, people who develop serious biochemical problems in the brain may actually have had quite pleasant childhoods, if that is possible.

However there is today an army of people who make their living from out-moded concepts about 'the mind'. And they cause unending guilt in the families of those who become mentally ill. The members of this army will, of course, vehe-mently be defending their patches and the terms of their training.

But we have had them with us in ever-increasing numbers since the 1950s, while both physical and mental health continue to deteriorate: more and more people are on drugs to keep them stable; hyperactivity in children escalates, and violence in adult males increases. In the US the annual costs of dealing with mental illness, which came to $20 million in 1966, had become by 1986 up to $40 million.[38] There are six million American children on the drug Ritalin; thousands in the UK, New Zealand and Australia. Just where are the gains from maintaining this army?

If we want a better society, a better way of life, we will have to create a new paradigm to understand the brain and how it works. The intelligent and flexible among this army will seek to cure in a different way. And they will be successful.

It is the opinion of Drs Gross, Torrey and many others that as there is no sci-entific or sensible basis for Freudianism, it will 'slowly fade from view just as the Cheshire cat once did, except that in this case the grin will fade first and the genitals last of all'.[39]

As we have noted, in every generation there are the brilliant few who see clear-ly what is wrong and who spend their lives proving superbly that there is a better way. Only to be cursed and reviled for their trouble by their fellows.

Thus did Galileo and Copernicus try to tell the people of this world that the planet was actually round, only to risk their lives in the attempt. For there is noth-ing more tragic in its consequences than the faulty paradigm, nor more vehement than the adherence of its supporters.

But just as Galileo and Copernicus are now respected by all who have grasped the revolution in thinking they brought, the exploration of the world that followed and the technological progress that was possible in the wake of that revolution in thought, so the people of our century who revolutionized the care of the mentally ill deserve the highest plaudits. The names of such doctors as Abram Hoffer, Humphrey Osmond and Carl Pfeiffer must one day be engraved in gold alongside those of Hal Huggins, Orion Truss and all the others who have seen the truth despite their faulty training. For the truth about how our brains function is, to me, quite as important as the roundness or flatness of the earth itself.

EMERGENCY ADVICE

If you wish to try 3 grams of vitamin B_3 (niacinamide) and vitamin C (in the ascorbate form to protect the gut lining), etc., please work up to these doses *slowly*. Some need up to 9 grams daily at the outset. The experts say that one must take B_3 until a slight nausea sets in, then slowly work back down. Be warned that B_3 will give one a magnificent 'hot flush' (both sexes), through the head and the rest of the body. Do not be alarmed. This is great! And temporary.

Also remove food allergens from the diet. Many people with schizophrenia and other mental illnesses have wheat allergies, or a problem with gluten in general. Milk, sugar and food additives may also be problems, in fact any substance frequently ingested.

To test an individual food or substance, eliminate it for one week (that is, every single molecule of it), then consume a big dose. If symptoms return, then that food is a problem and must be eliminated for three months.

One of the best sources of information on the nutritional treatment of mental illness can be found in a book written by Dr Melvyn R Werbach (Assistant Clinical Professor, School of Medicine, UCLA) entitled *Nutritional Influences on Mental Health: A Sourcebook of Clinical Research* (Tarzana, CA: Third Line Press Inc, 1991); a precise way of determining nutrient requirements is to be found in an article by Russell Jaffe MD, PhD and Oscar Rogers Kruesi MD, 'The Biochemical-Immunology Window: A Molecular View of Psychiatric Case Management', *Journal of Applied Nutrition* vol 44, no 2, 1992, pages 27–42. This approach leans heavily on advanced chemical and immunologic testing techniques to determine nutritional requirements.

⚠

24: SALT

'The salt of the earth! Great stuff!'

Well it would be, except that early in the 20th century it was discovered that if they took almost all the minerals out of the salt – that is, 83 out of the 84 nature puts there, they could produce a cheaper, easier to handle product. Salt is no longer anything but sodium chloride now, but it tastes good and therefore it sells well. It is also bleached and chemicalized (aluminium, implicated in Alzheimer's Disease, is added, for one, to make it pour freely.)[1] 'When it rains, it pours!' the advertisements used to proclaim. Indeed so.

Real salt is greyish and clumpy. It does not pour.

One of the reasons we have more mental problems today is that we lack many of the essential minerals and trace elements we need to stay sane. Similarly, as noted in Chapter 4 on aspirin, it has been found that in soft water areas, or among people who use water softeners, there is more heart disease, because the magnesium normally in hard water is low or absent in soft water.

Animals are given salt licks with the salt in its natural state, in recognition of their need for the minerals and trace elements that it contains. But then animals have commercial value. We humans have no commercial value whatsoever! And no one gets rewarded for helping us to be well. So in today's world there is no incentive anywhere to help us to be healthy.

Lithium is one of the vital trace elements necessary for mental health. In the past we used to get it in tiny amounts in our daily salt. We probably had very little bipolar illness (also known as manic depression) in those days, or possibly it did not exist. These days lithium is, in much larger doses of course, 'the treatment' for people with bipolar illness. In some it gets them nearer to normal. And those parts of the world where there are high levels of lithium found naturally in the water are those with the lowest levels of bipolar illness, or none at all. It is even possible it is one of those 'new' diseases that has occurred since the alteration of our foods.

The brain is sensitive to such losses as lithium. Apparently infants lacking this trace element tend to be restless and sleep disturbed, and develop into edgy, tense children and adolescents. It may be a factor in hyperactivity.[2] And all of it unnecessary if only the mother had had some decent salt, and after the birth also the child. The violation of our salt, that ordinary substance sitting on tables for centuries, providing people with a daily dose of essential minerals and trace elements, is just one tiny aspect of what could be termed 'the assault on our food', which of course in its entirely ultimately leads to the breakdown of our health and to premature ageing and death.

Another point: What effect then of the prescribed restriction of salt, now only sodium, for people with heart disease? Inasmuch as every cell in our body needs sodium – for one thing for the 'sodium pump' alone, which is how essential nutrients are carried into our cells – a no-sodium diet must be a death sentence in the long term. A study in the medical journal *Hypertension* would tend to bear this out.[3] Sodium restriction was associated with an increased risk of myocardial infarction (the sudden heart attack) in drug-treated men with high blood pressure.

Common sense should tell us that sodium in small amounts should be taken in, but – and here's the but – not in the form of the synthetic salt we most of us eat these days.

EMERGENCY ADVICE

Yes you can buy real salt in most health food shops. But remember, it's got to be GREY and CLUMPY. If it is white and flows freely, don't buy it.

⚠️

25: PROZAC

'Depressed? Try Prozac!'

In New Zealand, with a population of around 3.9 million, 10 people attempt suicide every week, or over 500 per year. That is, those which are reported as such. Of these, over 150 succeed in taking their lives.[1] In most cases, suicide is the last stage in depression, despair, and 'no way out.'

It is said in the media that we in the modern world are suffering from an avalanche of depression. In particular, that people born since 1955 have three times the rates of depression of those born earlier.[2]

As depression is difficult to measure, such statistics must come from calculations on the intake of psycho-pharmaceutical drugs like Prozac. And there can be no doubt that this intake has increased enormously in recent years.

According to Margo White writing in the *NZ Listener*,[3] New Zealand prescriptions for Prozac more than doubled between 1996 and 1997, rising 'a whopping 140%'. At the same time prescriptions for the other older antidepressants did not drop, implying that the Prozac prescriptions were for new cases.

The actual amounts of antidepressant drugs dispensed are similar around the English-speaking world – in the US, in Britain, Australia and New Zealand – implying a fairly constant pool of that which we label 'depression', as well as an upsurge of late. And that does figure, because the same pre-conditions occur in all these countries.

I would suspect that the figures on antidepressant consumption would be significantly lower in mainland Europe. In fact for many years the herb St John's Wort (*Hypericum perforatum*) has been used more often than drugs in Europe.

There will be several reasons for the phenomenon we label 'depression' and its treatment with drugs. One of them will have to do with medical practice. That is, that at this particular time in history drugs are now the accepted treatment for any patients who are 'down'. So if you go to a used car dealer, chances are you will come away with a second-hand car. Similarly, if you go to a doctor with 'depression' you will come away with a prescription for a mood-altering drug. It is perhaps of interest that the city in New Zealand with the highest number of psychiatrists and doctors per head of population is also the one with by far the greatest numbers of Prozac and other antidepressant users.[4]

In the obligatory 5 to 15 minutes in the doctor's surgery, it is difficult to get at the antecedents for the depression, for not only is there no time but most doctors appear not to have the foggiest notion as to what truly causes it. For, as with most human phenomena, especially those to do with the brain, the causes of depression are not a simple matter but probably a combination of factors.

Another reason for the upsurge in depression is what one could call 'the psychiatrization of society', or the 'Freudianization of society'. In other words, 'depression' often goes with the self-preoccupation that came with Freudian concepts, that constant taking of the inner temperature: 'How'm I doing?' 'Am I happy?' 'Why aren't I happy?' I call it 'the Woody Allen phenomenon', because he seems to exemplify it.

All this began to seep into the Western consciousness around the middle of the 20th century, beginning as a trickle and now a raging torrent. I get the impression that, before then, life was not necessarily easier, but that one tended to just get on with the job, without the constant angst. Or that one accepted one would be down at times, and did not seek instant solutions.

But it is not quite that simple. Also in the second half of this century began the serious decline in our nutrition, that fuel which feeds both body and brain. And the brain cannot function without the right minerals and trace elements. If even one is missing, our brains cannot function at an optimum level. And thus the decline in brain health began with the decline in our soils and what one could describe as the rape of our foods.

Also, consider Chapter 2 on the lack of Essential Fatty Acids (calculated as deficient in 80% of Americans, and probably similarly deficient throughout the English-speaking world). Consider what this lack does to our brains, especially the brains of infants and children. That word 'essential' is not used capriciously. Consider also the loss of essential nutrients from our daily bread, now 'refined' and chemicalized. Consider also that we have lost the lithium from our salt, and are unlikely to make it up from food grown on depleted soils. As we noted in Chapter 24 on salt, that tiny daily dose of Lithium could have kept us all mentally healthier, in combination with the EFAs and so many other nutrients lost to us. Also, as mentioned in Chapter 3 on milk, magnesium is extremely important in mental health.

Then too, there will be other environmental factors, such as the increase in electromagnetic fields, those invisible 'knockers' of the human immune system which constantly surround us. And of course there is the increased load of toxic sprays and heavy metals in the brain. In the US, the generation born in the fifties and sixties were those exposed to Strontium 90 both in the uterus and in their developing years. They are 'the depressed generation', and also the AIDS generation. We have in the foregoing chapters noted numerous other things in our environment which are 'immunosuppressive'. In fact the suppression of the immune system has negative effects not just on the body, but also on the brain and the entire nervous system.

There are also various illnesses which can cause depression: parasites, yeast overgrowth, metabolic dysfunction, thyroid and/or adrenal insufficiency; there are also pharmaceutical drugs whose side-effects may include depression.[5] These can be 'the Pill', Hormone Replacement Therapy, cholesterol-lowering drugs, cortisone and beta blockers against high blood pressure. Add a few more possible reasons: There is an enormous recent increase in the intake of dairy products, an increase which has contributed to lower magnesium levels, critical to mental health as well as to heart health and a thousand other things.

Food allergies, hypoglycaemia, excess caffeine, alcohol, tobacco, exposure to environmental toxins such as solvents, lead or perfume (which, as noted, is nearly always petrochemically based) and too little sunlight can each play a part; also the contraceptive Pill may create nutrient imbalances in folic acid, B_2, B_6, B_{12}, vitamin C and zinc,[6] all of which will reverberate in the brain.

Add the loss of community and the breakdown of the local support systems which used to keep us more secure in life. And a final but not least important reason for widespread depression comes from the political arena. In the English-speaking Western world we have in the past few decades seen the emergence of New Right governments, of which there is nothing truly new. For they are merely the Old Wrong dressed up by modern PR experts. These governments cause a deep insecurity in possibly two-thirds of the population – that is, among those who are *not* swept up in 'the good life', according to Milton Friedman, or among those who are barely there, hanging on by their fingernails.

Also with the massacre of the trade unions there is no longer true job security, which makes for more than a docile workforce. It makes for an insecure workforce, an insecure population; because one's mere survival becomes the main preoccupation. Moreover, almost every move made by New Right governments causes jobs to disappear with nought but a downward spiral indicated.

And then, in ever-heaping piles of injustice, the finger is pointed at those without jobs. They have to be 'responsible', they have to 'get back to work' in an economy which makes it almost impossible to do so.

It would be different if those unemployed and unemployable, those put out to pasture, those who were 'old brooms', were regarded with respect for their contributions, or their gift of a job to another (because today if one **has** a real job it usually means another must go without). And inasmuch as our way of showing respect means giving one the means to live in dignity, that would be a partial solution to the problem. But they are not given that respect and dignity. They are, in fact, hounded and abused in a clear case of 'we have put out their eyes, and accuse them of being blind.' So it is easy to explain the drastic and dramatic increase in suicide (and crime) considering all of the above.

The young are told today that they are lucky to inherit a brave new world of endless consumer goods, high technology and 'out-of-sight' expectations of personal wealth and the 'good things in life', all in a context of perpetual job insecurity. It has had a dramatic effect on the mental health of our people, especially the young. The suicide rate among them has soared to heights never seen since such things were recorded. It is the main cause of death in the young, after accidents; and some of those accidents, such as car crashes, can be seen as a kind of suicide also. For professional observers have taken note of a new kind of recklessness, a heedlessness of danger in youth. Youth, that is young males, have always been comparatively reckless. But there is a new kind of carelessness with personal safety, as seen in 'jumping down waterfalls', skiing down quite obviously dangerous mountain sides, 'flashing around' on the motorways at speed and other such high-risk behaviour. One is reminded of the final car race in Nevil Shute's novel, *On the Beach*.

If one can find no place for oneself in the world one lives in, no stable future; moreover, if one lives in a world daily distorted in all the media one encounters, a world which has become a hollow lie; what is there to live for?

Yes, there are plenty of reasons for the swelling tide of 'depression'. And it can be a very serious matter to those suffering from it. As Margo White says, these drugs may at their best be 'small mercies'. But are antidepressants the best solution? There is evidence that antidepressant drugs may be temporary solutions, and even necessary in emergencies, to get one through to where more rational treatment could make an impact. But where is that more rational treatment?

The chances are that drugs are not the best long-term solutions. And with Prozac there is even a chance it could finish one off.

In the late 1980s, when Prozac first came in, it promised to be a new kind of antidepressant: 'safe, effective and easy to use'. Whereas up till then the antidepressants carried the risks of 'hypertension, erratic heart beat, dizziness, sluggishness, constipation and weight gain, causing doctors to question whether the possible side-effects were worse than the depression the drugs were intended to treat',[7] Prozac promised to be an entirely new kind of drug.

One of the differences in 'then' and 'now' may be that today we are prepared to talk about our depression, whereas before it carried a social stigma and was kept quiet. In some circles it is now 'trendy' to be on Prozac, just as it may be trendy to drink the fashionable drink and dine out in the hippest restaurants. But that doesn't mean the depression isn't real. Elizabeth Wurtzel, author of the best-selling *Prozac Nation: Young and Depressed in America* (1994), describes herself as formerly a 'freakishly depressed person who scared the hell out of people for most of my life, with my mood swings and tantrums and crying spells'. She apparently is feeling better on Prozac.[8]

Indeed, to some it does seem to be the dream pill, the simple answer to all one's personal problems. They are happier, more self-confident, more relaxed. To others it creates a nightmare world of extreme tension (hyperactivity, or 'climbing the walls'), severe insomnia, hostility and madness. There is evidence that on Prozac, people have committed violent acts they normally never would. There is also the 'dangerous deed' response *('Look, I can fly!')* as people jump out high windows, the suicides and the murders. There may also be numerous other side-effects.

By the middle of 1991 in the US, 14,100 people had reported that Prozac caused them to behave in a manner unusual to them; there were numerous accounts of adverse reactions, and many lawsuits filed.[9]

Some commentators have gone so far as to suggest that Prozac may in fact contribute to the causes of suicide; these allegations remain thus far unproven.

In response to intense public pressure, in September of 1992 the American Food and Drug Administration held a special hearing on Prozac. According to Maureen Kennedy Salaman, then Vice President of the National Health Federation (now President), witnesses appeared before the panel 'pleading that Prozac be removed from the market'. It was claimed that among those who had taken their own lives following taking the drug, were those who had been given the drug for weight loss or to help them quit smoking.[10]

Many have not been as fortunate as Elizabeth Wurtzel. In the US, Prozac has been put forward as a defence in at least 60 murder trials. Few of these cases have been successfully defended on these grounds. Perhaps because if this became an acceptable ground for murderous behaviour it would open up the floodgates to numerous defences on biochemical grounds, and then where would we be?

However, several defendants have had murder charges reduced to manslaughter or suspended sentences by pleading self-defence against the violence aimed at them by someone on Prozac.

And one woman on Prozac who shot and killed her husband received a suspended sentence.[11]

According to Dr Gary Null,[12] the basis for the numerous recorded suicides in people on Prozac has been established by at least four studies on the suicidal impulses which can follow on from taking Prozac, studies conducted by academic psychiatrists:

In Feb of 1990, Dr Martin Teicher and several other Harvard Medical School researchers released a study entitled 'The Emergence of Intense Suicidal Preoccupation During Fluoxetine Treatment'. These researchers said, 'The purpose of this report is to suggest the surprising possibility that fluoxetine (Prozac) may induce suicidal ideation in some patients.' That is, they start thinking about suicide when it may not formerly have been a problem.

In February 1991, in a *New England Journal of Medicine* article entitled 'Suicidal Ideation Related to Fluoxetine Treatment', researchers from Syracuse University wrote: 'We report on two patients in whom suicidal ideation and fluoxetine treatment were strongly associated.'

There are other similar studies. From the Yale University School of Medicine came 'Emergence of Self-Destructive Phenomena in Children and Adolescents during Fluoxetine Treatment', reporting on a study of children aged 10 to 17. 'Suicidal ideation of self-injurious behaviour persisted for up to one month after the fluoxetine was discontinued.'

A University of California group found that Prozac could bring on a condition called akathisia (literally 'can't sit down'), a state linked to homicides and suicides: 'We have observed the development of agitation, pacing, an internal sense of desperation and suicidal ideation.'

Among the milder side-effects, one-quarter who take Prozac will experience nausea and insomnia.[13] But worse, it can act like a stimulant similar to amphetamines, or like about six cups of coffee in a row. A few years back, a letter from a friend in southern California told me of her participation in a particular support group. She said, 'You can always tell the ones on Prozac by their tapping feet.' They are restless and cannot keep still, just like the children we label 'hyperactive'. Apparently, studies show that 30–40% of people on Prozac get agitated or overstimulated.[14]

A friend of mine was almost 'climbing the walls', sleepless, agitated, strung out, with zero libido, on Prozac. She said she 'couldn't take it any longer'. Together we decided on St John's Wort (*Hypericum perforatum*) and minerals (in particular magnesium). Gradually she became better and made the decision to come slowly off the Prozac. She feels lucky to have survived the experience. And she was, for such overstimulation may lead to psychotic behaviour and worse.

According to Dr Peter Breggin MD, co-author of *Talking Back to Prozac: What Doctors Aren't Telling You About Today's Most Controversial Drug*,[15] the extended stimulation can definitely lead to psychosis: 'People become manic and do outlandish things, like directing the traffic naked or spending all their money.' It was Dr Breggin who acquired some basic information about Prozac under the Freedom of Information procedure. Following this it became clear that the manufacturers had, in fact, admitted in the records that Prozac could actually *cause* depression. But the US Food and Drug Administration removed that admission from the records, and it did not appear on the warning list of side-effects that go with the drug.

In other words, before the approval of the drug, the manufacturers of the drug had admitted that Prozac can actually *cause* the very thing it is supposed to cure.[16] Dr Breggin's exposure of these facts has never been challenged. He says of his findings, 'They've had me under oath in court. And they haven't contested a single word I've written in the book.'

Serious nerve damage leaving patients with permanent disabilities such as involuntary movement, tardive dyskenesia (so named because it is usually *late*-developing nervous system damage) has also been noted. However, of two Prozac users who have sued for this reason, one of them claims she suffered permanent neurological damage within 48 hours of taking two capsules of Prozac a day.[17] And sexual dysfunction is known to occur in half of those on the medication. Dr Breggin actually calls the drug, the 'anti-empathy drug' for the reason that it makes people less interested in other people.

There is no better evidence for the uniqueness of all human beings, the bio-chemical individuality of each one of us, than the differing responses to Prozac. That lesson at least, should be carried over into the rest of the world of prescribing.

Moreover, the other lesson we can learn from Prozac is that *if* it can cause hyperactivity in adults, as it does in some cases, there is no better proof that hyperactivity in children also may be caused biochemically.

It is clear that for some the drug is extremely dangerous. And when at length information on the original pre-marketing trials was forced out into the open under the Freedom of Information Act, it was found that the initial clinical trials to establish its efficacy and safety were both flawed and highly unethical, in my view. Dr Null has labelled these practices the creation of a 'bullet-proof' scientific data base.[18]

From a trial which began with 1,730 patients, only 286 remained by the end of the study, most having been removed or having removed themselves from the study.[19] Fewer than 300 subjects is not truly enough to investigate all possible side-effects.[20] Any remaining patients becoming excessively agitated on Prozac were put on sedatives. This fact alone should have invalidated the trials. If approved by the FDA, there should have been added a co-condition that Prozac must be given 'in combination with addictive sedatives'.

Even though the FDA was aware of the problems with the trials,[21] they still approved the drug for human consumption. By all the criteria for acceptability and ethical marketing, Prozac should never have been approved as a drug for human consumption. It should be removed from the market. But as of 1999 it is still there.

(Anyway, we live in a world today where most 'scientific' studies come up with the results desired by those commissioning the study. There is no reason to be brow-beaten into submission by 'science'.)

In an interview with Dr Null, Dr Breggin summed up what can happen to people on Prozac in his experience:[22]

People start taking the drug, and in the beginning they feel better. Maybe, after all, because it's just good to get a drug. They feel like, wow, I'm doing something for myself. Or maybe the drug gives them a burst of energy. Stimulants will do that. They will make people feel energized. Then they get more depressed. They get suicidal feelings. They don't know the drug hasn't been tested on suicidal patients. They don't know that Eli Lilly once listed depression as an effect of the drug. And so they end up thinking they need more Prozac, and their doctor agrees. When that fails to work, they end up eventually getting shock treatment, never knowing that if they hadn't been started on Prozac they might never have gotten so severely depressed.

It is plain that the clinical trials to establish both the safety and efficacy of Prozac violated the basic procedural requirements laid down by the FDA itself. Moreover, this should necessitate an investigation into the practices of the FDA and its possible collusion with pharmaceutical companies.

Prozac looks to me like the right drug to symbolize the corruption and the carelessness in both medicine and government, the 'anti-empathy' preoccupation with Self that characterizes the late 20th century, our *fin de siècle*.

But inasmuch as the use of the even more costly and ineffective 'talking type' psychotherapy has fallen somewhat, in favour of these mind-altering drugs, we have to see the trend as getting nearer to the actual causes of depression – that is, that it is often mainly biochemical with an overlay of response to social causation.

One has to hope that it will not be too long before the next step in understanding is taken. That we will, by improving the individual brain biochemistry in a rational way, make it easier for people to cope with their daily lives and be able to see more clearly the problems to which they react and to work to resolve them, rather than to escape into a world of chemicals unnatural to the brain.

The solutions to our widespread depression and mental malaise are the same solutions as for our widespread poor physical health. And we will have to come to these solutions sooner or later, which means either in time, or too late.

As to the taking of such drugs as Prozac and other 'antidepressants', studies are beginning to surface as to the long-term results of these mood-altering drugs. That if we take them we will eventually damage our brains, just as if we keep taking heroin or alcohol we will eventually damage our brains. One cannot expect to interfere so drastically with the normal functioning of such a complex and vital activity as the workings of the precious human brain with impunity, without doing some damage.

EMERGENCY ADVICE

See your doctor, of course, but also see your naturopath or herbalist. Know that we can expect to be shocked and depressed in certain life situations, that it is both natural and normal. That time often does heal.

The best antidepressant 'as established in orthodox controlled trials against pharmaceutical drugs' is the herb St John's Wort. This is safe to take according to the instructions that come with it. Another herb is Kava Kava, a mild relaxant. The mineral magnesium, also safe, aids against depression. St John's Wort, Kava Kava and magnesium should be taken in accordance with instructions. Unless one has diabetes, it is also safe to take supplemental amino acids, which can act as precursors to the brain's neurotransmitters, the substances that make it all happen in the brain. Among the best amino acids are tryptophan, tyrosine and phenylalanine. Tryptophan, which was banned owing to one contaminated shipment from Japan, can now be found in 5HTP and occurs naturally in goat's milk products and eggs also. Exercise can help against depression.

Ask your doctor to check your thyroid function. Take antidepressant drugs only for emergencies to get you through a difficult time. It is well to remember that both the drugs and the St John's Wort can take two to three weeks to kick in and relieve depression. Some of the supplements, such as Kava Kava and magnesium, may bring relief much sooner.

For legal reasons, some material published in the original New Zealand edition of this book has had to be deleted from this UK edition.

⚠️

26: THE AMERICAN FOOD
AND DRUG ADMINISTRATION

'The FDA is the guardian of our health.'

When the FDA sneezes, the rest of the world says 'Gezundheit!'[1] The FDA is of course American, but its decisions concerning food and drugs affect the rest of the English-speaking world, for if a drug or food is approved in the US it can usually be found soon after in other countries. That was how Prozac 'went around the world', and how 'life-long' tomatoes and 'pesticide-resistant' soy are rapidly doing the same.

However, if one assumes that such a government-supported (that is, taxpayer-funded) body is there to help ensure the good health of the American people and the rest of the English-speaking world, think again.

Politics and health make for strange bedfellows. No less than that exemplar of modern social concern, Milton Friedman, 'Father of the New Right', has called for the elimination of the FDA. It was, apparently, set up early in the 20th century at the request of several large producers who wanted to wipe out competition. It did that. And to this day it still plays that role. Through its regulations and drug policies which benefit certain established interests, it makes both food and drugs not only far more expensive, but riskier too. There is evidence that through FDA policies and practices it damages and even kills untold Americans and those in other countries affected by its decisions.[2] Worse perhaps, whether it is in the area of cancer treatment or for the creation or maintenance of human health in any modality other than drugs and surgery, it attacks anything that threatens the established practices of orthodoxy. In short, the FDA keeps the world safe for established medicine, the pharmaceutical companies, the giant food technology industries and other related businesses.

In practice, what these policies mean to the average person is that the FDA destroys the democratic choice of doctors, the ill and well people to involve themselves in other forms of health care.

But to focus on the drug aspect of the FDA, Prozac was not the first questionable drug to be approved by it. According to Dr Gary Null PhD, science researcher, author and journalist, there have been hundreds:

Hundreds of drugs that initially pass their tests end up having major label changes – i.e. a major new warning has to be made – or wind up being withdrawn. In the field of psychiatry, the rate is especially high. During the time Prozac was approved, about 16 other psychiatric drugs passed inspection, and nine of these have since had major label changes.[3]

In 1991, the US General Accounting Office (GAO) issued a report on the 198 drugs approved by the FDA between 1976 and 1985. Of these, 52%, or 102 of the drugs, proved to have 'serious post-approval risks', some of them causing disablement or death. Many of them had been withdrawn from the market for these reasons.[4]

For example, there were two other antidepressant drugs, forerunners of Prozac, which after being approved by the FDA for the market proved to cause severe anaemia and other 'side-effects' ('side-effects' being a euphemism for 'bad things that happen to you when you take a drug'). After several deaths they were taken off the shelves. The same doctors who had originally testified as to their safety were also there to testify as to the safety of Prozac.

Similarly, of course, there were always doctors willing to testify on behalf of cigarette manufacturers as to the safety of smoking, long after reasonable doubt had been removed.[5]

In 1989 a US Congressional investigation revealed that certain FDA officials had accepted bribes from generic drug makers to speed their new products through the agency's approval process. It has been alleged that many of these officials subsequently leave the FDA to accept better paid jobs in the companies they have formerly been ruling on, sometimes moving back to the FDA later on.[7]

Dr Peter Breggin MD (author of *Talking Back to Prozac*, as discussed in Chapter 25) tells how the FDA reveals truth to physicians but not to the public. He attended a day-long seminar sponsored by the FDA and found there displayed large black posters bearing the words:

ONCE A DRUG IS APPROVED,
IS IT SAFE?
NO IT IS NOT.[8]

They were making the point to the assembled physicians that many drugs turn out to be dangerous after approval. But how many doctors get to such a seminar, and how many patients have any idea that a drug approved for the market may not be safe? The reason for the post-release dangers lies in the fact that the numbers in the trials are usually too few and the timespan too brief to flush out all possible problems. Moreover, the trials are often conducted by the very companies which stand to profit by their release; hardly an assurance of an impartial trial.

Logic and human decency should dictate that, as lives are at stake with the introduction of chemicals foreign to the body, one would expect the FDA to lean heavily in the direction of safety. But clearly this is not the case.

A Dr Gambee and Pamela Hoffine, patient advocate, both of Oregon, looked over the transcript of a meeting of the Federation of State Medical Boards, April 1996. At one point in the transcript a Dr John Renner indicates how his priority lies with the FDA system, rather than for the welfare of patients in connection with drugs:[9]

The public doesn't understand that when a medication is put out on the market and then eventually withdrawn because of some new information, that that's a sign the system works. Patients interpret that as 'It should never have been approved in the first place'.

Of this comment, Gambee and Hoffine scoffed:

He must be referring to those silly, ignorant patients who don't want to suffer or die unnecessarily! Oops we better pull that one off of the market too, or there'll be too many lawsuits?

One could question why so many are cleared to go on the market in the first place. Surely the trials to test them must be about as effective as the one for Prozac was. There should be no such 'new information' as severe consequences and deaths.

No one has succeeded in bringing the FDA to court for charges of collusion with drugs manufacturers. We have noted that there is a group attempting to do so on behalf of those afflicted by the depredations of the neuro-excitotoxins MSG and aspartame. Also, 50,000 American women are engaged in a class action suit against the makers of the Norplant contraceptive, which they claim has caused headaches, weight gain, joint pains, strokes, paralysis and other health problems. And there are 'scores of lawsuits regarding food, cosmetics, drugs and dyes, filed against the FDA'.[10]

Even the conservative, business-oriented *Time* magazine has deplored the current state of affairs and has concluded that in the US science is beset by 'embarrassing cases of fraud and failure … US science, once unassailable, finds itself in a virtual state of siege.'[11]

Also, if we believe that the FDA exists to ensure fair pricing for a people over-burdened with excessive health care costs, think again. A few drugs such as antacids and anti-smoking gum have recently been taken off the prescription list and placed at the disposal of the public. They can now be bought 'over-the-counter' (OTC). When these OTCs were first announced people became excited about the possibility of getting them a little cheaper – that is, eliminating the middlemen – as well as having more personal choice. A pharmacist told one woman trying to stop smoking that the anti-smoking gum undoubtedly would become cheaper. But when they arrived, the price had gone from US$40 (from a doctor) to $60 for the same number of pieces of gum; proof, it would seem, that the FDA, supposedly existing to protect the public, is not doing the job. Over and over again there is evidence that the FDA does not appear to be there to protect consumers but to protect the profits of the pharmaceutical companies and prescribing doctors.[12]

There is also plenty of evidence that the FDA has no more idea of what constitutes real health than does orthodox medicine. It exists to support the technologized food industry as well as the pharmaceutical industry, as witnessed by their hasty approval of such questionable items as irradiated food and biogenetically-engineered food, on the one hand, and on the other their constant harassment of doctors who use vitamins and other supplements in their practices.[13] Dr Fred Shull MD is of the opinion that, 'The FDA exists to keep us sick and senile, although most establishment doctors take their word as God's truth'.[14]

In 1989 the World Medical Association released the Declaration of Helsinki, which stated that:

In the treatment of the sick person, the physician must be free to use a new diagnostic and therapeutic measure, if in his or her judgement it offers hope of saving life, reestablishing health or alleviating suffering.

In 1994 a German Federal High Court decision went even further: It ruled that 'A physician is under obligation to employ unconventional methods when conventional methods have failed.'[15]

These rulings were of course made with the intention of breaking down the current medical paradigm, the paradigm that says only drugs and surgery are acceptable. But under the FDA, such freedom of practice does not exist in the US. The FDA, through its links with powerful vested interests, the local medical boards and, above all, the media, has always attempted to belittle, persecute and bring to court any doctors who try to do things a little differently – in short, who try to deliver real health care in contrast to mere 'disease care' which is the hallmark of modern medicine.

There have been many doctors persecuted, raided by the FDA, their records and stocks of supplements and herbs confiscated, taken to court for fraud and repeatedly ruined. It is difficult for the average person to grasp the extent of FDA activities.

A recent example of this is the ongoing persecution of Dr Stanislaw Burzynski MD, who uses naturally occurring amino acids, 'antineoplastons', to reprogramme cancer cells to normal. With these he has successfully treated over 3,000 patients since 1977. Most of these patients had reached the end of the line with conventional chemotherapy and radiation before coming to him.[16]

The success of Dr Burzynski's methods has been recognized by the American National Cancer Institute, and aspects of his methods have even been *approved for trials by the FDA itself*, both for cancer and for HIV.

Nevertheless the FDA has repeatedly tried to shut down Dr Burzynski's Texas practice. There was considerable publicity when a little boy with multiple brain tumours, Jimmy Kilanowski, presumably near the end, met President Bush. After three months of Dr Burzynski's treatment he was, after PET scans, classified 'in complete remission'.

This kind of publicity must represent an enormous threat to the cancer medication industry. The FDA prosecuted Dr Burzynski in 1983, 1990 and again in 1994. Despite these raids, grand jury investigations always vindicated him. But he was raided again in 1995 and faced 290 years' imprisonment. The charges brought against him consisted of 'trafficking interstate' – patients were coming from other states (in fact they were coming from all over the world) and then leaving the state of Texas with his treatment. This of course is what happens when word of mouth from satisfied patients brings other patients from far afield. But this is the way the FDA 'breaks' doctors who try to be different. The repeated trials initiated by an FDA, with unlimited taxpayer funding, drains these good doctors financially to the point where they can no longer afford to practise even when the courts vindicate them, as they usually do. This has happened again and again with almost any doctors who seek for a better way. And it is always the most brilliant and the most compassionate doctors who appear to 'get it' from the FDA. For indeed, it is easier to 'make a buck' under the conventional system than to face the hassles of treating patients differently. But many continue to do so because they know it is the right thing to do, and they undoubtedly must get satisfaction from curing those patients others have failed with.

Dr Burzynski's supporters and ex-patients are many. Therese Emmanuel and Steven Mehler claim that: 'Never before has the FDA approved an experimental drug for clinical trials with cancer patients while simultaneously trying to destroy the scientist who discovered it.'[17]

As of June 1997 Dr Burzynski was once again vindicated by a higher court and free to practise, that is until the next FDA raid. The question is how long will he be able to continue, given the costs involved in defending himself?

The same thing is going on in Canada, with the recent harassment and trial of Dr Jozef Krop MD, a doctor who practises chelation therapy. And this despite an Alberta law, a unanimously passed private bill to amend that province's medical act permitting medical doctors to offer *any complementary medical procedure provided it cannot be proven to do more harm than conventional drug and surgical treatments.*[18] And that is certainly true of chelation.

Dr Krop and Dr Burzynski are just the most recent in a long line of brilliant and innovative doctors, persecuted, reviled and sued until they are broken by the powers that be. The FDA's operations include sheriffs with drawn guns arriving in doctor's consulting rooms, terrifying the patients, confiscating records and supplements and going on to jeopardize the doctor's livelihood and entire future.

Again and again this has happened, the dinosaurs attacking the mammals. And again and again the US Government does nothing. The FDA is almost a law unto itself. Repeated appeals over the years to Presidents and Congress from numerous groups and concerned individuals fail to reform this dictatorial body, such is the power of the huge industries behind it.

The *Well Mind Association Newsletter* (Seattle, Washington) published this in February 1995:

The following is a summary of raids made by the FDA on nutritionally-oriented laboratories, clinics, health food stores and even pet-supply businesses from 1985 to November 1994:

Burzynski Research Clinic, Texas, 1985, Cancer therapy.

Life Extension Foundation, Florida, 1987. Unapproved supplements.

Highland Laboratories, Oregon, 1990, Unapproved supplements.

Pets Smell Free, Inc., Utah, 1988, Unapproved pet deodorant.

Solid Gold Pet Foods, California, 1989: Labels on holistic pet foods. [I will discuss this in more detail later in this book]

Traco Laboratories, Inc., Illinois, 1988: Unsafe food additive (Blackcurrant oil).

H. A. Lyons Mailing Service, Arizona, 1990: Vitamin literature mailer.

Nutricology, Inc., California: Unapproved and unsafe supplements.

Scientific Botanicals, Nebraska, 1991: Alleged label violations.

Thorne Research, Idaho, 1991: Unapproved supplements.

Dr Jonathan Wright MD's Tahoma Clinic, Washington, 1992: Unapproved supplements.

Ye Seeker (and several other health food stores), Texas, 1992: Unapproved supplements.

Mihai Popescu, California, 1992: Sale of Gerovital.

Nature's Way, Utah, 1992: Unapproved food additive (vitamin E).

Family Acupuncture Clinic, California, 1992: Chinese herbs seized.

Natural Vision International, Wisconsin, Unapproved pin-hole glasses.

Tierra Marketing, New Mexico, 1993: Sale of Gerovital.

Kerwin Whitnah, California, 1993: Unapproved drug; deprenyl.

Waco Natural Foods, Texas, 1993: Unapproved drug; deprenyl.

International Nutrition Inc., New Mexico, 1993: Alleged misbranding of Neiper (German) supplements.

Hospital Santa Monica (Donsbach), California, 1993: A combination Mexican/US operation. Unapproved supplements.

Zerbo's Health Food Store, Michigan, 1993: unapproved supplements.

Life Extension Services, Maryland, 1994: unapproved foreign drugs.

The full descriptions of what happened in each of the above instances makes for sobering reading. Businesses have been destroyed; some are afraid to continue; some are in court at great personal expense; some are traumatized by the FDA's violent raiding tactics. A detailed account of all the above can be obtained from:

Life Extension Foundation, PO Box 229120, Hollywood, Florida 33022–9120 US. Please send a small donation to cover their costs.

As far as harassment goes, in order to choose a fairly neutral example of FDA activity and its drive to ruin anyone who threatens established interests, I reproduce in full an item by Dr Jules Klotter, in his column 'Shorts', as printed in the *Townsend Letter for Doctors and Patients*:[19]

FDA VS NATURAL FOOD FOR PETS

An astounding example of the FDA's misuse of power was revealed in April 1994, in a Gary Null radio interview with Sissy Harrington-McGill. In 1974 Sissy founded Solid Gold Health Products for Pets, Inc., a company that offers pet food made from organically-grown grains and herbs, and nutritional supplements for cats, dogs, and horses. Her interest in canine nutrition began when three of her Great Danes died from bloat, a condition caused by animal fat and soybean in dog food. In hopes of closing Solid Gold down, the FDA took her to court in April 1988, for violating the Health Claims Law. Sissy was told that this law categorizes vitamins, minerals, and herbs as drugs that must be prescribed by a veterinarian. At that point, Dr Null alleged that **no such law exists**…

Sissy ended up spending **114 days** in a maximum security federal prison for selling Solid Gold products to health food and animal supply stores.

Sissy told Gary Null:

In court, the FDA committed perjury many times, telling the Judge that I had refused to change the labels of the products. Well, I have

**changed the labels a total of 37 times ... the law says that you will not
say that you can treat, prevent, mitigate, or cure a disease. I never
said any of this on my [labelling]; I will see that it is corrected, updated
or improved upon ... the FDA says that they have control over literature put out with a project ... but a letter from the Federal Trade
Commission says very clearly the FDA has jurisdiction only over
labelling. But for anything accompanying that, they do not; the FTC
does.**

Apparently, Sissy had difficulty finding a lawyer willing to help her sue the
FDA. The group Independent Citizens Research Foundation for the Study of
Degenerative Disease alleges that 'suing the FDA incurs the wrath and atten-
tion of the IRS, who then investigate the lawyers for tax fraud'.[20]

It seems likely that Sissy had threatened the vested interest of the dog
food cartels.

On 15th January 1999, Sissy was at last vindicated by a 'landmark decision' when the US Court of Appeals for the District of Columbia held 'uncon-
stitutional' the US Food and Drug Administration's health claims rules to
labelling, one of the major ways it could harass those attempting to produce
and sell products outside 'the system'. The judges said, among other things:

**Although the government may have more leeway in choosing suppres-
sion over disclosure as a response to the problem of consumer confu-
sion where the product affects health, it must still meet its burden of
justifying a restriction on speech – here the FDA's conclusory asser-
tion falls far short.**

Jonathan Edmord JD, attorney for the American Preventive Medical
Association (APMA) who, with others, brought the case before the court,
said,

**This is perhaps the most significant labelling law decision handed down
by a court in over 20 years. This decision invalidates the FDA's entire
review regimen for labelling claims, on the basis that it is unconstitu-
tional, arbitrary and capricious.**

The APMA's president, Dr Ralph Miranda MD, said,

**This has been an expensive, six-year battle for us. For years, dietary
supplement companies have been afraid to challenge this agency, for**

fear of retaliation. Our members, practitioners who use and prescribe dietary supplements, felt the need to step into the breach and press the case for fairness and free speech ... Now, the FDA will no longer be able to get away with continually raising the bar for supplement manufacturers in an effort to prohibit the dissemination of truthful, scientific information.

Others involved in the case were the National Health Federation, Citizens for Health, Direct Aids Alternative Information Resources, People Against Cancer, and the Foundation for Advancement of Innovative Medicine. (A copy of the complete decision can be found on the website at http://www.emord.com.)

The Independent Citizens Research Foundation for the Study of Degenerative Disease would of course be finding the FDA among its main obstacles to progress. If medicine were doing its job, why should people find it necessary to form a citizens group to study degenerative disease? Why, in fact, the need for the proliferation of patient support groups all over the Western world, patients doing research into their own illnesses? If the normal channels of help and research were doing the job these would not come into existence, would not have to exist. It is extraordinarily difficult for ill people to fight for themselves.

It is clear that there is a life-and-death struggle going on in the English-speaking world between established medicine and those who would attempt to do better and do it more humanely. The FDA is determined to keep things in the dismal state they are presently in.

That is dismal for thee and me; safe for the making of billions by industry, and safe for orthodox medicine. Orthodoxy and the FDA appear to have everything on their side, but in fact people are turning away from orthodoxy. It is only a question of time before it is forced to make considerable modifications. However, in the mean time a lot of unnecessary harm will be done.

In Europe and Great Britain there seems to be more tolerance, more room for differences of opinion and practices. (New Zealand and Australia, more under the influence of the US, stand somewhere in between. These governments are presently poised to challenge our freedom of choice; **consumers should not allow it to happen.**) Meanwhile in the US, doctors, dentists and psychiatrists who do not 'toe the party line' are ridiculed, harassed, persecuted and prosecuted. They get drummed out of their home states and have to flee to more tolerant states or to other countries. Most of this is due to the appalling example set by both the AMA and the FDA, who lead the way in these matters. In fact the FDA is a law unto itself, and it is high time that US government took responsibility for permitting it to be so.

And thus the FDA goes cheerfully on its crooked way, ruining decent doctors and others, holding back decades worth of progress, and is never brought to account because no one has the guts to dismantle it or replace it. It is long past time something was done about it.

⚠

27: PRESCRIPTION DRUGS

'A prescription drug'll fix you up.'

New Zealand's official prescription drug dispenser, Pharmac, spent around $775 million in the year ending 1997.[1] Moreover, as in many other countries, **the major reasons for hospital admissions** here are related to pharmaceutical (that is, prescribed by doctors) drug problems, either from adverse reactions or overdoses.[2] Figures for these in New Zealand were published in the *New Zealand Herald* (June 26, 1995), indicating that 2,500 people per year die in New Zealand hospitals from drug errors and adverse drug reactions, most from preventable errors. (There are approximately 3.9 million people living in New Zealand.)

These figures do not, however, include those who may die prematurely from the effects of prescription drugs, taken long term, but who do not appear in the statistics because they may be said to have *acquired* heart disease or other serious problems. In addition there are 5,000 preventable injuries per year occurring in New Zealand hospitals. The NZ Nurses Society believes that some of these problems can be laid at the door of staffing shortages. That is, that overworked hospital staff cannot give the kind of care they would like to give; plausible given the state of New Zealand's 'health care' system, once the best in the world.

In Australia the Hospital Care Study came up with an estimated 10,000 to 14,000 preventable annual deaths, and 25–30,000 people permanently disabled in hospitals every year.[3]

In 1989 the American overall 'disease-care' bill came to 12% of the Gross National Product. By comparison, in Japan it was 6.8%; in Britain 6.1%.[4] Since then it has been rising every year. What this means in actual figures is that the total American health bill, which was $200 billion a year in 1979, today approximates **one trillion dollars per year.**[5]

Prescription drugs account for a major part of this horrendously huge American bill, and their cost is ever-increasing. In the 10 years ending 1990, inflation rose 54%, but the prescription drug bill rose 135%.[6] The costs have risen similarly all over the West. And this increase is reflected in the numbers of people addicted to prescription drugs, numbers which have increased by 500% since 1962, a situation which caused Deepak Chopra to declare that 'the number one cause of drug addiction is ... not street drugs from Columbia but legal medicine prescribed by doctors.'[7]

Americans spend nearly $2 billion a year on prescriptions, for drugs to treat injuries, for illness, and to kill pain.[8] And beyond that there is a $20-billion annual bill for hospitalization to repair the damages from all the drug-taking.[9]

A recent study (reported April 15, 1998) in the *Journal of the American Medical Association* was conducted by Dr Bruce H Pomeranz MD, PhD, and colleagues at the University of Toronto. They analysed 39 studies of Adverse Drug Reactions in the US to estimate the incidence of serious and fatal drug reactions in hospital patients, and came up with the sobering conclusion that there are 2,216,000 hospital patients who suffer these per year, and that these Adverse Drug Reactions cause 106,000 deaths per year, making this between **the fourth and sixth leading cause of death in the US**. So here is where that $20-billion bill for patching up comes in.

It is also well to bear in mind that the *JAMA* report contained the caution that in the reporting process, 'health care practitioners may miss or pass over many ADRs ... and even any fatal events.' Also these figure will miss the possible deterioration unto death of the long-term prescription drug-taker.

It is worth noting that Dr Pomeranz also initiated a study into deaths following *correctly prescribed* prescription drugs. As a result, the *Journal of the American Medical Association* reported that there are an estimated 100,000 deaths per year from these correctly prescribed drugs, and an additional 2.2 million hospitalized patients who've had a non-fatal reaction.[10] The top culprits were: painkillers (from narcotics which halted breathing to aspirin which created stomach bleeding), antibiotics and antiviral drugs (causing severe diarrhoea) and cardiovascular and anticoagulant drugs (causing a range of problems, including internal bleeding). This data puts deaths due to correctly prescribed drugs ahead of lung disease, pneumonia or diabetes as killers of Americans. And this study did not of course include those prescription drugs which were incorrectly prescribed, as in the studies mentioned earlier in this chapter.

Perhaps the most salutary point to make is that despite the enormous costs of drugs and the cleaning up after them, according to the annual disease statistics this massive expenditure has not overall resulted in improved health. Hence the World Health Organization's dire predictions as to heart disease and cancer mentioned in the Introduction.

As noted, Milton Friedman has called for the disbanding of the American Food and Drug Administration, because it kills competition. He argued that there are many drugs/substances available in Britain, Switzerland or Germany that are outlawed in the US. Friedman believes that the free market and the common law would provide far more protection than this government body, without hindering new and helpful treatments. I'm not convinced that we don't need something to care about us. But clearly something needs to be done about the current control by unbridled monopolies. Another study, by Dr Sam Peltzman of the University of Chicago, established that past and current FDA drug policies have caused hundreds of thousands of deaths and massive amounts of human suffering.[11]

One could also add that millions and billions are spent on drugs to attack various diseases, but little or nothing is spent on that far less lucrative endeavour, the prevention of disease. And why should there be? There is no incentive to prevent disease; no billions to be made.

Prescription drugs are, of course, the mainstay of modern medicine. But not all doctors use them. Dr Victor Penzer MD, DMD, FASCD, is of the opinion that 'there is no known disease caused by a deficiency of synthetic pharmaceuticals in the body, yet this is what most doctors prescribe ... most of the time.'[12] Many would agree with Dr Penzer, but to do so requires a definitely different way of looking at human health, how it is maintained – or regained once lost. When we look at Chapter 32 we will see how these differences have arisen.

The traditional, the natural, the so-called 'alternative' view is that the symptoms, which are what orthodox medicine attempts to treat, *are not the disease*. The symptoms are the visible or felt *signs* of disease, the body's attempt to correct a problem. For example, fever is the body's way of coping with proliferating germs. To tamper with fever, unless dangerously high, is to tamper with the body's defences. Dr Luc De Schepper MD, PhD, writes of studies showing 'that children's diseases are prolonged when anti-fever drugs are given'.[13]

One account that would confirm this viewpoint was presented by Dr Bob Witsenberg, describing his experiences working in a hospital in Ghana during the measles epidemic of 1967–68. Hospitalized children who were treated with cough-suppressants, fever-reducing drugs and sedatives to suppress their symptoms sustained a 35% mortality rate. But those children whose fever and rash were not suppressed by medications sustained a lesser 7% mortality rate, and this despite (or because of) experiencing fevers of 40–41°C, and subjectively appearing to feel much worse than the other group.[14]

A rational view of health sees the body as a marvellous collection of trillions of superb little chemical factories driven by the blueprint which is our DNA. When we become ill, the dis-ease will have arisen from an imbalance or deficiency in that which the body needs to repair itself, and/or a toxicity (or poisoning) in the body, accrued from an overload of substances it cannot deal with. As such, treatment aimed at obliterating the symptoms may temporarily relieve those symptoms, but the ongoing disease process is maintained, while at the same time, in the attempt to cope with the unnatural, or even poisonous (to the body) substances which constitute most pharmaceutical drugs, the drugs themselves will draw further on the body's declining resources.

The fact that drugs can adversely affect one's nutritional status, and hence one's health, has been well established. This happens because nutrients and drugs share common routes of absorption and compete for transport mechanisms. Also because the molecular structure of some drugs is superficially similar to the structure of some vitamins, the drugs can significantly interfere with the absorption of these actual vitamins; they may cause a greater need for enzyme systems that require vitamin cofactors; and they may interfere with the synthesis of vital nutrients, for example antibiotics interfere with the synthesis of vitamin K.

The oestrogen-containing oral contraceptives can cause folate deficiency, which may be the reason for the greater risk of vaginal and endometrial cancer on these drugs. They also interfere with vitamins B_6 and C.[15] Even aspirin can reduce the uptake of vitamin C and the protein-binding ability of folate.[16] And in Chapter 4 we noted all the other possible sequelae of taking that simple drug long term.

All drugs have to be detoxified or go through some biochemical transformation before they can be excreted. And this process involves using vitamins and minerals as cofactors. As noted, the main difficulty may be that it is those already suffering nutritional deficiencies who become ill, and who are therefore prescribed drugs, which will further deplete their nutritional stores.

(See the chart on pages 206–07.[17])

As we noted in the chapter on aspirin, both prescribed in various forms or obtained over the counter even that 'homely' drug can be dangerous if used over time; it can go beyond interfering with our nutrients. But there's more: Dr Alfred Pischinger, Professor of Histology and Embryology at the University of Vienna, made a special study using iodine uptake methods of the largest functioning system in our bodies, that is the extra-cellular matrix.[18] Our cells do not float around in a vacuum. There is a liquid milieu which bathes and nurtures all our cells and tissues. All cells are embedded in this matrix. Every brain and nerve cell relies on it for its integrity. And whereas the behaviour of the cells is fixed, the matrix must adapt, accommodate and control all the major systems of the body in relation to what fluids and substances it encounters.

It is a communications system, bio-electrical as well as biochemical. Professor Pischinger's extensive studies have shown that natural therapies promote healing functions in this matrix, but that synthetic drugs always have a shock effect upon it even though specific symptoms may be improved. As such, Professor

Pischinger's work provides a scientific basis for the traditional approach to health care followed for centuries. His book has, of course, been ignored.

Another expert who has extensively studied the effects of drugs is Dr Ernst T Krebs Jr, DSc, of the John Beard Memorial Foundation. After years of studying the question, he made the following comment: 'Almost every drug is totally dispensable; every micronutrient is indispensable.'[19]

Udo Erasmus has likened the effects of drugs on the precisely coordinated human biochemical 'symphony orchestra' to the introduction of badly trained musicians or the at-will use of strange instruments such as a bongo drums, hammers or a cannon during an internationally acclaimed top-level classical performance.[20] The discordant sounds are then written off as 'side-effects,' but is it what the composer intended?

In any event, while individual drugs may alleviate (or suppress) individual symptoms, it is clear that the billions of dollars a year spent on drugs has not improved the overall health of the American people or those of us in the rest of the English-speaking world. When we consider the question of drugs what we need to ask is, 'Are they truly effective and safe in the long run?' In several parts of this book we have looked at the answer to the safe part; the answer to the 'effective' part is difficult to come by.

When we looked at the chapters on Prozac and the FDA we saw that a drug's approval for distribution and sale is not necessarily a testimony either to its effectiveness or its safety. One of the reasons is that the FDA does not do its own research on each drug before it is unleashed upon the world. It is dependent upon the pharmaceutical companies to do their own trials and report them. But as we have seen these trials may be neither honest nor reliable. Such research cannot be other than self-interested, and moreover evidence obtained through the Freedom of Information Act indicates there may be cooperation between some FDA officials and the manufacturers of these drugs. As we have seen, when drugs are approved they often have to be withdrawn within a year or two of release, occasioned by the serious outcomes and even deaths.

But we need also to look at the method of prescribing drugs. In an individual doctor's practice how can he or she, in 5 or 10 minutes, find out much about one's health? And do doctors even ask the right questions? Furthermore they will know even less about whether their prescriptions work or not. In an entire lifetime, during short periods of which I have had some association with orthodox medicine, I only once had a physician ring me up to see how the treatment, the drug I had been prescribed, worked.[21] Other things they could do is arrange for a nurse to ring, or ask patients to fill out and return a questionnaire so as to determine whether the prescribed treatment was of the slightest use, or worse, had done any damage. I would submit that anyone truly interested in healing people has to do this.

Drugs	Vitamins	Possible mechanisms	Possible Manifestations
Anticonvulsants	Folacin	Decreased absorption Competitive inhibition of vitamin co-enzymes Enzyme induction	Megaloblastic anaemia
	Vitamin D	Enzyme induction Enzyme induction	Rickets, osteomalacia Neonatal haemorrhage
Cholestyramine	Folacin Vitamin B$_{12}$	Complexation of the vitamin Inhibition of intrinsic factor function	
	Vitamin A Vitamin D Vitamin K	Binding of bile salts	Osteomalacia
Colchicine	Vitamin B$_{12}$	Absorptive enzyme damage Damage to the intestinal wall	
Courmarin Anticoagulants	Vitamin K	Unknown	Haemorrhage
Estrogen containing oral contraceptives	Folacin	Inhibition of absorptive enzymes Increased synthesis of folate binding macroglobulin	Megaloblastic anaemia
	Vitamin B$_{12}$	Change in tissue oxygenase distribution	
	Vitamin B$_6$	Induction of trytophan enzyme Competition of vitamin binding sites of apoenzyme	Depression

	Riboflavin
	Thiamin
	Vitamin C
		Unknown
		Unknown
		Decreased absorption
		Increased ceruloplasmin
		   concentration
		Increased concentration of
		   reducing compounds
		Changes in tissue distribution	

Glutethimide	Vitamin D	Enzyme induction	Osteomalacia
Hydralazine	Vitamin B$_6$	Increased excretion; vitamin- drug complex	Peripheral neuropathy
Irritant cathartics	Vitamin D	Increased peristalsis Damage to the intestinal wall	Osteomalacia

Isoniazid	Vitamin B$_6$	Increased excretion; vitamin-
		   drug complex
			Peripheral neuropathy
			Generalized convulsion
			   infants
			Anaemia

Drugs	Vitamins	Possible mechanisms	Possible Manifestations
	Niacin	Competitive inhibition of vitamin co-enzymes Secondary to Vitamin B_6 deficiency	Pellagra
Methotrexate	Folate	Inhibition of dihydrofolate reductase enzyme	Megaloblastic anaemia
Mineral oil	Folate Vitamin A Vitamin D Vitamin K	Lipid solvent	Rickets
Neomycin	Vitamin B_{12} Vitamin A	Damage to the intestinal wall Inhibition of intrinsic factor function Damage to the intestinal wall Inhibition of pancreatic lipase Binding of the bile salts	
Para-amino Salicylic	Vitamin B_{12}	Decreased absorption	Megaloblastic anaemia
Pencillamine	Vitamin B_6	Increased excretion, vitamin-drug complex	periperhal naturopathy
Potassium Chloride	Vitamin B_{12}	Decreased ilea pH	
Pyrimethamine	Folacin	Inhibition of dihydrofolate reductase enzyme	Megaloblastic anaemia
Salicylates	Folacin Vitamin C Vitamin K	Decreased protein binding Decreased uptake in thrombocyotes & leukocytes Unknown	
Sulphasalzine	Folacin	Decreased absorption	
Tetracycline	Vitamin C	Increased absorption	
Triamterene	Folacin	Inhibition of dihydrofolate reductase enzyme	Megaloblastic anaemia
Trimethoprim	Folacin	Inhibition of dihydrofolate reductase enzyme	Megaloblastic anaemia

Does the fact that doctors do not 'follow up' in this way mean they just assume their 'remedy' is appropriate and safe? Does it mean that they are not aware of how different people may react uniquely to different substances? (As we noted in an earlier chapter, the phrase 'side-effects' is a euphemism for 'bad things that happen to you when you take a drug'. And there may be plenty, both short term, which are obvious, and long term, which are not so obvious.) Does it mean that the 5 or 10 minutes doctors give us is all they are prepared to give? Does it mean that they have implicit faith in the hype, the promotion, the often questionable trials and studies which go both to prop up and to promote the billion-dollar pharmaceutical industry? Or does it mean that they don't *want* to know if their remedies don't work?

One cannot assume that because a patient does not return it is because he or she has been cured. That is only one possibility. It could be that the patient did not get better and went elsewhere. It could be that the patient tried the medication and had such negative effects that the rest went down the toilet (or preferably, for the environment's sake, into the rubbish). It could be that the problem resolved itself before the drug was even started. It could be that the patient was too embarrassed to say that the remedy had not worked. In today's irrational climate, many feel inadequate about their ability (or inability) to heal. There are numerous possibilities.

How can doctors, people who pride themselves on their 'science', actually function the way they do? Someone from Mars, or that person from the middle of the next century, would say that this is a practice based on faith and/or carelessness. But it cannot be a practice based on 'science'.

When considering efficacy, or whether drugs work, the treatments for rheumatoid arthritis come readily to mind. In 1993 Dr Alan Gaby MD[22] pointed out that the *Family Practice News* of October 1992 had published a debate on the efficacy of the so-called 'anti-rheumatic' drugs. These would be prednisone, gold injections, methotrexate, sufasalazine or hydroxychloroquine, all designed to halt the joint destruction and deformity associated with rheumatoid arthritis. But there was in fact no evidence that any of them did any good. *Family Practice News*:

Ten years after initiating treatment, virtually no rheumatoid arthritis patients still take these medications, either because they do not work or because of side effects. A recent international medical congress held in Europe proposed that none of the drugs used for rheumatoid arthritis should be classified as disease modifying.

In plain language, they are all useless.

And yet still the rheumatologists go on prescribing them, for lack of anything else to do. Dr Gaby calls it 'an epidemic of quackery'. Dr Gaby himself has seen many complete remissions from rheumatoid arthritis, but not from the above-mentioned drugs. He eliminates allergenic foods from the diet and uses appropriate supplements. He says,

I would agree that these treatments are also unproven, but I would rather achieve remissions with relatively safe unproven remedies than not achieve remissions with relatively toxic unproven remedies. It is the height of hypocrisy for ... apologists for the ineffective and dangerous conventional approach to call these alternative methods 'quackery'.

One of the arguments they use is that patients lose valuable time pursuing alternatives, while their joints continue to deteriorate. That argument would not be so ludicrous if the arthritis establishment had a clue about how to arrest or retard joint destruction.

There is other evidence that the usual anti-inflammatory drugs for all kinds of arthritis may initially help with the pain, but the long-term effect is to make things worse. The gut will deteriorate and the body will overall decline further under the toxic load of the drugs. As we noted in the chapter on aspirin, the *New England Journal of Medicine* reported on a study which revealed that aspirin is implicated in the development of emphysema, or lung disease.[23] And there are several other possible problems.

The world's best anti-inflammatory substance is, in fact, fresh ginger root, and it can do no harm in either the short or the long term. Cultures which use ginger often, fresh and in their cooking, seldom suffer arthritis (provided other foods are not faulty). As in the discussion at the end of Chapter 3, one can take it in *very* tiny pieces, washed down with water, if necessary. Or add it grated to other beverages, for example with a tea.

And there are numerous other substances which have anti-inflammatory effects without the serious long-term problems that drugs may pose. For example: bromelain from pineapple (taken between meals); zinc, creatine, D-phenylalanine; L-tryptophan; DL-valine; vitamin E; querticin; chromotrypsin and several herbs, including feverfew (taken with meals).

Sometimes drugs and procedures are used for decades because of medical habit rather than as a result of sound studies. For example, it was standard procedure for many years to administer lidocaine in hospital when someone had a heart attack. But after decades of this, 14 controlled trials revealed that those patients receiving lidocaine had a significantly higher death rate than those not receiving it.[24] (I would like to see a controlled trial of cayenne, magnesium and vitamins C and E immediately following heart attack. What are my chances?!)

And as mentioned, similarly, for decades full mastectomies (breast removal) were done for breast cancer, including often the nodes under the arms, to the subsequent severe discomfort and misery of the patients. Then, after over 50 years of doing this, they finally tried removing only the lump. The consequences were about the same for each procedure (that is, not often a good long-term outcome). But clearly there had been nothing we could call 'science' involved in the mastectomy procedure. Just as with the bypass procedure, someone started doing it, and because it called upon skills and was well paid, it was continued on through time.

In the chapter on cholesterol we looked briefly at the fallacies in connection with health and cholesterol levels. There were, of course, and still are, widespread attempts to lower cholesterol with drugs, despite the trials that revealed that total heart deaths were about the same in the drug-treated and non-drug-treated groups, and further evidence that lowering cholesterol increases one's risk of cancer, impotence, suicide and the likelihood of violent behaviour developing.

There were various other disasters as well: In the gemfibrozel test, there was vertigo (dizziness), skin problems and a decrease in the white cell counts. On the drug cholestyramine there was a 700% increase in colon cancer. On clofibrate there was an increase in total deaths of 36%, half of them from cancer. There are 12 such trials discussed in the book *The Cholesterol Conspiracy*,[25] none of them reassuring. But owing to the faulty idea that cholesterol causes heart attacks, there is always another, 'better, safer' cholesterol-lowering drug coming along to make its creators millions. The latest are now being advertised in news magazines for lay people.

By 1997 $1.93 billion was being spent annually on this direct-to-consumer marketing.

One of these anti-cholesterol wonder drugs, pravastatin, has actually been shown to reduce cholesterol and even heart attacks. That is, there were 50 deaths out of 3,302 in those taking the drug, or 1.5%. And there were 73 deaths among the 3,293 not taking the drug, or 2.2%. That is, the drug is claimed to have reduced deaths at the rate of 30% of those taking it vs those not taking it.

But even supposing the trials were performed correctly and the subjects selected appropriately, the *Physicians' Desk Reference*, the physician's bible, warns of 'serious side-effects'. Governments are now trying to finance huge populations taking this drug. The costs are over US$500 a year per person, plus the costs of all the 'side-effects' which could add considerably to the cost when people are hospitalized. One has to ask whether it is worth it for the claimed 30% reduction in deaths, given that it still leaves 70% unimproved, especially considering the 'patchup costs'.

And as Bill Sardi of Eye Communications says, 'The body threatened with heart disease does not have a shortage of pravastatin; it has a shortage of antioxidants.'[26]

Apparently, even the esteemed *New England Journal of Medicine* once reported on a study establishing that vitamin E reduced the risks of heart disease by 45%. Garlic, niacin, flaxseed oil and magnesium can also reduce the oxidized kind of cholesterol which can become a problem when hardened in the arteries. But over-all, as we have noted, it has been well established that seriously reducing choles-terol levels in the long run increases cancer levels. So what will be the total cost of the drug pravastatin in the long term?

It has been established that these anti-cholesterol drugs actually reduce the body's production of Coenzyme Q10 (that is, ubiquinone), essential for cardiac function. This finding was presented at the Spring 1994 Conference of the American College of Advancement in Medicine held in Minneapolis by Dr Folkers from the University of Texas. His research established that congestive heart fail-ure's main symptom was a CoQ10 deficiency.[27] Dr Warren Levin MD of New York recommends that CoQ10 should always be given with anti-cholesterol drugs. One is tempted to suggest that CoQ10 and other nutrients be given *instead* of these drugs.[28]

When we look at the long-term results of taking drugs it should give us pause as to the whole concept of putting 'foreign materials' into our bodies. The market-ing of HRT, or hormone replacement therapy, will probably be seen by future generations as the classic example of the primacy of the lust for money over the welfare of women; women's health, women's lives. Oestrogen (either synthetic or from undoubtedly disgruntled, if not long-suffering, mares) has been prescribed for menopausal symptoms since the 1970s, and is a multi-million dollar industry.

There is no question that in many, oestrogen helps with menopausal symp-toms. But Dr Michael T Murray ND, author of numerous books, lecturer, and edi-tor of the *American Journal of Natural Medicine*, when researching this topic[29] found evidence in the most prestigious and respected of medical journals (*The New England Journal of Medicine* and the *Journal of the American Medical Association* to name but two) of associations between HRT, oestrogen therapy, and an increase in the risk of endometrial cancer (in the lining of the womb) and breast cancer.[30]

Thus these studies and the associated implications of risk have been in print in the most reputable medical journals, starting in 1988. But the HRT prescrip-tions to women continue. The massive Harvard Nurses Health Study (of 85,095 nurses)[31] established that the risks of breast cancer increase in women taking HRT. A recent article in the *Lancet*, based on even more recent studies, warned that the risk of breast cancer increases after five years of usage.[32] In fact this leading medi-cal journal advises '*these findings create an ethical responsibility*' for physicians to advise women of this risk. But not to worry, for the most part doctors and women have been advised to continue on as usual and await the major study on women's health presently being conducted by the American National Institute of Health, the results of which will be available in the year 2007! Meanwhile no one's profits will be affected.

However, the truth about oestriol, synthetic oestrogen, did not need to be established with human guinea pigs. It had already been established in the laboratory by 1977:

When added to long-term culture of human breast cancer cells, estriol stimulated their growth, and overcame the anti-oestrogenic effects of tamoxifen, even at concentrations hundreds of times lower than that of tamoxifen. The data do not support an anti-oestrogenic role for estriol in human breast cancer.[33]

But it is not only oestrogen that has been implicated in breast cancer, but also beta-blockers and antidepressants.[34] And as we went to press, the *NZ Herald* published an account of the latest study on oestrogen replacement therapy (from the University of California, San Francisco). These drugs have also been recommended for the prevention of heart attacks in women. But this study found that women on HRT actually suffered more heart attacks during the first year but had fewer heart attacks later. Make of that what you can.

In Europe, where doctors are not quite as subservient to the great pharmaceutical companies, menopausal women are more likely to be prescribed the far safer and just as effective herb black cohosh (*Cimifuga racemosa*).[35] The BGA, the German counterpart to the US Food and Drug Administration, has approved this herb as *Remifemin*, for menopausal symptoms. But in the English-speaking countries only herbalists, naturopaths and innovative doctors know how to cope with menopausal symptoms without risky drug-taking. (In fact, taking in phyto-oestrogens, that is plant based oestrogen-like substances such as soya, is another way of resolving these symptoms. Asian women have been doing this for centuries and they hardly know what 'the menopause' is.)

However, unfortunately medical journals garner considerable revenue from carrying advertisements for drugs (just as they once did for advertising cigarettes). They are therefore not likely to give much consideration to safer and cheaper alternatives.

The whole concept of drugs goes well with that of conquering and controlling Nature, like the idea of bombing and blitzing the land into submission with pesticides and fertilizers. It is a way of seeing both nature and the body as machines to control, instead of something almost sacred to work with gently, to encourage the body's own healing systems. We can do this only with herbs, homoeopathy and other traditional remedies, or by making up our numerous dietary deficiencies.

However, inasmuch as there are **fallacious stories or gross exaggerations planted at regular intervals in the media** about the alleged 'risks' of herbs (actually less than 1% as risky as drugs), people have been denied these safe and simple remedies. In the US during the seven-year period from 1983 to 1989 there were

2,069 reported fatalities resulting from legal pharmaceutical drugs; in the same period total fatalities from use of vitamin and mineral supplements amounted to one (later deemed a reporting error.)[36]

For 1991, a characteristic year, the actual numbers of poisonings between drugs on the one hand, and herbs and vitamins on the other, as recorded by poison control centres in the US were as follows[37]:

Herbs		Supplements	
Ginseng (Ren Shen)	0	Vitamin A	0
Echinacea	0	Vitamin C	0
Dandelion	0	Vitamin D	0
Astraguli	0	Vitamin E	0
Angelica (Dong Gui)	0	Iron	0
Rehmanniae	0	Zinc	0
Bupleuri	0	Vitamin B, B Complex	0
Polygoni Multiflori	0	Calcium	0
Goldenseal	0	Magnesium	0
Hawthorn	0	Potassium	0
Total	**0**	**Total**	**0**

Pharmaceuticals*	
Analgesics	2,669
Antidepressants	517
Antihistamines	412
Antimicrobials	953
Asthma Therapies	257
Cardiovascular Drugs	370
Cough and Cold Preparations	1,526
Gastrointestinal Preparations	619
Hormones and Hormone Antagonists	488
Anti-Anxiety/Anti-Psychotics	888
Topicals	1,106
Total	**9,805**

* Some of the poisonings were considered suicide attempts. The US Poison Control Centers do not differentiate such factors when gathering yearly totals. Presumably no one attempts suicide with herbs and vitamins; or if they do, do not succeed.

But apart from the deaths there are other kinds of damage drugs can do. Ten thousand children paid the lifelong price of dreadful deformity because the drug thalidomide was declared 'safe' by the FDA. And some of *their* children are now paying a similar price. That is, thalidomide may have caused a permanent alteration in the DNA.

After the disaster became apparent, the manufacturers of thalidomide were **acquitted on the grounds that research on animals could not reliably predict how a drug would affect human beings.** And still the animals are experimented on, tortured, often at length, and later 'sacrificed', as they say. Animal experimentation is a multi-billion dollar business.[38] And will someone please tell me what is the point of torturing and killing all these animals if drugs are to be released on the basis of trials with them, and then when disaster strikes the manufacturer will be excused on the grounds that the drug had been tried out only on animals?

Sometimes, as with HRT prescriptions, it can take a while to learn the disastrous consequences. With DES, diethylstilbesterol, it took a whole generation. This was a synthetic oestrogen used for all 'female problems'. When I was living in the US and expecting my second son, large-scale double-blind studies had already shown that DES **did not prevent abortion and premature birth**, but the FDA took no action. I was prescribed huge doses of the stuff because I had formerly had a premature birth. In fact the FDA permitted it to be used for that purpose and many others for **another 20 years.**[39] How's that for kind consideration to the pharmaceutical manufacturers and absolutely no consideration for the lives of the women involved, or for their offspring?

The story of the failure of the FDA to act in an appropriate manner over this drug is outlined in a book already mentioned, *Our Stolen Future* by T Colburn *et al.* (NY: Dutton/Penguin, 1996).

As a consequence of the FDA's delinquency, thousands of female infants who had been exposed to DES in the uterus later died as young women, of vaginal cancer. Fortunately for me I had a son who, as a male, was not obviously affected by the DES, or at least not physically so far. However, I do not believe I escaped without consequences myself. Other women given this drug have suffered cancer, infertility, miscarriages and blood clots. And no one can predict the total long-term effects. While as for the offspring, exposed in the uterus, there has been cancer, infertility and deformities even unto *their* children – that is, in the grandchildren of the women who were given the drug.[40]

DES was also a major food additive in the US at the time, because we all got it in milk as well as meat and chicken, it being fed to farm animals to fatten them up. DES was not effectively banned until 1973, but other synthetic hormones have since taken its place.[41]

As a consequence of the DES experiment on women like myself and our children, at least we now have the understanding of 'hand-me-down poisons' –

that is, an awareness that they can cause damage through the placenta, across the generations. Awareness yes, but are we acting upon that awareness?

Dr Raymond Peat is one who believes that **those who do such great harm with drugs should not get off scot free with their billions in profits, but should be held responsible**. He believes that the deaths from DES and other drugs should be regarded as 'aggravated homicide'. He says,

If those who kill hundreds and thousands for the sake of billions of dollars in profits are not committing 'aggravated homicide', then it must be that no law written in the English language can be objectively interpreted, and the legal system is an Alice in Wonderland convenience for the Corporate State.[42]

I would agree with this view, because if both the drug companies and the FDA were held responsible they would perhaps then be more careful with people's health, people's lives. And moreover, this should also most emphatically apply to the food industry and others.

Another aspect to consider and a reason that drugs are a major cause of death in the Western world: often with drugs, the dangerous or lethal dose is sometimes too close for comfort to the safe dose. Dr Alan Gaby MD, writes about such dangers inherent in prescribing:

In a letter to the *New England Journal of Medicine* (May 27, 1993), Dr Klaus D Hoffman MD, pointed out that a previous article on cancer chemotherapy contained an important dosing error. Instead of recommending that a certain combination of drugs be given '*every three to four weeks*', the article recommended that the treatment be given '*three to four times weekly*'.[43]

The former dose was 'medically appropriate'; the latter would have been a lethal dose.

Another article pointed out that 'more than 40% of nursing home patients were receiving at least one inappropriate medication, and 10% were receiving two or more inappropriate medications concurrently.'[44]

As we have noted, drugs are often withdrawn within a year of clearance owing to the disastrous side-effects and even deaths that follow. According to Dr Brian Strom, Associate Director of Medicine and Pharmacology, University of Pennsylvania School of Medicine:

10 to 20% of all drugs cause adverse side effects, ranging from nausea and skin rashes to fatal outcomes ... Every year in the US they put 1.6 million people in hospital and kill up to 160,000 Americans at an annual cost of over $20 billion.[45]

Dr Strom continues, 'No drug is absolutely safe. Among older Americans who use 40% of all prescribed drugs, the problem of drug-induced illness is especially severe.'

Further facts on prescribing for the elderly are as follows:

More than 240,000 older Americans are hospitalized annually and hundreds of thousands more are subjected to dizziness or fainting spells due to drug reactions.
From a total of 200,000 hip fractures annually in American senior citizens, among these are approximately 32,000 attributed to drug-induced falls, and many of these hip fractures lead to death. One study for the National Institute of Aging found that people on long-life tranquillizers (prescribed for 30% of geriatric cases) had a 70% greater risk of hip fracture than those on short-life tranquillizers or no drugs at all.[46]
More than 163,000 older adults suffer from memory loss or impaired thinking from prescription drugs, and another 61,000 develop drug-induced Parkinson's disease.

A 1987 US Government survey reported that 'nearly one fourth of elderly patients were taking prescription drugs that, according to many experts, were generally unsuitable for their age group.' This study did not include potentially dangerous drug interactions, or incorrect dosages.[47] A 1992 study found that 17.5% of 30 million Medicare recipients was on at least one unsuitable drug, when safer alternative drugs could have given them the same benefits with fewer side-effects. Even the conservative FDA has estimated that the annual cost to the US of inappropriate prescription drug use is $20 billion in hospitalizations.

There are figures from three different countries to show that when the drug-prescribing doctors go on strike, the death rates actually go down,[48] while, as mentioned above, the overall figures from the effects of drugs and from incorrectly prescribed drugs are horrendous. We delude ourselves if we think prescription drugs are safe. And all the time the medical mafia which controls the media is spreading fear and misinformation about the terrifying effects of herbs and vitamins!

And if one has the temerity to mention to most doctors anything as a remedy that is not a prescription drug, one will more than likely hear the tired old chestnut they get at medical school, about 'the toilets getting all the expensive vitamins'. Just what on earth do they think happens to most of their far more expensive drugs? The body secretes anything it does not or cannot use. **The major part of every drug we take ends up in the toilet**. And if we were to ask the planet which it would prefer its waterways to be polluted by – herbs, vitamins and homoeopathic remedies or drugs – I think we know what the answer would be.

I am reminded of the quotes I put at the head of one chapter when I wrote *The Mile-High Staircase*.[49] At the time I was speaking of I was sceptical of the effects of drugs, having already had several unpleasant experiences with them.

Learning the truth about DES was only one. So in my chapter about drugs, 'The Magic Bullet', I prefaced it with the following quotes:

'No families take so little medicine as those of doctors, except those of apothecaries,'[50] (Oliver Wendell Holmes, *Medical Essays*); while Dr Richard Clarke Cabot writing in the *Journal of the American Medical Association* said,

I believe that we not only feed the public demand for useless and harmful drugs, but also go far to create that very demand. We educate our patients and their friends to believe that every or almost every symptom can be benefited by a drug.[51]

In Cabot's day there was still debate over the nature of human health. You would not find these remarks in the *JAMA* today.

'Half the modern drugs could well be thrown out the window, except that the birds might eat them.' (Martin H Fischer, *Fischerisms.*)

'Some drugs have been appropriately called "wonder drugs" inasmuch as one wonders what they will do next.'[52]

And someone who dared not give his name wrote, 'A drug is a substance that, when injected into a rat, produces a scientific paper.'

Much earlier, Molière most tellingly wrote: 'Nearly all men die of their medicines, not their diseases.'

Most important of all, George Bernard Shaw had the most positive comment:

Nature has provided ... in the phagocytes ... a natural means of ... destroying all disease germs. There is at bottom only one genuinely scientific treatment for all diseases, and that is to stimulate the phagocytes. Drugs are a delusion.[53]

What Shaw meant by 'phagocytes' was essentially our immune system. That is, he was saying in 1913 what many have not yet caught up with today, 86 years on. It is my belief that he was absolutely right. The future belongs to those healers who can assist and strengthen this system, our natural defence against all problems.

In any event, that chapter in *The Mile-High Staircase* described my experiences of being terribly ill in a Sydney hospital where I was regarded as quite mad because I had a drawer full of supplements, and because they did not know what was wrong with me. Of course the supplements didn't do me any good, either, because what I desperately needed at that time was to be 'detoxified' but 20 years ago I knew nothing of that, and today, possibly only 1% of the medical profession does. Drugs are the thing. In most cases, the only thing. Meanwhile the World Health Organization calculates that 33% of all disease is caused by medical treatment.[54]

Robe Carson believes that the long-term taking of drugs can cut 20 years off our lives.[55] In fact the most pessimistic view is that the chemical, heavy metal and food industries pollute our environment and damage our foods, which deadly combination subsequently afflicts our health. And then medicine creates toxic drugs to 'cure us' of the ensuing ravages.[56]

For rational health care and the welfare of millions, it is long past time that proper studies were done to test the overall effectiveness and safety of all drugs presently in use. They should be done in comparison with the safer, more natural methods and they should be done by those with no vested or personal interest in the outcome. At the present time, only small-scale trials of herbs and supplements can be undertaken because of the costs involved. And as Dr Gaby says:

Many effective, safe, and inexpensive natural treatments are frozen out of the market, because no one is willing to put up $231 million to develop an unpatentable product. The FDA approval process has caused American medicine to fall further and further behind.[57]

The question we all should be asking is, **WHY does it cost $231 million to test these substances?** Is not human health, are not human lives at stake? It is quite clear that no one is going to put up $231 million to establish that magnesium or B_6 is kind to the heart and could possibly compete and win against all drugs for the cardio-vascular system, because no one will make a fortune out of it. And it is plain to see why drugs are so expensive.

But people are dying unnecessarily because of such greed and ignorance.

Dr Alan R Gaby says this: 'As multi-billion dollar drug companies become ever more aggressive at marketing their overpriced and sometimes dangerous drugs, informing the public about safe, effective, and inexpensive alternatives becomes increasingly important.'[58]

There is no doubt in my mind as to where the truth lies about drugs vs more natural methods, despite the tight control on health information in the media exerted by those interested in keeping things the way they are. For in my own experience it is possible to improve the health of almost anyone with a health problem *without using prescription drugs*. I have done it many times. As we will note in Chapter 32, severe pain is always best dealt with by orthodox medicine; advanced diabetes would be another exception, and a few acute or rare diseases, but even those situations can be improved with appropriate nutrition, herbs, homoeopathic remedies and supplements.

Moreover, despite the control of the media by pharmaceutical and medical interests there is widespread dissatisfaction with drugs at some levels of the population, mostly the better educated, and a turning back to older, safer methods. Professor Edzard Ernst of the University of Exeter recently reported that (despite massive 'anti-herb propaganda') between 1990 and 1997 there was a 380% increase in the use of herbal treatments in the US. While in Germany total annual sales of herbal medicines are calculated at \$3.4 billion and \$1.1 billion in France.[59] These sales are primarily among the better-educated who are growing cautious about the use of prescription drugs. And they would hardly be buying them unless they worked.

In response to this, some of the big pharmaceutical companies can see the handwriting on the wall. One has recently bought into a major producer of supplements. When people make their preferences known, the big boys will of course go where the money is. And we should be sending them in the right direction.

The most commonly treated problem in medicine today is hypertension (high blood pressure) which is widespread and tends to be a harbinger, a forerunner of heart disease. In 1986 Dr N M Kaplan MD had calculated that over 30 million Americans suffer with hypertension.[60]

The American National High Blood Pressure Education Program was begun around 1973. Since then the number of patients with hypertension has increased from 51% of a doctor's practice to 84%.[61] This means either more awareness or more high blood pressure. Whichever it is, the percentage of patients with high blood pressure taking medication has increased in this period from 36% to 73%. Thus the most frequently prescribed drugs in medicine today are against high blood pressure.

Most doctors today have simply no idea *what actually causes* high blood pressure or heart attacks in the first place, the 'unexplained being the unexamined'. Thoughtful people, prepared to seek for these answers with open minds, might point to the fact that the world for the most part had no significant problem with high blood pressure or heart attacks until around 1926. And that the significant increase occurred soon after the changes in our fats and oils.

Others might see that there was another surge soon after our milk was homogenized. But despite the evidence in the medical journals, and we looked at this evidence in the first three chapters, most doctors do not look to the environment, the terrain, for the reasons. For when the world contains primarily drugs as a means of 'cure', many categories of causation are simply ignored. And one has to realize that it will not be just purveyors of fats and oil and homogenized milk who will be affected if people change their habits and cure their long-standing heart and blood pressure problems. There is no money to be made either by medicine or the pharmaceutical companies in that.

So what has happened to this problem of high blood pressure? The drugs taken in their millions have at the very least not resolved the problem they are given for. For in only 21% of those who take these drugs is the blood pressure brought close to the ideal of 140/90 or below.[62]

As of 1993, there were 68 drugs in eight therapeutic classifications used for this problem.[63] In 1995, 6 million Americans took 87.3 million prescriptions for **calcium channel blockers** to treat high blood pressure and angina. In 1992 the journal *Hypertension* had actually put forward the view that these FDA-approved drugs may actually *cause* heart attacks: 'They may adversely affect carbohydrate and/or lipid metabolism in such a way as to increase the risk of atherosclerosis or heart disease.'[64] (We had a look at calcium and the medical advocacy of *taking it in*, in Chapter 3, with reference to the epidemics of osteoporosis, PMS and heart attacks in women.)

In any event the heart attacks continue unabated. Almost half of us are dying from heart disease. Almost all of us know someone who has recently died of a heart attack, and the chances are she or he was, at the time, on prescription drugs to prevent it.

⚠

28: MAMMOGRAMS

'The answer to breast cancer!'

In little New Zealand, approximately 600 women die every year from breast cancer.

There is a common fallacy that goes: 'The earlier we catch cancer, the more likely we are to survive.' But under the present methods of diagnosis and treatment there is no study, not a statistic anywhere to prove this shibboleth.

In fact, in the case of mammograms at least, there is evidence that a diagnostic technique may actually *increase* cancer deaths.

On June 2, 1991, the *London Times* headlined: **BREAST SCANS BOOST RISK OF CANCER DEATHS**.

There had been a Canadian study, a gigantic effort to establish that mammograms would increase life expectancy by diagnosing women earlier. In this study, 89,835 women were *randomly assigned* to either the group receiving regular mammograms or the group receiving none. But after only 8 years it was clear that the women in the group receiving mammograms had 50% *more* deaths from breast cancer than those not receiving them. The possibility exists that screening detects precancerous conditions that would not otherwise turn into cancer without the exposures to radiation,[1] and/or that the subsequent 'treatments' are killing women *more so than if nothing is done*, or possibly both.

There were strenuous attempts to suppress the findings of this study. But fortunately there are always those who care more for their fellows than they do for profiteering.

As early as 1985 the phenomenon had already been written up from other studies in Britain's most prestigious medical journal, the *Lancet*.[2] And whatever the cause, the incidence of breast cancer has increased by at least 30% in the US since the 1970s when the National Cancer Institute *began* the mass screening programmes.[3]

In Britain the medical community was sufficiently alarmed about the lack of progress in the diagnosis and treatment of breast cancer that in 1993 the *Lancet* called an international conference – 'The Challenge of Breast Cancer' – to be held in Brugge, Belgium, in 1994. The *Lancet* editorial announcing this said of screening tests:

'There are no reliable data to suggest that screening reduces mortality in the youngest or oldest age groups,' while it continued to advocate testing in the middle or the 50-to-64 age group.

As the probing type of studies, like the Canadian one mentioned, are seldom done, the situation may be that we cannot truly know whether more modern screening techniques are safer or not.

Back in 1978 I was working with health statistics. After looking over the cancer statistics and finding not an iota of true improvement in breast cancer deaths in 40 years, it looked to me as though people were in more recent times being diagnosed two years earlier and that those two years were being added on to alleged survival time. But it could not mean that women were living longer. It just meant they knew about the cancer which would change their lives two years longer. As mentioned in the chapter on root canal-treated teeth, I also noticed the astounding fact that middle-class women had more breast cancer than so-called working-class women. I therefore wrote to New Zealand's feminist journal, *Broadsheet*, imploring women to avoid high-tech medicine, to stop the worrying self-examination and to concentrate on preventive measures. I advised them to eat less meat and dairy, to increase fruits and vegetables, to take more exercise and so on.

As a result of this letter there were terrible outcries over the airwaves, and everywhere my name was mud. 'Early diagnosis' was critical, said my opponents. Clearly my letter had been addressed to those who did not have breast cancer, and I had foolishly not foreseen the effect it would have on those already diagnosed. I knew then that if I entered the debate I would have to point the finger at the efficacy of conventional cancer treatment, to the distress of many involved in it. I would sow doubt, but I could in the long run make no impact. It was a battle no individual could win, no matter what the statistics. Hence I did not reply.

But of course the statistics that so worried me in 1978 and ever since have been available to the entire medical profession. Either they do not look at their own statistics, read their own literature, or they wish to have 'something to do' for cancer, even if it is useless. But they must face up to the fact that *most* medically-approved cancer treatment, for *most* conditions, is *worse than useless*. In fact, *it is often harmful, and accelerates death*. (More on this in the next chapter.)

I still stand by every word I said in my letter of 1978. Since then the incidence of breast cancer has increased by 30%, and the death rate *still* has not improved since the 1930s.

Today in the face of ever-increasing assaults on our immune systems it is even more important now than it was in 1978 to live our lives with the goal of nurturing this all-important defence system against cancer. This book suggests many things *to avoid* – and there is, of course, a more pro-active approach which I will write about later.

In the mean time, for treatment suggestions, see page 238 at the end of Chapter 30.

⚠

29: THE BRA

'A brilliant invention that gives women a lift
both physically and mentally. It is also perfectly harmless.'

You may not believe this one, but two medical anthropologists went to a lot of trouble to establish the fact that wearing a bra for long periods will actually increase a woman's chances of getting breast cancer. They interviewed 4,700 women, with and without breast cancer, in five major US cities, with startling results.

When they had put all their statistical data through the computer, they then established the fact that women who wear a bra more than 12 hours per day are 19 times more likely to develop breast cancer than women who wear a bra fewer than 12 hours a day.

Moreover, women who wear their bras all the time, even to sleep in, or virtually 24 hours a day, have a 113-fold increase in breast cancer incidence when compared with women who wear their bras fewer than 12 hours a day. Moreover, in the 'braless' countries such as among African, Asian, Egyptian and Native American people, there are far lower rates of breast cancer.[1] Of course there would doubtless be other reasons also, such as much lower levels of sugar in their diets, no TFAs, etc.

The possible reason breast cancer increases with bra wearing may be that by artificially constricting the breasts the bra suppresses the body's lymphatic system for flushing accumulated wastes from the body, causing toxins to accumulate in breast tissues, creating an environment ripe for a host of health problems.[2] Well, it is also a fact that if men wear their jeans too tight they can get cancer in some vital part.

If you'd like to check up on this, the researchers Sidney Singer and Soma Grismaijer have written a book entitled *Dressed to Kill: The Link Between Breast Cancer & Bras*.[3]

So perhaps we weren't so crazy to 'burn our bras' in the early seventies? Not that we really did. Vanity usually came before ideology, unless one was rather on the thin side.

Of course when this study first came out early in 1996 I wrote letters to all the papers to warn women. But none of the papers would print them. Wonder why?

More along these lines in the body torture department, the Harvard Medical School has just released the results of a survey to do with the effects of wearing high-heeled shoes. They cause a strain on the knees, in fact on the whole muscular-skeletal system. The result: eventual arthritis in the knees and elsewhere.[4]

Well, what to do? Barefoot and braless?

30: CANCER

'So now you've got cancer ... we'll fix you up
with surgery, radiation and chemotherapy.'

I'm trying to remember a terrible old joke about cancer. I think it goes: 'Saliva causes cancer, but only if you swallow a little now and then.'

It's difficult to find anything to smile at about cancer. It's the curse of the late 20th century, after heart disease. It did, of course, exist before, but it was rare. I remember my old doctor friend telling me, speaking of the period 1940 to around 1970, that he hardly ever came across a cancer patient. He was, perhaps, trying to reassure a worried mind, but whereas cancer deaths in 1900 were one in 50, today's estimate is nearly one in three women,[1] and one in four or five men, and that is increasingly the situation almost all over the English-speaking world.

In New Zealand, 'cancer is a growing disease, with death rates rising faster than in other countries.' Dr Brian Cox of the Otago Medical School says that the incidence of diagnosed cancer is expected to increase by 40% in 2005, relative to 1990. Moreover, in this period there will be a 27% increase in deaths from cancer.[2] To put it in actual numbers, each year in a country of 3.9 million, 6,200 women and 6,100 men develop cancer, while 3,280 women and 3,750 men die from it. However, the actual cancers which are increasing most are prostate cancer in men and lung cancer in women. But the overall rates of increase are 'more pronounced in women than in men'.[3] What is worse, of the 12,000 cases[4] developing each year, over 100 are new cases in children.

Meanwhile, in the US there is one death from cancer every minute, and the disease accounts for $200 billion of the nation's nearly trillion-dollar-per-year disease care bill.[5]

In particular, the enormous number of victims of breast cancer constitutes an epidemic far greater than AIDS and many other diseases. There is some disagreement over the statistics on this, but they range from a projected one in nine to one in seven women to get breast cancer, with one-half of those affected dying from the disease within a year of diagnosis.[6] The incidence has actually increased by 30% since mass screening began.[7] (See Chapter 28 on mammograms).

According to Liane Clorfene-Casten, who wrote the book *Breast Cancer: Poisons, Profits and Prevention*,

Fifty years ago, a woman's chance of getting breast cancer in her lifetime was one in 20. Thirty-five years ago, it was one in 15. A few years ago, when breast cancer began to garner some publicity, the chance was one in nine. Now it is one in eight.[8]

Whatever the figures, it is a rising epidemic and should be considered as such.

In fact, these statistics don't really tell the story. Let's look at the actual numbers: Today, there are 130 million women living in the US. Of these, more than 16 million will develop breast cancer. There are 300,000 new cases per year, and 150,000 deaths.[9] In fact, only lung cancer kills more than breast cancer. It should therefore receive at least the kind of media attention and research funding as do far less common diseases.

When we look at the situation with prostate cancer, the male counterpart of breast cancer and the most common cancer in men, the incidence also continues to rise. In 1991 in the US there were 22,000 deaths from prostate cancer.[10] Among men aged 40 to 60, 55% will have some form of prostate problem.[11] A 1982 study at St Bartholemew's Hospital in London showed that 'No therapy yet has been found for prostate cancer that gives a survival rate greater than no treatment at all.'[12] In fact it is possible that no treatment may bring a *greater* survival time.'[13] And this is the same almost right across the board with cancer. (As mentioned, I prefer the use of saw palmetto and sunflower seeds, to prevent it happening in the first place.)

For perhaps the primary aspect to focus on with all cancers is the fact that despite all the horrifically expensive and cruel 'procedures' which have been devised as 'treatments' for cancer in the last 40 years, apart from two uncommon types of cancer (a percentage of those suffering from Hodgkin's disease and childhood leukaemia) the overall mortality rates from any cancers have not changed for the better from 1930 to the present. Quite the reverse.[14] (As far as I can determine, childhood leukaemia is being treated by a plant-based drug, *Vinca rosea*, the Madagascar Periwinkle.) And this despite the fact that if you happen to live five years after diagnosis you are classified as 'cured', which is unfortunate if you live five years and one day. So inasmuch as there was scant treatment in 1930, we have to ask the question, 'Does modern cancer treatment do any good?'

In 1993 Britain's top medical journal, the *Lancet*, with superb honesty answered this question in an editorial on breast cancer:

Some readers may be startled to learn that the overall mortality rate from carcinoma of the breast remains static. If one were to believe all the media hype, the triumphalism of the profession in published research, and the almost weekly miracle breakthroughs trumpeted by the cancer charities, one might be surprised that women are dying at all from this cancer. Most patients with clinically overt breast cancer will die of their metastases if followed for long enough. So if we acknowledge the failures of primary therapy and secondary prevention ... we should not be surprised by the static overall mortality from carcinoma of the breast.[15]

However, despite this frank acknowledgment of failure the whole business of screening and 'treatment' continues. And thus women with breast cancer are victims of a cruel hoax. Cancer is an industry; breast cancer its star performer. In the face of all the above, I find it difficult to believe the New Zealand claim that breast cancer deaths are declining there.

But speaking of cancer in general, the public is urged to seek early medical treatment for it – yet Dr Joseph Beasley MD (Director of the Institute of Health Policy and Practice, Bard College Center; former Chairman of the Department of Demographics and Human Ecology at Harvard University; former Dean of the School of Public Health at Tulane University; and member of the National Commission on Population Growth and the American Future) has established with a study of three decades that **untreated cancer victims tend to live up to four times longer than treated ones**.[16]

This was also reported to the American cancer Society by Dr Hardin B Jones, Researcher at the University of California Department of Medical Physics:

My studies have proved conclusively that untreated cancer victims actually live up to four times longer than treated individuals. For a typical type of cancer (for example of the breast), people who refused treatment lived for an average of twelve and a half years. Those who accepted surgery and other kinds of treatment lived on the average only three years. Beyond a shadow of a doubt, radical surgery on cancer patients does more harm than good.[17]

Dr Beasley adds:

The 'cure' rates most often cited are based only on conventional treatment of the most favourable cases. If the less 'curable' cases are included, therapies are seen, overall, as having little, or even negative impact on cancer patients.[18]

Al Schaefer of International Cancer Victims and Friends says the term 'proven' means 'proven to kill you sooner than the cancer does.'[19]

Oncologists know that 'radical surgery does not extend the life of the patient, but they have nothing else to offer.'[20] Surgery, even a biopsy, can release cancerous cells into the bloodstream. And thus they metastasize – that is, they migrate to other parts and start up other cancerous colonies. This must be how the cancer cells get to the spine in breast cancer patients and cause such an agonizing death. (Of course if a vital function is being cut off by a tumour then the surgery should be received with gratitude, if one wishes a little more time; just as pain relief should be received with gratitude.) But it can never be a solution to the basic problem, because **the tumour is not the problem**. The state of one's immune system is.

Orthodox medicine regards 'the tumour' as 'the disease', a pernicious invader in an otherwise healthy body, to be repelled and demolished; whereas traditional or natural medicine has always regarded it as a total body or systemic problem. For example, radiation weakens the tumour, while at the same time it weakens the body's ability to fight off the tumour. German scientist Dr Joanna Budwig has found that radiation 'destroys membrane integrity'.[21] That is, it destroys the outer wall of our body cells.

Chemotherapy was derived from wartime experiments with nitrogen mustard gas, designed to disable and wreck the enemy. It is immunosuppressive – that is, it weakens one's defences against cancer, and clearly will shorten one's life. It initially appears to help because it shrinks tumours. But the tumour is an adaptive mechanism, the body's way of isolating and encapsulating a very toxic problem. And when we break down that tumour we send the problem all over the body, precipitating the victim's end.[22] In 1990 *Der Spiegel* recorded the German cancer statistician Dr Ulrich Abel's findings on chemotherapy. His conclusion: '**Reduction of tumour mass does not prolong ... survival.**'

In the US, chemotherapy costs an average of $100,000 per patient, and appears to be 'effective' in 2–3% of cancer patients.[23] Moreover, chemotherapy is so very poisonous that some might prefer to die of cancer rather than by such poisoning.

There have been several articles critical of chemotherapy in the medical journals since 1975, but the public does not hear of them.[24] A report in the *Journal of Clinical Oncology* discussed the side-effects of chemotherapy. In the medium dose range, 50% of the patients suffer central nervous system and lung complications. In the high dose range, 61% suffer liver damage, 81% ear damage, 70% kidney damage, 92% 'adverse pulmonary events' (lung damage), and 94% are left with damaged hearts.[25]

From a five-year study of thousands of women taking tamoxifen, a chemotherapeutic agent claimed either to prevent or cure breast cancer, it has been claimed that it could actually *cause* both cancer and blindness in formerly healthy women.[26] This was reported in 1993. More recent studies conflict entirely with each other. Early in 1998 the *Scientific American* triumphantly proclaimed that in trials tamoxifen had decreased breast cancer by 45%. However, within months, reports on studies emanating from Britain and Italy declared not only that it had been useless in preventing breast cancer, but that there had been serious long-term 'side-effects' to the drug. Overall the only true long-term assessment of any modern 'treatment' will lie in the mortality figures. And, once again, in attempting to assess the worth of any study, we must ask the question, 'Cui bono?' Who stands to gain?

Dr Barbara Joseph MD was a practising obstetrician and gynaecologist when she was diagnosed with breast cancer. She was thus a conventional doctor. And yet in her book *My Healing from Breast Cancer*[27] she states unequivocally that she saved her life 'by stepping out of the medical model' and into a different kind of treatment.

She says that self-examination and mammography are useless, as are current treatments:

We are being misled by the medical approach to illness that worships the magic bullets of surgery, radiation and chemotherapy. Cancer is not a deficiency of the latest generation ... antineoplastic wonder drug. Cancer is an end product of a thwarted biological process, a process which is uniquely individual. There are many roads to breast cancer.

Dr Jules Klotter writes,

Doctors often tell people that cancer is due to a genetic predisposition, that it's out of anyone's control, and that the patient can do little to alter the course of the disease outside of accepting chemotherapy, radiation and/or surgery.[28]

While it is true that there are genetic 'markers' or predispositions that appear to go with certain cancers, such as breast and colon cancers, there must be an interaction with other factors taking place, otherwise the incidence would be the same all the time, and that is not the case. With breast cancer always on the increase we have to look to an environmental factor, or factors, for the cause. Barbara Holt, President of the New Zealand Breast Cancer Action Group, said recently at the World Conference on Breast Cancer in July of 1997:

The breast cancer epidemic is spreading and worsening ... some scientists as well as those industries that profit from poisoning the earth deny that there is any environmental connection to cancer. We must remind them that there has been a 350-fold increase in the production of synthetic chemicals in our life-times. Their production and manufacture went from one billion pounds in 1940 to more than 400 billion pounds annually in recent years, with just 10% of new chemicals adequately tested for carcinogenicity.[29]

Dr Peter Greenwald, Director of Cancer Prevention at the US National Cancer Institute, would also challenge the genetic/fatalistic view of cancer. He says that 70% of all cancer can be prevented, that the predominant factor is 'environmental'. He says that 30% are due to smoking; 35% are due to poor diet; and that occupational hazards, pollution, alcohol, prescription drugs and so on take care of the rest. In other words, he believes in a predominantly environmental view of cancer causation.[30] The World Health Organization issues bulletins very much along these lines and declares that cancer is 90% environmentally caused; in other words, cancer is predominantly 'man-made'.

In the *British Medical Journal* of June, 1923, there was a letter from a British doctor who had been practising medicine in Nigeria for 23 years and had found no cancer among his patients.[31] Following this letter there were several letters of concurrence from other long-serving doctors in Africa.[32] Then in 1931, Albert Schweitzer, who had founded his hospital in Gabon in 1913, recorded that he had found no cancer among the native Africans there.[33]

These natives were grain vegetarians (their staples were cassava and millet) who had a minimum of polyunsaturated fats in the diet, certainly no hydrogenated ones. Today there is a group living on a similar diet in the south Philippines islands who have almost no cancer.[34]

In 1960 the Irish surgeon Denis Burkett, working in Uganda, noted the freedom from colon cancer there and attributed it to the high fibre content of their diet. This is in part why we have heard so much about fibre since then. And we noted in Chapter 3 on homogenized milk that there is possibly a correlation between eating red meat and colon cancer.[35] Most groups of vegetarians are nearly free of colon cancer. Unfortunately, after the African natives came into contact with Europeans and adopted their eating habits, they also began to die of cancer.

In 1983, Dr David Horribin of Scotia Pharmaceuticals and Dr Stephen Seely of the University of Manchester reported on a worldwide study on sugar in the diet and breast cancer: the more sugar in the diet, the more breast cancer. For example, the UK has both the highest sugar consumption in the world and the highest death rate from breast cancer; the US has about 80% of the sugar consumption of the UK, and 80% of the breast cancer of the UK; Greece has one-third the sugar consumption and one-third the breast cancer; Japan has one-quarter the sugar consumption and one-quarter the breast cancer.[36] Also, 'Japanese women used to be very free of breast cancer, but when their children grew up in the US, their incidence of the disease became like that of Americans.'[37] So there is plenty of evidence that diet is critical. Why don't we hear more about these studies?

The problem is that most modern doctors give scant recognition to environmental influences on health. And we will be looking at the reasons why this is so in the next chapter. The US doctor-oriented and -controlled Cancer Society was woefully late in coming out against smoking as a cause of cancer, just as the Heart Foundation is and continues to be woefully late in telling the truth about our fats and oils. To this day, the Cancer Society has yet to say a word against a whole range of environmental causes of cancer, many of them quite sufficiently studied. It is only recently that it has started talking about eating fruits and vegetables, which is an admission, at least, that diet can be a factor.

There is nothing mystical about cancer. It is the perfectly logical result of the way we live.

The aforementioned enormous increase in cancer in children (over 100 new cases per year in little New Zealand[38]) has not come about from a wicked fairy at the christening. It is caused by what the children are exposed to from even before conception, and thereafter. This could include: pesticide residues in either partner before conception; mercury vapour from the mother's amalgam fillings; toxic infectious material from root canal-filled teeth; phthalates from PVC plastics which are in just about everything; X-rays and possibly ultrasound of the foetus; diets deficient in Essential Fatty Acids and numerous other nutrients. Some of these are factors which grow cumulatively worse by the generation as more and more carcinogenic substances cross the placenta. And no one can know the synergistic (combined) effects of so many substances we were not designed to cope with.

In the first few chapters of this book we looked at the story on our fats and oils and the fact that there is evidence that hydrogenated polyunsaturated oils, those convenient oils in the clear glass bottles we buy in the supermarket, will actually suppress the immune system, our defence against cancer.

Dr Robert Kradjian MD, author of a best-selling book on breast cancer,[39] is of the opinion that these oils are among the main causes for the soaring breast cancer rates. The intakes of this dangerous substance dramatically increased from the 1960s on, the increased incidence of breast cancer following on behind. These deformed fats may in part be causative factors, in combination with others such as pesticides, sugar consumption, root-canalled teeth and cumulative radiation from fission products.

A British study, the UK National Case Control Study, analysed women diagnosed with breast cancer before the age of 36 and found that the contraceptive pill was correlated with a 40% increase in the risk of developing breast cancer. After eight years the increase in risk rose to 70%. The *New England Journal of Medicine* also reported that post-menopausal women who had taken an oestrogen-only form of Hormone Replacement Therapy had a 30% higher risk of breast cancer.

Those who had taken a formula containing both oestrogen and progestin had a 41% increased risk. Overall, ingesting oestrogen for over five years increased the risk of death from breast cancer by 45%.[40]

As we noted in Chapter 21 on pesticides, there was also a major study on breast cancer carried out in Israel and reported on in the 1970s. It seems that young Israeli women were twice as likely to die from breast cancer as comparable women in other countries. In the course of this study, 'the major modern cause of breast cancer was identified as being the organochlorine group of pesticides (DDT, lindane, chlordane, etc.),'[41] which in Israel was found to be very high in dairy products.

After these substances were banned, the death rate in pre-menopausal Israeli women declined by 34%. And significantly, **Israel in the only country today still experiencing declining death rates from breast cancer. Everywhere else they are soaring.**

Unfortunately, that huge study on the 85,095 nurses we noted in Chapter 1 and elsewhere was looking at heart disease in relation to fats, and bowel cancer in relation to beef consumption.[42] It would have been an ideal time to determine whether those consuming the suspect oils had more of other cancers, particularly more breast cancer. What we need to do is to go back to that study and assess it for cancer deaths in relation to types of fats and oils consumed. And better still, in addition, to suspend all consumption of suspect fats and oils in one group, sugar in another, both in a third group, and see whether the statistics improve. That way we could probably reduce heart disease as well as cancer.

It looks as though many have come up with evidence for numerous environmental influences on breast cancer. Chances are these influences are all contributors. It may be that cancer can follow very large doses of a toxic substance, but also that some cancers are not caused by any one thing but by an accumulation of several substances the body's detox systems cannot handle. It is possible that just about everything we have looked at in this book can cause cancer if the immune system is not up to defending the body, if the body's defences are overwhelmed.

It is often the case with older people that both the wife and husband will get cancer around the same time. There is nothing mystical about this either. Generally the two have been exposed together to the same diets and to many of the same environmental hazards. So it should not be surprising.

But the wife will use cosmetics, hair dyes and take more prescription drugs. She will wear a bra which restricts the flow of the lymphatic system (the system which carries off wastes throughout the body), and she will have more invasive procedures like mammograms. Many of these items are carcinogenic. So she is the one generally more at risk of cancer. (He used to be more at risk of heart disease. But no longer, as we noted in Chapter 3 on milk, the rate of heart disease in women has recently caught up with that in men and surpassed it, probably due to the bad advice to 'eat more dairy for your bones.')

So to refine it still further, anything we were not designed to cope with can cause cancer, depending on how good we are at detoxifying, excreting what we cannot use. And when we consider that we were designed to live in fresh air – which no longer exists any more now that we are down from 30% oxygen in the air when we evolved to 12% oxygen in the worst hit cities today – that we should be living in caves or tree houses, without all the man-made chemicals polluting our living environments; that we should be drinking pure fresh running water (which does not exist anywhere anymore except frozen in the glaciers laid down before the world went mad with poisonous sprays, etc.); and eating fresh uncontaminated fruits and vegetables grown on natural soils (along with nuts, seeds and a little fish and game perhaps), it is plain how far we have strayed from the original 'design'.

The surprising thing to me is not that so many of us get sick with cancer, heart disease and a host of other degenerative diseases, but that any of us stays well at all.

It is as if we were to put treacle, poisons, sugary soda drinks and heavy metals into a thorough-bred Ferrari racing car, and expect it to perform. We, of course, have more leeway than a mechanical marvel, but neither can we 'run as well' on the wrong fuel. It will eventually shorten our lives. And is a Ferrari more precious than a human being? It would seem so.

Nearly three decades ago we had in the US the presidential announcement of a 'War on Cancer' launched with much patriotic and military fervour. Since then, nearly one trillion dollars have been spent on cancer research. And every year since then we have had big media promotions about the latest medical research discovery. Always with hope for a cure 'just around the corner'. But there has in fact been not an iota of progress, and every year the carnage from cancer not only continues, but increases.

I have read numerous accounts of people who have beaten cancer, but it has seldom been done with the recommended conventional medical treatments. Dr Joseph, who cured her breast cancer and restored herself to health, is only one example.[43] Nor, as we have noted, is there any evidence anywhere that these outrageously expensive and destructive orthodox 'treatments' do much good. Quite the contrary. They do however cause a great deal of unnecessary misery, and in some countries they manage to drain people financially in the process of making them miserable before they die.

In fact anyone going through this personally and financially nightmarish ordeal would be justified in deciding that 'Cancer care is a trip to the dark side of the moon.'[44]

Chuck and Lisa Winther, who spent some years researching the outcomes of cancer treatment declare,

Nearly 90% of the calls we received were from family members of cancer patients. They reported negatively on their experiences with medical treatment.

All of the patients said that once they left the hospital, the doctor stopped support. They were not told how to live so that the cancer would not recur.

I would suggest that that is because doctors do not know that. Advice is not given because there is none to give, doctors having such a narrow knowledge or vision of what constitutes human health.

If the medical hierarchy were truly serious about curing cancer, then they should all be fighting for everyone to have the kind of environment which will not cause cancer, or even better will strengthen the human immune system to resist it.

It is a similar story with the war on AIDS. Millions of dollars and not an iota of progress, and for the same reason that there is no progress in cancer. Health and sickness are being looked at with entirely the wrong paradigm. It is as though the blind men looking at the elephant saw only the backside of the elephant and decided that was what the whole elephant was like.

One can predict that, until medicine looks elsewhere, there will be no progress. But what the medical hierarchy has also been doing for most of this century is to persecute and hound anyone who claims to have a cancer remedy that is neither a marketable drug nor conventional high-tech medicine. They use the FDA to do this. It is a situation which has brought forth the hollow American joke, 'Cancer? See your travel agent.' A reference probably to Mexico, where the alternatives thrive.

In Chapter 26 we looked at an example of this in the persecution of Dr Stanislaw Burzynski MD. His successful method was recognized by the American National Cancer Institute, and part of it had even been approved for trials by the FDA itself, for cancer as well as for HIV.

Nevertheless, the FDA has repeatedly tried to shut down Dr Burzynski's Texas practice. They prosecuted him in 1983, in 1990 and again in 1994. Despite these raids, grand jury investigations always vindicated him. But Dr Burzynski was raided again in 1995 and faced 290 years' imprisonment on charges relating to 'interstate trafficking' – that is, people were coming from outside Texas and carrying away the substances he was using, a situation that is *absolutely inevitable* given that word of mouth advice from people overjoyed with his treatment will travel, and people seeking help will come from everywhere.

'Never before has the FDA approved an experimental drug for clinical trials with cancer patients while simultaneously trying to destroy the scientist who discovered it.'[45]

As I mentioned before, these courageous doctors are invariably vindicated by the courts, but the FDA with its bottomless purse keeps taking them to court until the brave ones are financially ruined and simply cannot carry on. How the American people and its government can permit such a situation to continue is beyond my comprehension. The 'something is rotten ...' has to be much worse than we can imagine. (But of course in the UK, New Zealand and elsewhere when it comes to concern about the welfare of people it is almost as rotten. And we seem to be equally helpless to correct a bad situation.)

The failure to cure is a remarkable situation because neither chemotherapy, nor coronary bypass, nor psychoanalysis, all permitted in a very big way, have ever been proved effective by the least of standards required, or rather demanded of, so many traditional/natural therapies. (The costs of establishing such effectiveness is in the millions, and could in fact be borne only by huge pharmaceutical companies in anticipation of big returns.) This permissiveness towards those within 'the establishment', and the harsh persecution of those without, could be the main reason why after all these years and all these scientists spending all these billions of dollars, there is still **'no cure for cancer'**.

However, not all doctors remain silent. The best will be inclined to attack the establishment on this in any possible way. Dr Irwin Bross MD, former statistician for the US National Cancer Institute, has publicly charged the NCI with *criminal fraud and genocide*, and supported these charges with statistics. He wrote: 'There is solid documentary evidence that the fraudulent claims concerning reduction in cancer mortality have been used to obtain taxpayer dollars under false pretences.'[46]

Besides the fact that medicine is 'looking in the wrong place' – that, is for a marketable drug which can never work – one must ask the question 'Could it be that the present multi-billion dollar cancer industry is too good an "earner" to be jeopardized with any substantial "cures"?' Because, as noted, cancer 'treatment' accounts for $200 billion of America's annual trillion-dollar disease care bill.[47]

Among several books published recently questioning the benefits of conventional medical treatment, Dr Ralph W Moss PhD, formerly a science writer on the staff of the Sloan-Kettering Cancer Center in New York, has written *The Cancer Industry*, the classic exposé of the cancer establishment,[48] and *Questioning Chemotherapy*.[49] He points out that in any given situation it is relevant to ask 'Cui bono?' (Who stands to gain?). Clearly in the 'War on Cancer' it is the same as in all wars: it is the arms manufacturers and the dealers – in this case the dealers in chemotherapy, radiation, surgery and the rest – who stand to flourish and grow wealthy from the continuation of the present cancer industry. Future critics looking back will note the extraordinary fact that the oncologists (cancer specialists), like the cardiologists and others, made excellent livings despite the general inefficacy of their treatments.[50] That is, despite, as Dr Moss points out, the fact that survival rates for most common cancers, 90% of them, have remained unchanged for the last 45 years. Cancer treatment is therefore largely a ritual medicine goes through, but unlike the African witch doctors who may wave coloured feathers in the air or shake a rattle, those who give this treatment inflict agony on the patients, both to their persons and in many cases to their wallets.

When remonstrated with about the inefficacy of modern cancer treatments, one doctor was quoted as saying, 'If we don't give them something, they'll go to the quacks.'[51]

Inasmuch as a quack is, according to the dictionary definition, 'an ignorant pretender to medical skill', someone who promotes, uses and personally gains from an unproven remedy, then, except for those two mentioned (Hodgkin's disease and childhood leukaemia), we must classify doctors who promote conventional cancer treatments as 'quacks', because in most cases they neither cure nor heal, and every doctor knows it, or should know it.

In fact, clearly it is better to go to the kind of 'quack' who costs less anyway. Moreover, the 'something' you get from the 'officially condoned quacks' may leave you a lot worse off physically. It could shorten and make miserable your remaining life.

As we have noted, both Dr Joseph Beasley and Dr Hardin Jones claim, based on decades of research, that untreated cancer patients live four times as long as treated one. Breast cancer death rates have not changed since 1930, when doctors could do very little. The situation is identical today. But the trouble is they don't 'do very little'. They must intervene, and so intervene they do, at the cost of unnecessary additional suffering and in some countries enormous expense on the part of breast cancer victims. Breast cancer is an industry that supports numerous people – in fact everyone involved but the victims themselves, it appears.[52]

So long as we go on putting brains and resources into the search for 'a cure for cancer', just so long will we be delaying the day when we must take a hard look at the many environmental causes of cancer. For cancer is inevitable unless we get rid of the many poisons and other hazards in our environment. On an individual basis we must also strive to boost the immune system, the whole human organism. This is in fact the way we *must go* if the human race is to survive.

Having said all that, at last we are beginning to see signs that the best minds in orthodox medicine, after decades of cancer research to no avail, may at last be beginning to realize that they are on entirely the wrong track. Currently, doubts are being raised in more advanced orthodox circles (the *Lancet* medical journal) as to the wisdom of the traditional model.[53] In this new model, cancer is seen as a process. Amazingly, it is speculated that treatment should be directed towards strengthening the normal body systems. This is a radical departure for modern medicine. It means it has at last joined with a traditional natural healing approach.

It is a great breakthrough in changing the approach to cancer and towards a weakening of the entire incorrect medical paradigm, which we will be looking at next. However, we have also seen over and over again that articles in medical journals, vital knowledge, can be ignored for many years, in fact for generations. So don't anyone hold their breath. Also, any change from the current system threatens the livelihoods of perhaps millions of individuals – in fact, chances are a real breakthrough in prevention or treatment would not be warmly received by those making their fortunes from the current situation.

It is my belief that in the end it will be the insupportable costs and costs alone which will alter this situation. Future generations will look back aghast on the barbarism that is cancer treatment in our century. It will be regarded as on a par with the treatment of the mentally ill in our century. How could anyone supposedly helping their very ill fellows have done such things to them? And how could people have put up with it for so many generations, in the absence of any proof of efficacy?

EMERGENCY ADVICE

We should live every day as though we have cancer, because we have. At least 300 cancer cells form each day. But if all is working well, our immune system knocks them off as they emerge. To strengthen and support our immune systems we need excellent nutrition – that is, food grown on real soil without sprays, these days hard to come by. And there are a whole lot of other things we can do which I will be writing about later.

Till then, Dr Sherry Rogers MD, environmental doctor *par excellence*, recommends, both as a preventive measure and possibly a cure: CDG (Calcium D-glucarate), 3 to 4 500-mg capsules twice a day (if suffering with breast cancer, 4 to 6 500-mg capsules twice a day). Note: This is quite different from the ordinary form of calcium. Also vitamins A, C, E and CoQ10[54] (but please note: ***Vitamin E should not be taken by any woman with breast cancer***) plus large amounts of organically grown fresh fruits and vegetables.[55] I would also add magnesium, selenium, turmeric and flax seed oil; lots of fresh juices from organically grown vegetables.

If one is so unfortunate as to receive a diagnosis of cancer, ask to see the studies establishing the efficacy of the treatment that is recommended. (One could also ask to see the manufacturer's warning for the product being promoted.) If they are not forthcoming, then why accept useless treatment? Spend your money on a better kind of 'whole-body' treatment where there is some hope of restoring you to health. And live longer. At worst one would 'go more gently into that good night,' far from the torture chambers of modern medicine.

PS When I rang up the Auckland Cancer Information Center to check on NZ statistics, there was a kind and very cheerful nurse to assist me. Yes, the numbers were appalling. Over 12,000 New Zealanders newly diagnosed each year. Over 100 were children. 1993 was the most recent year they had figures for.

Cancer was caused by 'old age ... We've got to die of something.' It was 'inevitable'.

(I forbore to ask why so many children and young people are victims today.) And the treatment was very successful, 'At least half went into remission.'

I did not envy her her job.

31: ANTIBIOTICS

'The greatest thing since sliced bread!'

Yes, they are. Well, they could have been if used wisely. Unfortunately they have not been used wisely, so there is definitely a down side to antibiotics. They might even harbinger the end of the human race.

I remember how aghast I was some years back when I read the autobiography of Virginia Woolf.[1] When she was 13, her 49-year-old mother died from 'a chill'. By the time she was 24 she had also lost a brother, Toby, from typhoid fever contracted in Greece, and her half-sister, Stella, had died of a respiratory infection of some sort. Thus, out of five young adults, two were lost. They had died from the kinds of ailments which we would today resolve with antibiotics. Similarly, a President of the United States, Theodore Roosevelt, lost a son from a mere blister on his heel, a blister which became infected. And in 1915 Rupert Brook died during the First World War from an infected mosquito bite. Earlier, Queen Victoria's husband, Prince Albert, had died from an infection (typhus?) incurred owing to blocked drains.

When the antibiotics were discovered in the early 1940s, it must have seemed like a dream come true; like the dawning of a new millennium in human health. We noted in Chapter 7 on root canals that, on the announcement of the discovery of penicillin, a huge research programme dealing with the effects of infections in the mouth was simply abandoned, and all 60 scientists dispersed, to our subsequent sorrow. But as we will see in Chapter 32, the antibiotics did much more than offer the hope that man could conquer bacteria. The discovery or creation of these new life-saving drugs strongly reinforced the direction in which medicine had gone since the early part of the century. Moreover, the fortune that was to be made from drugs, and the power that went with that fortune, were to cement that narrow pathway in so deeply that nothing but the path mattered, certainly not the trees and shrubs, the flowers on either side of the pathway.

But we are not in this chapter doing a history of medicine. We'll be looking at that soon. Here we will just look at the part the antibiotics have played, and what they are doing to the human race – in the short term, the medium term and in the long term; for each one presents a problem of differing and cumulative magnitude. If there is a life at stake, then the use of antibiotics on a particular occasion is a wonderful thing. They have saved lives. But if a life is not at stake, we have to ask, is it worth these other consequences?

1. THE SHORT-TERM EFFECTS

Dr Harold E Buttram MD has done considerable work and writing on the subject of the effects of antibiotics.[2] His research indicates that the immediate consequence of the ingestion of antibiotics is a reduction in one's own white cells – that is, those cells which are there to defend us.[3] Of this Dr Buttram says,

This immuno-suppressive effect of antibiotics may explain a commonly observed pattern in patients treated for minor respiratory infections. Although the patient may feel better while on the antibiotic, symptoms of infection soon return after it is discontinued, perhaps requiring a second and even a third course.

As we have seen throughout this book, there are numerous other substances that can also knock back our immune systems. For example sugar, vaccinations, pesticides, fluoride and mercury.

In 1991, both the *British Medical Journal* and the *Journal of the American Medical Association* reported on a Dublin study which revealed that antibiotics used in children's ear infections were no more effective than a placebo, or no treatment at all, for children over the age of two. Moreover, those who took the antibiotics had more re-occurrences than those who did not.[4]

A second short-term result of antibiotics is an overgrowth of potentially harmful bacteria. In the digestive system, we live with a multitude of micro-organisms we call flora, gut flora, or gut bacteria. These serve us well through life by keeping potentially harmful others at bay. But when we take antibiotics, these more beneficial flora get killed off along with 'the baddies' we are trying to get rid of. Thus we lose another line of defence against disease-causing bacteria and fungus. Food allergy and eczema in childhood have been directly linked to this phenomenon.[5]

Then there is the problem of parasites. Dr Buttram believes also that the overuse of antibiotics and the subsequent immuno-suppressive effects predispose us to the spread of parasites. They may be there in our water and in raw foods. Highly sensitive tests such as the RST (Rectal Swab Test) are needed to spot these parasites in us. They can interfere with the absorption of vitamin A, B_{12} and folic acid, and cause tissue damage. Symptoms in association with these parasites may be fatigue, muscle weakness, 'flu-like symptoms and swollen glands, all of which may unfortunately be diagnosed as stemming from a bacterial infection, resulting in the prescribing of even more antibiotics.[6]

A 1990 sampling of the upper-income town of Elmhurst, Queens, New York City, found that 74.5% of the people tested were infected with intestinal parasites. That is, 51 out of 67 had *Blastocysts homis.*[7] One cannot be truly well while harbouring these parasites. There may be diarrhoea, abdominal cramping, bloating, gas and many other symptoms. Without tests for parasites, all sorts of incorrect diagnoses and treatment may be instituted, even surgery. The problem is more widespread than many would suspect. And most of it can be laid at the door of antibiotics. (The centuries-old custom of 'purging in the spring', for example the taking of sulphur and molasses and other ghastly mixtures, was of course the way to go. Few of us have this annual 'spring clean' these days.)

Also, Salmonellosis outbreaks have become increasingly frequent since the 1970s. Apparently the use of antibiotics 'usually causes chronic carriage' if given for salmonella bacteria.[8]

2. THE MEDIUM-TERM EFFECTS

Also a serious matter is the fact that antibiotics can produce antibiotic-resistant micro-organisms either directly or indirectly. We have noted that in the presence of mercury, most bacteria die. But a few always survive and these have or acquire a genetic resistance to mercury. People with these resistant bacteria will also have bacteria resistant to antibiotics,[9] a phenomenon studied by a group of microbiologists, statisticians and medical physiologists, and reported in the April 1993 issue of the journal *Antimicrobial Agents and Chemotherapy*.

Then there is the indirect way of acquiring resistant micro-organisms. The Centers for Disease Control in Atlanta, Georgia found that antibiotics used in animal feed can affect those who eat the meat from such animals, in a process known as 'jumping genes'. In this manner, antibiotic resistance can be transferred from one species of bacteria to another. Thus the continued use of antibiotics may favour the emergence of an array of resistant species.

For example, the London *Times* (March 19, 1998) reported on a clear link between the use of antibiotics in animal feed and the emergence of 'superbugs' in hospitals. For some years now antibiotics have been given in animal feed because they can increase the animals' growth rate by 5%. But research carried out by Henrik Wegener of the Danish Veterinary Laboratory indicates that a common type of bacterium found in the intestines of people, pigs and chickens, enterococci, had by 1986 developed resistance to a major antibiotic, vancomycin. In other words, these recent gene tests revealed that the resistance had moved from animals to humans.

If you're wondering why doctors have of late become reluctant to prescribe antibiotics, here's another reason. Like many official health departments, the Washington State Department of Health sent out a letter (in September of 1998) which called for new limitations on the prescribing of antibiotics. The grounds for this were that whereas between 1992 and 1996, 3% of isolates of Streptococcus pneumonia were found to be highly resistant to penicillin, by 1998 11% were highly resistant, with a further 25% found to show a decreased response to penicillin.[10]

But perhaps the worst medium-term effect of antibiotics is that they can bring about the transformation, or more accurately speaking the transmogrification, of an innocuous yeast, Candida albicans, into a dangerous monster. The ordinary Candida albicans is a single-cell yeast that is always with us and can be regarded as a fairly harmless passenger through life. But under the influence of antibiotics it changes from a harmless tiny sphere-shaped organism into a much larger branching fungal form (mycelia) which invades the tissues of the digestive system and the vagina. The longer this continues the more serious the consequences, especially if the immune system is compromised by other factors, many of which we have noted in other chapters.

The first reports on the adverse effects of antibiotics were recorded by Mildred Seelig 33 years ago.[11] And there are, of course, more recent ones.[12] About 20 years ago I spoke to an older doctor about the prevalence of vaginal thrush. On this he said, 'When I was first in practice, you might see two cases a year. But now, you'll get six or more a week.' It was a 'sign of the times', because the thrush (the fungus, the Candida) follows in the wake of antibiotics.

This monster, Candida albicans in its mycelia form, let loose upon our bodies is just about as dangerous as the other monster, Trans Fatty Acids, only it gets around more. In one study, 86% of a group of antibiotic-treated animals had Candida spread to the liver, the spleen and the bowel.[13] Also, in the late 1960s a Japanese bacteriologist discovered that this virulent organism produces a potent toxin (its excreta) which he called canditoxin and which has adverse effects on the immune system.[14] It can also produce LSD-like substances such as a mania-inducing excitotoxin. People suffering from Candida overgrowth tend to have difficulty relaxing; they may seem constantly over-excited, even when weak and exhausted.

Worse, this transmogrified mycelia version can actually burrow through fairly solid tissue. And thus the integrity of the gut wall may be breached. Through it goes! A gap is formed. And thereafter we have undigested food particles leaking through and into the bloodstream. When these particles get into the bloodstream they are interpreted as the only thing they can be – foreign invaders. And thus we develop both food allergies and sensitivities and nutritional deficiencies. Overall, the effect is a further weakening of the immune system.

An American researcher in this field is Dr Steven S Witkin PhD, (Director, Immunology Division, Department of Obstetrics and Gynaecology, Cornell University Medical School, New York). During the last 15 years Dr Witkin and his associates have produced many publications on the results of their work, 'Defective Immune Responses in Patients with recurrent Candidiasis,'[15] to name only one of many. However the problem is not confined to women, despite its research origins in gynaecology. Children and men are also victims.

The effects of Candidiasis are multiple, affecting the intestines and genitourinary systems, the nervous system, the immune system and the endocrine system.[16] It can cause irritable bowel, multiple allergies, depression and irritability, vaginitis, menstrual problems and even infertility. There can be symptoms of spaciness, inability to concentrate, poor memory and disabling fatigue. In children there may be hyperactivity and learning disabilities. Asthma, eczema and hay fever may get worse with Candidiasis. Extreme sensitivity to chemicals and inhalants of any kind may arise. Candida also secretes a number of human-like hormones which cross-react with human tissues and trigger the production of anti-ovarian and anti-thymic antibodies, and thus autoimmune disorders increase with Candida overgrowth. Candidiasis can also lead to arthritis.[17]

If all this is Greek to your doctor it is probably because: a) the profession as a whole does not want to know about Candida because it threatens the free use of antibiotics, the mainstay of modern medicine (any talk of Candida is dismissed as 'faddish'); b) as I have said before, doctors do not appear to read the brief indications that have appeared in the medical literature; and c) it is difficult to prove this scenario because most laboratories are not up to proving it. As we know, the laboratory always has the last word. No matter how many new discoveries are made, or new techniques devised to measure them, at any one given time what the laboratory says is gospel. Overall it is medical intransigence, medical obtuseness that denies this dangerous phenomenon. The presence of Candida albicans in its more dangerous form can actually be confirmed by a testing technique known as ELISA, only it is not available in very many laboratories.

The brilliant Dr Buttram has this to say on the subject:

Few medical issues today have been more controversial than the Candida Syndrome, probably because no one fully understands its nature. It probably involves far more than just the invasive overgrowth of Candida in the digestive tract and vagina. It may in part be caused by direct injury from antibiotics to the intestinal immune system (the secretory IgA system), sometimes referred to as 'antiseptic paint' coating the intestinal lining. It may also involve overgrowth of other pathogens as well as Candida and a reduction of beneficial intestinal microorganisms. The overall result may be an increased intestinal permeability, (the so-called leaky gut syndrome) leading to an increased propensity to food allergies and other sensitivities.[18]

Apart from Dr Seelig, there are two others who have made significant research contributions in this area: Dr A Constantini PhD at the Mycotoxin Collaborating Center of the World Health Organization, and Dr Mary Matossian, author of *Poisons of the Past*.[19]

It has been found that a high percentage of people suffering from the so-called 20th-century diseases EI (Environmental Illness), CFIDS (Chronic Fatigue Immune Dysfunction Syndrome), MCS (Multiple Chemical Sensitivities) and so on have a yeast or Candida involvement.[20] How can doctors assist even those with vaginal thrush coherently, let alone CFIDS, etc., if they do not care to study this phenomenon?

From all of these medium-term effects, Dr Buttram finds evidence that many children today, compared to children of earlier generations, are showing 'an increasing pattern of immunotopic derangement'. By that he means the dramatic increases in the incidence of allergic phenomena, the asthma, the eczema and other allergic problems.

3. THE FINAL AND LONG-TERM EFFECTS

The final and possibly the worst effect of antibiotics is the overall decline of the immune system in combination with ever-more-resistant microbes. 'Frequent or prolonged courses of antibiotics depress the immune system.'[21]

There is also the fact that by the 1980s it was becoming apparent that the microbes were mutating faster than we could make drugs to oppose them. Sometimes they didn't work at all. Hospital infections are most acutely affected, of course. Thus by 1992, in the US, 13,300 people had died of infections that resisted every antibiotic tried.[22] In New Zealand, according to the *New Zealand Medical Journal*, 3,049 bloodstream infections were recorded at the country's 23 hospitals, and up to 800 people die every year from 'hospital bugs' – that is, they are victims of antibiotic-resistant bacteria.

According to *Time* magazine (12 September 1994, in an article entitled 'Revenge of the Killer Microbes: Are we losing the war against infectious diseases?') 'every disease organism known to medicine has become resistant to at least one antibiotic and several are immune to more than one.' And even the French, who overall have better luck with health than all other Western countries, have calculated that in Paris 5% of patients entering hospitals left with a disease they did not have when they checked in to hospital, resulting in 350–700 deaths per year, or around 10,000 in the whole of France.

But the pharmaceutical companies go valiantly on concocting their new antibiotics. As they must.

In 1986 Marc Lappée, author of *When Antibiotics Fail*,[23] explored the multiple abuses and overuses of antibiotics, especially in animal husbandry. Also the practice in hospitals of giving antibiotics 'just in case', as well as in the ordinary consulting situation.

Apparently the great Sir Alexander Fleming, inventor of penicillin, warned early on against the indiscriminate use of his miracle drug. But no one listened to him. Lappée says that the great weakness of our century has been our uncritical acceptance of technological breakthroughs and a lack of recognition of possible harmful side-effects. Because, as we have noted, when the benign travellers are destroyed by antibiotics their place is taken by the new harmful antibiotic-resistant microbes. And there is a minority of specialist scientists in this area now suggesting that *our survival is related to the survival of our 'good bacteria'*.

The worst possible scenario is that the antibiotic resistance is fast spreading into other bacteria, and that we face a prospect of antibiotic resistance throughout the entire bacterial world. At the present time, sexually transmitted diseases such as syphilis, gonorrhoea, chlamydia, genital herpes and staphylococcus aureus, once killed off by penicillin, are now thumbing their noses at it. And despite the fact that over 250 articles on this problem were published between 1960 and 1982, little has been done to prevent the spread of these resistant infections.

Had antibiotics been reserved for life-threatening situations, we could perhaps have counted on them for centuries. But alas! For 50 years they have been dished out indiscriminately, almost like sweets, with the bacteria we seek to control getting ever more resistant, and plenty of evidence that the human immune system is getting weaker and weaker. So it is only a matter of time before antibiotics will not do the job. And we will be back to the situation in Virginia Woolf's day, *only we will be far worse off*.

Future medical historians will look back on 'the time of the antibiotics' as a brief time in the history of the world when we *could* have made it, but instead *we blew it.* For just as the drug quinine caused the malaria protozoa to mutate into ever more horrific and more resistant strains now impervious to any drug, so all of them will go. And thus, the future of the world, the human race, is not reassuring. It is possible that by the end of the next century only those people with extremely strong immune systems will survive. But in the mean time we are doing nothing to strengthen our immune systems, in fact many things in our lives, including just about everything mentioned in this book, tend to weaken them!

There is plenty of evidence that the immune system is being compromised at every turn. We eat food lacking in nutrients because it is produced on depleted and poisoned soils. We have to cope with vast amounts of toxicity we were never designed to cope with. The human immune system is undermined by the antibiotics, by vaccinations and by the heavy intake of sugar in the modern diet which, as we have noted, depletes the body's white cells. At the end of the 19th century we were eating 10 pounds per year; today it is 100.

But there is another factor people do not appear to be considering, perhaps worst of all. It occurred to me many years ago when I was reading that autobiography of Virginia Woolf that in saving most of those who are born on this earth in the West we have violated the most basic biological rule of life on this planet, the rule that says 'The fittest will survive and reproduce themselves.' It is a harsh dictum but it has been a fact of life on our planet since the beginning of life. What our antibiotics have done is to promote 'the survival of the unfittest'. And the long-term effects of 'the survival of the unfittest' is that a lot of us have swum out of the shallow end of the gene pool.

Let us suppose that those people who survive to adulthood without antibiotics have good strong immune systems. Let's call them 'As'. Those with the weaker immune systems who have been saved by antibiotics let us call 'Bs'. In the next generation, when the Bs marry Bs, do they produce another 'B', or could that child perhaps be a 'C'? Nobody knows! But we must consider the possibility that, generation by generation, we are declining. An analysis of childhood health, in fact overall health, would bear this out.

What happened in Virginia Woolf's time was tragic for those involved. But, speaking not in individual terms but in terms of the human race, the death of those who could not fight off marauding bacteria, often before they reproduced themselves, meant that the human race as a whole was stronger. Because only those with strong immune systems survived and reproduced themselves.

(If your life has been spared by antibiotics please do not be offended or feel in the least bit guilty. I am not at all implying that any human being should not live, or use all available means to do so. What I am saying is that we need to be aware of what has happened, and to plan for it. But are we? There is no long-term planning anywhere! Or short-term planning, for that matter.)

There are a number of alternatives to antibiotics, and these should always be used first, unless a sick person is at a critical point where it is quite plain they will die without them. I will be discussing these alternatives in a later book. But because modern medicine is so myopic about drugs, and that is all it knows, the antibiotics have been unnecessarily overused. Already in some people, in some situations, they do not work.

We can see the day coming when they will not work at all, and we will be back to the situation of Virginia Woolf's family only we will be far worse off because of the other repercussions we have noted: the more powerful bacteria we will face with weaker personal defences to fight them.

Had the many alternatives been continued and the antibiotics been regarded as BIG GUNS for BIG DISEASES, to bring up only in life-threatening situations, we would all be in a much safer position. We must give medicine its due and concede that no one could have predicted the way the handwriting on the wall would be writ, but what is happening today is becoming quite clear. (Of course Alexander Fleming, Rene Dubos and others predicted as much. But then, who listens to geniuses?) There is no excuse for medicine to continue on in this way. But how many orthodox doctors know what the alternatives are, or would dream of using them, such is the barrenness of a medicine that uses exclusively pharmaceuticals? For that is what they are trained to do and they can think of nought else.

If you have read thus far in the book you will have noticed how many times I have had to say the chilling words: THIS DAMAGES THE HUMAN IMMUNE SYSTEM. So it is not just the saving of people with inferior immune systems we have to worry about, but also what the entire environment is doing to us all, after what we have done to it.

If the 1918–20 influenza pandemic, the so-called 'Spanish 'Flu' which killed so many then were to return today, or something like it (and why should it not?), how many of us would survive? (The English used to call venereal disease 'The French Disease' while the French used to call it 'The English Disease'. And when this annihilating influenza was racing around the world, the French and the English got together and called it 'The Spanish 'Flu', or usually 'The Spanish Lady'. Yep! It was too awful to be male.) For that 'Spanish' 'flu, even in a 'slow transport' age, went around the globe and simply wiped out over 20 million people. And that was in a period when people had better air, cleaner water and far better soil, which means infinitely superior food, more vital nutrients than we have now. Most people consumed fats and oils that had not been altered and distorted. In addition, if they had survived to maturity their immune systems were doubtless far stronger than today's, on average. Thus they were better able to cope with infections than we are. Presumably that was why *some* of them survived the plague of the influenza epidemic.

How many of us today have strong enough immune systems to survive such a plague?

We have, with our drugs and our mercury and our fluoride, our poisoned earth, our toxic fats, our massive intake of sugar, our vaccinations, created a world wherein unless we pull up sharply and bend all our efforts, EMERGENCY FASHION, to the strengthening of the human immune system, we must contemplate a horrific vision of a world 30 years or so hence where the microbes have become stronger and stronger and the human defences against them weaker and weaker. We could be unarmed, defenceless, vulnerable to every passing malevolent microbe. We could simply be wiped out.

One has at times a horrific vision of a world 30 years' hence where the microbes have become stronger and stronger and the human race weaker and weaker, both of which are happening at this very moment. The privileged go around in portable glass bubbles frantically imbibing their antioxidants. All too late!

As T S Eliot said:

**This is the way the world ends
Not with a bang, but with a whimper.**

Observers from another planet may find some amusement in the fact that so many of us who cared enough to fight were so worried about 'the bang' (perhaps we had to be and still should be) that we did not worry enough about 'the whimper'.

It is my belief that only a massive effort to clean up our world can save us at this point. Only a concerted drive to clean up our air, our water, and above all, our soil, can save the human race. And we will have to put right every one of the problems posed in every chapter in this book.

EMERGENCY ADVICE

Antibiotics should never be taken, except in an extreme emergency, and not without the protection of plain *Lactobacillus acidophilus* yoghurt (that is, yoghurt containing the live form of this beneficial bacterium). That is, twice a day, all during the ingestion of the drug, and for two weeks thereafter. Also another benign bacteria such as Laterosporus should be taken to fight off the Candida, etc. and restore the gut to health. If you are both brave and sensible, put the good bacteria directly into the bowel, as in suppositories or as an enema.

⚠

32: THE MEDICAL PROFESSION

'Modern medicine is the greatest for our health.'

Just for a moment let us forget our individual kindly doctors who doubtless deserve gratitude for doing their very best for us. It cannot be easy dealing with sick people and their woes all day long. However, nor can it be all that bad, because our medical schools continue to turn out more and more doctors, and they do not appear to drop out of the profession very often. So it must be a better way to earn a living than most. And having said that, let us try to look at the entire medical scene objectively, if that is possible.

First, there is nothing like modern medicine if we're in crisis. Any kind of accident – a life-threatening infection in the appendix, heart or kidney failure, severe pain – and modern medicine comes into its own, doing what it does remarkably well. There is also a considerable contribution in the ability to relieve symptoms, and the immediate reduction of suffering in a crisis.

Provided there is a hospital or a casualty department/emergency clinic nearby, provided they are not short of staff or other resources, no one can detract from the remarkable work done in the area of accident and crisis-care. Also the rehabilitation from these health crises is often superb, as people are brought back from the brink of the grave, or from certain disability, often able to function once again as viable human beings.

No one can take from modern medicine this remarkable work, the shattered lives which have been saved. So it is certainly not the 'crisis care' one could quarrel with.

But can doctors prevent the health crisis from occurring? Can they truly produce real health with their methods? The answer has to be an emphatic 'No.' For it is in the area of 'health care' that modern medicine has failed us, and failed us monstrously.

According to the *Journal of the American Medical Association*,[1] 40% of Americans (approximately 100 million) suffer from chronic ailments such as diabetes and asthma, at a cost to the nation of $425 billion per year. By the year 2000 the number is expected to rise to about 148 million, at a cost of $800 billion. It is primarily 'diseases of civilization' which swell these numbers. Moreover, there is an enormous toll in 'iatrogenic disease' – that is, doctor-caused disease: Dr Robert Wilner says these iatrogenic diseases cause 120,000 deaths annually, which is 10 times the number of AIDS deaths per year. Most of these would be from drugs, and from medical mismanagement.[2] The World Health Organization estimates that 33% of all disease is caused by medical treatment.[3]

If you have read thus far, you will know something of the numerous hazards which can wreck us and cause us to die prematurely. And these are causes of ill-health on which modern medicine has either remained resolutely silent or is completely ignorant. For when it comes to that environmental impact on health, orthodox medicine is like the three thoroughly uninterested monkeys – they see no evil, they hear no evil, and they speak no evil. For not only is this kind of concern not in their territory, it threatens their territory!

We have also seen that there are numerous individual doctors (and a few dentists), mentioned in almost every chapter in this book, the extremely brilliant and courageous few who have tried to warn us about these dangers, who speak out on behalf of suffering humanity. They are doctors and dentists who practise a different kind of medicine, and who continue to do so despite, as we have noted, severe punishment and adverse effects on their careers, their livelihoods. Sometimes they are hounded to other countries or into the grave. It is THAT bad. But for all their efforts they are as one grain of sand in a bucketful. They have little impact upon the professions as a whole, although that impact is increasing as the more intelligent seek them out.

Why do the mass of doctors ignore the absolutely vital and critical effects of the environment, the air, the water, our food, upon us? And why is their record in health so very dismal?

The extraordinary reason for this state of affairs – that we haven't got a health care system at all, we have only a 'disease care' system and not a very good one at that – lies back in the mists of time. Well, not so misty as all that. Only back to the end of the 19th century.

But if we wish to understand what has happened to cause medicine to 'go wrong', we have to go back to the past, just as we had to in the chapter on mental health to understand Freud's negative impact in that field. There are at least two distinct historical reasons for the state of affairs today in modern medicine.

First, we do not need to know all the details. Suffice it to say that towards the end of the last century there was a great controversy about the nature of human health, between two opposing forces. It was a titanic and epic struggle, quite like that mythical titanic and epic struggle between the forces of good and evil up in heaven. But unfortunately for all of us throughout most of this century, unlike the outcome of that struggle in heaven, when it came to medicine, 'the baddies won.'

One of the leaders of the two opposing forces was Pasteur, the one whose name was given to the process of boiling up milk (pasteurization). This is perhaps ironic, considering that so many nutrients are lost in the process. Pasteur had become famous for his work with a vaccine against rabies. More recently the world's foremost Pasteurean scholar went through Pasteur's notebooks (specified by Pasteur before he died that they were never to be made publicly available. However, an uncooperative grandson donated them to the Bibliothèque Nationale in Paris) and found evidence of shady dealings such as manipulated data (not uncommon among scientists[4]) and 'ethically dubious conduct' surrounding Pasteur's highly publicized vaccination experiments.[5] In other words, he fraudulently published results not borne out by the experiments described in his notebooks. Dr Lancetot, MD, would deny even that lives are saved with Pasteur's rabies' vaccine.[6]

I have to say at this point that such 'fraud in science' is not unusual.

I think what started me off on a 'life of crime' (that is, my tendency not to believe everything I am told), was reading the book *Fraud in Science*, now probably out of print, when I was around 20. There have been numerous other books since, all worth a look.[7]

Anyway, whatever the truth about his accomplishments, Pasteur, like many of his day, had spent hours peering into microscopes; thus he believed that all disease came from invading forces outside the body. That is, that we are all your standard issue human being. That one can be peacefully minding one's own business when along comes a foul beast in the form of a microbe; you are attacked and you become ill. QED.

This was somewhat understandable during an age when most of the health problems of the day had to do with infectious diseases, diseases which appeared to stem from outside the patients. The doctors of this world being slow learners, it had taken them many years to accept what one Dr Semmelweiss more or less gave his life to tell them: That they should wash their hands between going from the mortuary, where they dissected dead bodies, to delivering babies in the 'lying-in hospital' and performing operations.

It was the custom for doctors in those days to wear long black frock coats, and they wore them for their dissections of corpses, their operations and their work in the wards, including delivering babies. The bloodier these black frock coats became the more the doctors liked it, because it was a status symbol to have a coat which showed the rigours of one's work. Florence Nightingale used to try to persuade the doctors to wash these ghastly objects by telling them they need not hang them up, they could just stand them up in the corners.

But what doctor would listen to a mere nurse? They went on wearing these blood-stained status symbols and not washing their hands for some years. They also used the same sponge in surgery, over and over again until it fell apart, resulting in a 50% death rate from infection following surgery.[8] Meanwhile, one-fifth of the mothers in the delivery wards died of 'puerperal' fever, which means that 20% of the infants born in hospital in those days went motherless. The midwives were not so germ-laden, and it got so that women were afraid to go into hospital and preferred to have a midwife, because they knew that with midwives they were less likely to die.

Semmelweiss, who knew exactly what was causing the deaths, ended up half demented with anxiety, demanding, begging and imploring his fellow doctors to wash their hands before surgery and delivering infants. Arrogantly insulted, they resisted and resisted this plea, leaving virulent and deadly germs from the rotting carcasses they dissected in their surgical patients and among the women giving birth, hence the 'puerperal fever', which terrible ending was to the doctors entirely a mystery.[9] Semmelweiss, devoted man, knowing so well what was happening, went quite mad in the end and, one could say, died in the attempt to get his fellow doctors to stop killing. **The whole terrible story is a classic example of how an entire profession can *ignore* the truth it does not want to hear.**

So it was ironic that about the time this point finally made it into doctors' obdurate and self-satisfied skulls and they stopped killing unnecessarily, enraptured at finally understanding this point they went overboard and became convinced that it was microbes that *caused all disease.*

(We have therefore to give Pasteur the credit for eventually persuading doctors to wash their hands *and* their bloody black frock coats, which is why today the event which seems to symbolize medicine in 'the soaps' is the elaborate procedure for 'scrubbing up'. Pasteur, in fact, became quite serious about 'germs' and refused to shake hands with anyone, a view some of us can find sympathy with today after reading about the studies on the lack of hand-washing in public toilets!)

Opposed to the idea that all illness came from outside the body, was another Frenchman, Bechamp, whose name most of us do not even know. However, in this great controversy he was the one who was right; it was Pasteur who was wrong. For Bechamp said that it was not the force of the invading microbe that was important in disease, it was the strength of the organism attacked, its power to resist that was important. In other words, continuing with the language of warfare, the Europe of that day being divided into armed camps, it was the strength of 'the terrain', and not that of the invader, that either won or lost the day.[10]

And if we take a moment to consider that influenza germs can charge around any group of people, say in the home, at the office, the factory or school, but that only a proportion of people exposed will actually succumb to that germ, then we can understand one of the reasons why Bechamp was right. At the time of this great controversy there were young supporters of Bechamp who tried valiantly to prove his point by publicly drinking down beakers full of cholera germs and remaining healthy. But apparently there is something about the process of becoming a doctor which addles the brain of most. Even these dramatic demonstrations had no impact on the argument.

So Pasteur won. And we all lost. It is salutary to discover and contemplate the fact that the very basis of modern medicine lies deep in the work and the personalities of two very clever yet misguided men – Pasteur and Freud.

For from then on nothing mattered in human health but worrying about invading organisms. The body thus came to be seen as a battle ground, a concept that was reinforced by the aforementioned political atmosphere in the Europe of that day. And, as we will soon note, it is still regarded as such in the language of 'health care'.

But an interesting fact about all this is that Pasteur, like Freud, recanted on his deathbed.[11] He had had a while to think about it all, and he was not stupid. So when he lay dying he said he thought that, after all, perhaps *it was the terrain that was important*. 'The presence in the body of a pathogenic agent is not necessarily synonymous with infectious disease.'

I suppose that for these 'great men' it is too difficult to make such announcements until their last hour. But of course, when the world has gone off half-cocked on one's earlier stupidity and made their personal fortunes too, nobody wants to hear it. And thus it was that nobody listened to Pasteur's last words, just as nobody had listened to Freud's. So unfortunately these deathbed recantations appear to be quite useless. However, for people later seeking after truth they do rather tend to put things into perspective.

The name is not important, but the doctrine that conventional orthodox medicine still revolves around today is known as 'The Doctrine of Specific Aetiology' or the 'Germ Theory of Disease' – that is, that all problems of human health are caused by one thing, one invading thing from the outside, and moreover there will be one thing to cure it, usually one pharmaceutical drug. Yes, this is the way your doctor is trained to think: One cause, one drug to cure it. And it was one Rudolph Virchow who solidified this theory, and named it.

And that is why doctors are comfortable mainly with one symptom only, and become uncomfortable and suspicious (you are in a psychological category) if you are unfortunate enough to have several symptoms. But more on this in the next chapter.

However, as a postscript to this section we should note that Rudolf Virchow, the scientist who originated the Germ Theory, in his later years also underwent a complete reversal in his beliefs and said, 'If I could live my life over again, I would devote it to proving that germs seek their natural habitat, diseased tissues – rather than being the cause of disease.' Unfortunately, mainstream medicine **has not yet caught up with** the 'born-again' Virchow. Because to do so would turn all of medicine upside down. (Had Pasteur and Virchow etc. 'seen the light' earlier, and Freud stuck to the weird and supernatural, as he later regretted he had not done, then perhaps we'd all be in clover.)

Fifty years after this epic struggle between those two great scientists, Bechamp and Pasteur, came a brilliant young scientist named Enderlin who seemed to have worked mostly on his own. He spent many hours with his microscope observing people's blood. He was particularly interested in the workings of fungi such as Candida albicans, *its capacity to transmogrify* (alter for the worse), Aspergillus, etc., for Enderlin found that almost all humans harbour the Candida albicans fungus but that most remain without symptoms from it. Bechamp before him had already established that the form of microbes is determined by the environment in which they feed, grow and multiply in the body, just as our 'form' is similarly influenced by our environment!

But as we have noted in the chapter on antibiotics, the increase in the prevalence of this organism, *its alteration*, and the symptoms of Candidiasis appear only when the immune system is significantly weakened. Enderlin would have been astonished to find it so widespread in our world today. He thought he was dealing with something rather rare. But then he was working before the discovery of antibiotics.

The situation with tuberculosis and pneumonia is similar. The organisms responsible are said to reside harmlessly in the lungs of most healthy individuals. Symptoms occur only when the defence system is weakened.[12] I have a special interest in this, of course, having contracted tuberculosis at the age of 10. And it happened soon after I was sent away alone mid-winter to a far-off place with a much colder climate than I was used to. There were very cold nights and few bed coverings, with inferior food (boiled-to-death cabbage, no fresh fruits or vegetables) and a great deal of personal suffering behind me and always with me. I had been an unloved and neglected child, and worse, since before I was two.

No one else at this institution had tuberculosis, but within weeks I had all the signs of it: the weight loss, the constant coughing, the lack of strength and the pale thin face and body. And that went on for nearly four years unrecognized and untreated until somehow I got on top of it. I very nearly did not.[13] So I know today that Enderlin was right. And of course in more recent years, again with a severely weakened immune system, I succumbed in a very big way to disseminated Candidiasis.

But because the brilliant Enderlin's findings, like Bechamp's (*that it is **the body**, the strength of the terrain that is important*) went against the medical paradigm that organisms invade from the outside, and that is all that is important. Thus he *could not get published in the appropriate medical journals.*

And this is *still* the fate of any who would attempt to defy the faulty paradigm. You cannot get your average GP to accept the concept of disseminated Candidiasis! It has not been published as such in the medical journals. And the medical journals will not publish anything about it because it goes against their rusty old paradigm. It threatens the very foundation of modern medicine. And this despite all the women with their vaginal Candida albicans. And many far worse than that.

In more recent years, despite the brilliant advance work of Dr Mildred Seelig published in three major journals (*The American Journal of Medicine, Medical Times* and the *Bacteriological Review*) as referred to in Chapter 31 on antibiotics, Dr Orion Truss MD, one of the great doctors to whom this book is dedicated, could not get his vital findings as to the consequences of what Dr Seelig had noted, the Candidiasis, into *any* conventional medical journal.

The fact that he managed eventually to get it into an obscure (not in knowledge, but in fame) Canadian journal, the *Journal of Orthomolecular Medicine*, saved my life. For I had lost far too much weight to continue in that way much longer, until someone thoughtful handed us that hard-won article and we obtained the appropriate anti-fungal treatment. (Incidentally, the first anti-fungal drugs were created by two women scientists who gave them to the world, asking no royalties for themselves. This in sharp contrast to the money-hungry approach of most today. Thus I owe my life to extraordinarily good people, always including, of course, the partner who nursed me so devotedly through many years of agony.)

It is still this faulty paradigm, this idea that we are fighting something *from outside our bodies*, that influences all medical thought today, all action. And it is also why we have the language of violence within medicine. It is the reason why we have presidents of the United States declaring 'War on Cancer', 'War on Diabetes' (considered necessary because the incidences of these diseases are constantly increasing). It is the reason why medicine is so violent in its response to illness, why *'if thine eye offends thee, pluck it out'*. Why we have surgery, chemotherapy and radiation to bombard the aliens causing cancer and just about everything else. Never mind that these treatments seldom work in the long term. For not only does medicine believe that it is useless to attempt to strengthen the body to oppose these scourges, they wouldn't have a clue as to how to go about doing it.

One wit said that disease is seen as 'a wild and hairy monster'. We do not pause to wonder why some people get ill and some do not. What we do is wait until signs and symptoms appear and then we attack with all guns blazing. And we can be sure that those more knowledgeable people from the future will, with the perspective of hindsight, see our medicine in those terms. We seek for healing and we get ... the Wild West.

A classic example of this concerns a friend who about three years ago went to his doctor with a slightly enlarged prostate and severe frequency (of urination) problems. He was advised to 'come back in three months, and we'll have another look at it.' Presumably then it might be up to the stage where medicine **could attack it**. But because I am in Bechamp's camp and not Pasteur's, I strongly advised him to increase immediately his organic zinc intake with sunflower seeds, oysters and other things. And to take the herb Saw palmetto (*Serenoa repens*), established in trials to be more effective than the prescription drug prescribed for prostate problems.

Then too, because it is only something from the outside that is a problem, medicine does not see the body as a whole, as a series of interrelated parts each affecting the others. That is why we have specialization, a carving up of the body: the handing over of our teeth to the dentists, the joints and muscles to the rheumatologists; the eyes, the ears and the mouth to the ENT men; the nervous system to the neurologists; the brain to the psychiatrists, and so on.

The body is carved up thus because it is simply not important to learn how the general body health, the biochemistry, the interaction between the various parts is affecting all these bits and pieces, or to improve upon it. For in terms of medicine's paradigm, its way of looking at health, it cannot be important. There is no realization that it could be. But in terms of true human health it has been disastrous to do this. For it is plain to some of us that what goes on in the mouth, for example, can affect the state of one's immune system, the breast, or even the big toe. That one's brain is affected by the state of one's digestion. And all the rest.

But of course when you provide a 5- to 15-minute consultation and you have only pharmaceutical drugs to offer, how can it matter anyway whether you divide up the body so? And you do not have to know anything more about your patient but a brief description of the problem. You get that and you search for the one best drug. QED. How the patient got this way or what can be done to correct it does not matter. The symptoms ARE the disease.

But **symptoms are not the disease**. Symptoms are Nature's way of *coping with disease*. And when we knock out the symptoms we have not necessarily coped with the cause of those symptoms. We have merely driven them underground for a time.

The business of maintaining or regaining health is complex and can be highly individualized. How can anyone worthy of the name of 'healer' do it in 10 minutes? It cannot be done. And clearly it is not being done.

It is plain that modern orthodox medicine has developed entirely from the study of disease, and not at all from an understanding of what constitutes health or wellness. Without that perspective orthodox medicine has no answers to numerous health problems, in particular to the virtual plague of chronic illnesses which today beset us. For doctors are working with an outmoded and narrow paradigm or perspective on human health.

Which brings us to the next point. The second historical reason for this perversion of health care into 'disease care' lies back in the realm of the vast petrochemical empire of John D Rockefeller. Towards the end of the 19th century, through the single-minded accumulation of power over one of earth's great resources, petroleum, it became possible for Rockefeller to amass a fortune of billions in today's terms.

There are a few people, quite wicked of course, who would put forward the notion that anything within the earth's crust should belong to all of us. These miscreants believe that those who exploit these resources are entitled to a good return for their efforts, but that basically such resources belong to the peoples of the area or of the world. They would say, how can one individual 'own' a coal mine, or all the oil resources in an area, *or even the water, our most sacred resource?* But surely, this is an extreme position, and these people must be misguided.

Anyway, Rockefeller with his personally-owned oil wells had so much money 'he didn't know what to do with it.' So the burgeoning medical profession with its faulty paradigm suited him as an area to take over. He became the scion of the new pharmaceutical industry, where it was all done properly, with the proper standardized ingredients and the proper hygiene. So of course it had to be good. He was doing a public service. (Ironically, it is said that Rockefeller, for himself, relied primarily on homoeopathy.)

When the antibiotics came in and performed their wonders, well, that reinforced utterly the concept that only the invading force mattered, because here was a way to *really* blast the hell out of anything that had the temerity to crawl into our bodies! And as we noted, they ignored the inventor of penicillin, Sir Alexander Fleming, when he warned that antibiotics were to be used with the greatest of care. With the result that, since the arrival of antibiotics, the microbial world has been infinitely strengthened, not to mention transmogrified, to the detriment of generations to come. With even the possibility that humanity could be wiped out entirely.

At the same time, all the traditional methods of healing were driven off or underground: the herbs, the homoeopathy and numerous other healing modalities people had relied on for centuries. 'Many people may be unaware that herbal medicine served as the primary mode of medical practice in the US until almost 1935 ... for perhaps 2,000 years physicians had used them.'[14]

In order to make the world secure for pharmaceutical medicine and the Rockefeller billions, these alternative healing modalities had to be driven out. This was quite easily done, for by that time the Rockefeller billions not only controlled all the medical schools and the medical journals, the funding for research, but they also controlled the mass media.

How this has been attempted and to an extent accomplished in the UK, has been carefully documented by an investigative medical journalist, Martin J Walker, in his book *Dirty Medicine*.[15] The book describes the campaign to destroy the alternatives, and establishes links to this campaign from orthodox medicine, industry, government and the media, in many cases all of them working together. This campaign originated in the US, where of course it is even better organized. In *Dirty Medicine* Walker names the people and the organizations which have harassed and ruined several British, European and American medical practitioners who had the temerity to find ways of treating ill-health not acceptable to the medical/industrial establishment.

As recently as 1987 in the US, 'the American Medical Association was convicted of conspiring to destroy chiropractic medicine.'[16] It would take a courageous journalist indeed to write a similar book about the US. And the result would doubtless be even more horrifying than the British story.

And thus, all through recent history they managed to accomplish the task of making pharmaceuticals pre-eminent by spreading fear and anxiety about 'the dangers of herbs, homoeopathy and so on' or of their 'inefficacy', by harassing individual practitioners as 'quacks' and by a constant proclaiming of the wonders of pharmaceutical drugs.

They are still doing it today. Every few weeks there is yet another article against natural healing methods. The fact, as we noted in Chapter 27, that there is substantial evidence (from hospital records and costs, from poison centres, from WHO figures) that quite clearly pharmaceuticals are far more dangerous than the alternatives, is not mentioned. As to the relative efficacy, how can we know? Clearly the orthodox have not brought us to a nirvana of general good health.

There is a most interesting book, *Medicine and Culture: Varieties of Treatments in the United States, England, West Germany, and France* by Lyn Payer.[17] In this book the author, a medical journalist and biochemist, looks at the influence of culture and belief on medical practice in the countries mentioned in the title. We learn that in England there is 50% less of the major surgery carried out in the US, and there is considerably more restraint in drug-prescribing practices. The British complain of long waiting lists. However, they live longer than the Americans.

The French have the longest lives of all. Their medical practice is closest to the ideals of Bechamp. After all, he was French. And thus there is more emphasis on 'the terrain' in France. The emphasis there is on the liver, for that is the main organ of detoxification. French eating habits (fresh foods, far fewer processed, butter, eggs, olive oil, i.e. cholesterol galore), alcohol primarily with meals (mostly wine) and medical attitudes undoubtedly go to explain why the French people live the longest in the Western world, and have the lowest rates of heart disease and cancer.

A number of French drugs, from aspirins to antibiotics, come as suppositories, which bypass the gut and show a respect for the liver also. Anaemia is treated with organic B_{12} from liver extracts, instead of inorganic B_{12} from iron as in the US and elsewhere. Iron overload is now implicated in several degenerative diseases. With the French the emphasis is on boosting and strengthening the body with tonics, vitamins and ways of stimulating the immune system. French doctors recommend rest, just as did Hippocrates, and send patients to spas with water treatments (hydrotherapy) and use herbs, homoeopathy, and aromatherapy as well as immune system therapy. Mental illness is likely to be treated with spa therapies and enemas to detoxify. They are of course on the right track in everything. Their longer lives and fewer drugs taken, especially tranquillizers and drugs for depression, are testimony to that.

Apart from the French, it is a fact that modern medicine is a constantly changing scene, so much so that a doctor trained even 10 years previously is out of his depth and should be retrained. This sounds good, but in fact it is not. It is because modern medicine, unlike homoeopathy, herbalism, naturopathy, has no fixed laws of health and cure, no reference point apart from the faulty paradigm. It may recharge itself with new drugs and new procedures, but they are always designed to prop up, to fix-up, and never do they create real health.

We have looked at the danger and the inefficacy of orthodox cancer treatment. We have looked at the farce that is bypass operations. We should also note the caprice that renders American women twice as likely to have their uterus removed as British women. And we have to face up to the fact that many of these 'procedures' are done because they pay well.

There is massive stupidity and indifference to the obvious environmental causes of heart disease and cancer, the total inability to deal with 'new' health problems, with the chemically sensitive, with the chronically fatigued, and with AIDS; questions we will be looking at in the next two chapters. Because, above all, when there is a problem there is always the Freudian fallacy to fall back on: 'It's all in your mind,' or the Pastaurean fallacy, 'It's a virus.'

There are also the defeatist judgements: 'It's your age'; 'You're *allowed* to have that'; 'You must *learn* to live with it'; or, 'You have six months to live.'

Above all there is the fact that medicine is entirely under the thumb of the great pharmaceutical companies, the food technology industries and others like the petrochemical industry. Why else would 6 million American children be taking a powerful drug, Ritalin, when there are far better and safer solutions to hyperactivity?

Why have most doctors been reduced primarily to the role of 'drug pushers'? And pushers who create the most addicts?

How many health consumers are aware of a US Office of Technology Assessment on orthodox medicine; that its report concludes that 'Only 10 to 20%

of all procedures currently used in medical practice have been shown to be effica-cious by controlled trials'?[18]

Moreover, we have been led by an excited media, and media 'plants', to believe that the many technological advances made by medicine – the dialysis, the trans-plants and all the other tricky surgery – all are evidence of the wonderful advances made in the field of modern orthodox medicine. In the West we clamour for them, we demand them. But what we must come to see is that *all these things are signs of failure*. Medicine has failed to keep people well enough to avoid these vast-ly expensive high tech procedures. With a proper 'health care' system rather than a 'disease care' system, they should not be necessary.

Perhaps most ridiculous of all, we must be aware that doctors (and occasion-ally lawyers) are the only ones in the world rewarded for failure. The sicker we are, the more they are rewarded. In other words, if you go to a doctor with a heart con-dition he is rewarded by the state (and in most countries by the patient also) and sometimes in addition by insurance companies – that is, rewarded for his failure to prevent that heart condition. And the longer it goes on, with you getting worse and worse, the more he is rewarded by the fees your advanced condition brings in. And as we will see in the next chapter, only around 15% of those who visit a doc-tor are taken seriously anyway. In what other walk of life could one succeed with this attitude?

This is not to say that the best of doctors are unaware of this situation. The bril-liant Dr William B Kannel MD, Professor of Medicine at Brown University, address-ing the American Heart Association in 1994 said this, 'The day must come when we consider a heart attack in our patients not as the first indication for treatment, but as a medical failure.'[19] In his talk he stressed dietary factors and urged physicians 'not to rely on pills'. He is definitely on the right track. But is he being listened to?

In no other walk of life can one succeed so much by failing. If the car doesn't run you don't pay the garage. If the shoes don't fit you don't buy them. If your house falls down you demand compensation from the engineers, the builders or the city council.

In no other walk of life do we reward people for failure. But that is how mod-ern medicine flourishes at present. It runs on health disasters and failures. This must be the reason why medicine does not look beyond drugs and surgery for the most part, despite the very obvious failure of medicine to heal, to assist people to get well. We must face up to the fact that there is no incentive to get people well. We must by now be long past the time when we could regard doctors, *most of them*, as doing what they do solely for the love of humanity. The world doesn't work that way any more. Nor should they have to.

And no society in the world can, in the long run, afford a health care system with costs ever-spiralling upwards, a 'disease-care system' that both promotes ill-health and prospers by it. The most recent figures put it at a trillion dollars a year for the US,[20] depending on how one figures it, with the rest of the English-speaking countries running at lesser amounts. But still it is a monstrous expense.[21] And there is no evidence whatsoever that it creates health.

We have looked at the what and the how this has happened, but now we need to look at the reasons why such obviously disastrous concepts of human health remain largely unchallenged, why they continue on through time. We need to understand why, despite the massive evidence right under our noses, medicine continues to embrace two incorrect paradigms, the Freudian and the Pasteurean fallacies. We need to look at what happens in every profession in every walk of life, in every century of recorded history.

Each profession perpetuates itself through a system of indoctrinating each new generation enlisting in its ranks. This applies to doctors, dentists, lawyers, engineers, the ministry, nurses and, to a lesser extent, teachers. Each profession is a great fraternity with its own distinct language and terminology, its rules and regulations, its mores and conventions. Each is sustained by professional journals and clubs. Each of the professions involves a long indoctrination process. If you approve of how people emerge from this process you call it 'education'; if you don't you call it 'brain-washing'. It is perhaps a combination of the two.

Alan R Gaby MD, a doctor so brilliant that even many years of 'brain-washing' couldn't fool him, likens what happens to medical students to what happens to people drawn into a cult. He calls the system 'the cult of modern medicine'[22] Cults have a method of indoctrinating their members. And once we understand this, and how effective the process is, we need not wonder why people will hole up in a mountain with an arsenal of weapons and refuse to come out. Or why they will kill themselves en masse to join up with a spaceship, even though they all appear perfectly sane. For cults manage to indoctrinate people in such a way that they cannot see truth even if it is handed to them on a gold platter.

And the way they do it is quite straightforward. You have an older and wiser member of the cult with a charismatic personality, the guru, or several gurus everyone already in the cult regards as all-knowing, all-wise. You have those gurus believing earnestly what they are telling you. You keep the new recruits in confined quarters for many hours, doing endless learning in a repetitive way ('a constant bombardment with information, the truth of which cannot be independently verified'), with scant sleep and rations, often trying to manage on food so depleted that it cannot nourish and sustain either brain or body. And after a few days (that's all it takes for some cults), or weeks, months, years of this, there is no resistance left.

Eventually you discover that the path of least resistance is to change your view of reality. You have given up. You now believe that what you are learning in medical school is the best way; indeed, the only way. At that point, one might conclude that you have snapped.

Thus concludes Dr Gaby. The all-powerful, the all-controlling cult has won!

Dr Gaby says quite humorously, but at the same time seriously, that whatever it is that does it, most of those who experience this four- or six- or eight-year process will come out thinking alike, and they will not question the basic paradigms on which rest their professional futures, their livelihoods, their social life, their everything. Because that is the way groups work. No reason to wonder why it took centuries to get any admission from science, religion or the state to the effect that the earth was actually round; it was part of the official position of all those powerful groups that the earth was flat. And thus today, most of the belief system of the medical profession rests on assumptions that will one day be seen as the equivalent of **'the earth is flat'**.

Another doctor, Christopher Bird, agrees with Alan Gaby:

As a template for regimenting attitudes, the paradigm, by definition a limited set of boundaries, essentially places constraints against free-thinking. The stricture is not so much dictated by human fiat as it is imposed by a somewhat indefinable consensus, in the same way that human culture imposes correct table manners or appropriate styles of dress for an occasion. The implication is that scientists within a given discipline are no more free to oppose the stricture of the paradigm than are the rest of us are to appear nude, or eat with our hands, in a public setting.[23]

It is as though each person emerging from a professional occupation is issued with a special pair of glasses. They are donned, and from then on the world is viewed through that particular pair of glasses. But what happens when the paradigm is all wrong? The glasses the wrong prescription? Only a few exceptionally brilliant members of that profession are capable of taking off the glasses and having a real look at the world and the role of their profession in it. And these are generally the few who have had significant life experiences that make them question everything.

In the medical profession, it is also those who are extraordinarily brilliant or who have had personal health crises and have learned from them who may go on to question the faulty paradigms. The rest 'appear perfectly rational'. But future generations will come to see that they are not at all rational. The only way they can continue with the failure of the past and current medical paradigm is to be somewhat **irrational**, and they will be judged so by future generations.

The esteemed British medical journal, the *Lancet*, proclaimed in an editorial which had to do with breast cancer: 'The most important lesson we need to learn

... is the extraordinary capacity of the profession for self-delusion.'[24] Future generations will doubtless agree whole-heartedly with that admission.

The failure of modern medicine is not only reflected in the ever-worsening health of both adults and children, but also in the fact that the costs of all this virtual disease care spiral upwards every year. They are completely out of the stratosphere, and cannot be borne much longer no matter how many fancy insurance schemes are dreamed up or how much 'managed care' is instituted (which is of course at heart 'managed profits').

It is of the utmost significance that today, *despite* the massive influence of the media directed into this area, by 1993 the esteemed *New England Journal of Medicine* went on record as saying that 'Americans utilize alternative practitioners more than conventional primary care physicians.' They are choosing to go outside the realms of orthodox modern medicine, either to doctors who practise a different way, or to lay people one could call traditional or natural healers.[25] The false paradigms are beginning to break down.

But unfortunately medicine does not give in quietly to those doctors who have seen the light and who wish to practise a saner kind of medicine. As we have seen, many of America's most brilliant and innovative doctors have been persecuted, insulted, derided, sued, had their consulting rooms invaded by FDA agents with drawn pistols; their records, their stocks of food supplements and other substances confiscated. Over and over again this has happened, because orthodox medicine now has its back to the wall and the only way it can survive is to persecute and try to drive out the new and the enlightened (in this case the old and enlightened), just as has always happened right throughout history.

In the US there are today at least 2,500 orthodox physicians who have rejected the faulty basic paradigms and who practise a different kind of medicine. They have recently been placed on a 'quack' list, put together by the 'quack-busting' National Council Against Health Fraud as part of its crusade against the inroads being made into orthodox medicine by practitioners of natural and traditional healing methods.[26] Most of the doctors on this list, of course, take the best from many different systems, including orthodoxy.

Orthodox medicine can fight on for its exclusive overlordship to 'health care', which in truth is solely 'disease care', but it cannot in the end win because throughout history, although it can take many decades, even centuries, the truth does eventually come out. As one very great human being particularly gifted with words once said, 'You can fool some of the people all of the time. And you can fool all of the people some of the time. But you cannot fool all of the people all of the time.' And that is why truth eventually wins.

Or, as the perceptive John Robbins says, 'The medical establishment will get off its pedestal as soon as we get off our knees.'[27]

But we have to realize that orthodox medicine's traditional livelihood is at stake. Until it can see a new way to earn a living it will cling to what it has. It will not go down to defeat without an almighty struggle. And we must remember that through the power of the great pharmaceutical companies and the gigantic food technology industries, it controls the media.

So unfortunately, unless we have the knowledge to take charge of own health, our own lives, we are doomed to shorter, less healthy lives than we might have were we more enlightened. Hence this book.

There is currently some dispute about the length of doctors' lives, a statistic which should have some relevance to this chapter. Someone took the obituaries in the *Journal of the American Medical Association*, averaged out the age of doctors at death and came up with 57.6 years. This information was posted on the Internet under the heading, 'Dead Doctors Don't Lie.' But this figure is disputed by others. Dr Morton Walker has come up with a 70-year average life expectancy. But even if this is correct it is still five-and-a-half years fewer than for the average American citizen.[28] It is not a good advertisement for modern medicine, for one would expect that if anyone could take advantage of 'the best' that medicine has to offer, it would be those who practice it.

Dr Robert S Mendelsohn MD, after practising medicine for years in his own way, reached the conclusion that: 'Modern medicine cannot survive without our faith, because Modern Medicine is neither an art nor a science. It's a religion.'[29]

The French scientist Jean Tissot, in the Preface to his massive three-volume, 1,179-page magnum opus, published between 1926 and 1946, summed it up in these words, still entirely sound:

Pasteur's false dogmas have been nefarious in completely falsifying the reasoning of scientists and starting them up blind alleys of research. By arrest of scientific progress they have for three quarters of a century directed medicine into a situation of incredible ignorance and incoherence and led bacteriology into a decline.[30]

The fallacious paradigm on which rests modern medicine is now over a century old, and we will see no improvement in health until medicine gets rid of both the Pasteurean and the Freudian fallacies.

Future historians will note with a smile that in our time those doctors who call themselves environmental doctors or clinical ecologists were the only ones on the right track. But they were persecuted and derided by the rest and called 'quacks', just as those who knew that the earth was not flat were abused in their day.

Most of the doctors who do become aware of the influence of the environment on human health have themselves been very sick. Hence their understanding. But everything they say threatens the existing pharmaceutical, food and other industries. Because, understanding the concept of toxicity, they tend not to recommend drugs or prepared foods.

All one can say is 'How long, oh Lord, How long?' How much more cancer, heart disease, diabetes, Alzheimer's Disease and so on must the world endure before the penny drops?

The brilliant Thomas Kuhn argued that scientific revolutions come about when existing paradigms have ceased to function adequately.[31] A pervasive sense of the inadequacy of the paradigm must exist. I would suggest that many people are well into that stage with both fallacious paradigms, the Freudian and the Pasteurean. The problem is to break the stranglehold held by those institutions which insist on the perpetuation of such devout beliefs.

The most likely solution will come, and is coming, through the fact that people are getting less and less satisfied with modern medicine, its ever-escalating costs and the lack of good results. Medicine may have to reform in the face of this dissatisfaction.

Beyond this, short of dynamiting the medical schools, the only solution I can personally dream up is that concerned people get together to finance some really bright young people to be trained in France, at the most Bechampian medical school they have. Then on their return they will be patronized more enthusiastically than their fellows, and they will get better results. If enough people were to keep doing this, the situation would have to change. But also we need an entirely different structure to our health care system, the achievement of which would require the existence of far more concerned and enlightened governments than those we are faced with today.

33: 20TH-CENTURY ILLNESSES

'All those people lying around for years!
Bunch of hypochondriacs!'

It is advisable never to utter these words. Because you never know when it will be you and not just 'those people'.

Starting in a small way around the 1950s people began to become ill in a way seldom seen before in our century. And as the century progressed there were thousands of people experiencing fatigue, exhaustion, malaise and severe allergic sensitivities to many things in their environments, as well as experiencing numerous other unpleasant symptoms. This whole body sickness had been noted by the perceptive before. In the late Victorian period both the inimitable Florence Nightingale and the great Charles Darwin were chronically ill in the same way. So even in that time there may have been other 'lesser mortals' (I mean less famous) similarly afflicted. As it happens, there were.

Both Nightingale and Darwin were extraordinarily brilliant and productive people, as an examination of their lives will reveal. Florence Nightingale, on her return from the Crimean War where she had organized the care of the wounded and dying from that war, became chronically ill and mostly on the horizontal for the remaining 40 years of her life. But even though so terribly ill she managed to play a part in reorganizing the War Office, designing hospitals, organizing the new profession of nursing and so on. In other words, she did far more ill and in bed than the majority of people do well.

Similarly, Darwin was never the same after his return to Britain after his trip around the world on the *Beagle*. He suffered 40 years of extreme frailty, as one can deduce from his wife's letters about him. And yet he managed to overturn the entire Western world's view of reality. Then he quietly wrote an enormous tome, the world's definitive work on the earth worm. It had to be worms because it did not require much energy to deal with them and observe them. (He did not, how-ever, mention how worms reproduce themselves, presumably an act too horrible for an English gentleman to contemplate, let alone write about!)

The reasons why both Nightingale and Darwin acquired this lifelong debilita-tion are easy to deduce once one understands what is going on. I will doubtless write about them at greater length elsewhere. And of course they have both been psychoanalysed to a fare-thee-well by retired doctors with nothing better to do. It is a quaint little hobby I call 'psychoanalysing the dead', and of course it is extrava-gantly wrong and entirely ridiculous. Such brilliant people, such forceful geniuses, did not lie around ill for upwards of 40 years because they hated their mothers or some such nonsense.

They were not, of course, as I have hinted, the only ones to suffer in this way. Every century has its examples. In the late 19th century, around the time of Nightingale and Darwin, there was an illness that affected mostly young upper middle- and upper-class Englishwomen. It was called *the green sickness*, strangely enough. These victims just lay around, pale and without energy. Perhaps they turned a shade of green towards the end. It is even possible that despite the name, most ironically, few in that time worked out what caused 'the green sickness': It was undoubtedly caused by a combination of arsenic in the wallpaper and corsets that were too tight. (I am not truly serious about the latter. But assuredly they did not help.) The wallpaper in question was expensive to make and required lavish quantities of arsenic to get the fashionable, just right shade of green. In truth it was women who spent the most time at home; and when they became ill they took to their damp bedrooms where a fire was lit to keep them warm. This heat undoubtedly caused even more arsenic to 'outgas' from the wallpaper.

Earlier on, Napoleon in exile on his damp island was possibly similarly 'done in' by this green wallpaper. On his damp island, under the influence of heat, just as in Britain, the fungus on the walls would exude arsenic, which poison gradually killed those who slept in the room with the wallpaper. At the time of Napoleon's death it was not possible to test for this. But more recently a piece of his hair (thoughtfully saved) was tested and found to contain traces of arsenic.

This same phenomenon almost killed Clare Booth Luce, American Ambassador to Italy in the 1950s, so many years on from Napoleon. But the cause was the same. To be terribly chic they had resurrected the old green wallpaper in Luce's elegant Rome apartment.

When people become ill *in a way one does not understand*, it is best to look to environmental toxicity. Today's almost total medical blindness in this area is particu-larly strange because in old textbooks of medicine and homoeopathy, poisoning is frequently described. Those poisonings were considered to be due to an accidental ingestion of something nasty, or to someone's deliberate attempts to 'do in' another.

Apparently these things simply **do not happen today**, let alone the effects of the vast quantities of poisonous substances we encounter in our daily lives!

But here is where Freud comes back into our story. As we have noted, Freud gifted his murky view of humanity to medicine. It was murky because it was vague, ill-defined and definitely unprovable. But it was a great convenience to medicine. It made it possible for medicine never to be wrong, never to have to say the words that arrogant, narrow-minded people loathe to have to utter, 'I don't know' or 'I was wrong.' And that was why Freud was not laughed out of court.

His murky ideas were used to prop up medicine in places where *it should never have been propped up*. These ideas enabled medicine to transfer back to the patient any problems it could not deal with. 'You have a personality problem.' 'You just think you're ill. All the tests show you're perfectly normal.' 'You're just trying to get out of doing the housework.' 'There's a reason why you're ill, but you don't know about it. We'll see what doctor Shrink has to say' and 'Don't take up my valuable 5 to 10 minutes with something I do not understand, nor do I want to understand it.'

After all, we should be aware that in our simple-minded medical tradition one is generally permitted a maximum of three symptoms. (In fact I know one woman doctor who claims proudly that her patients 'are allowed one symptom at a time. We deal with that. And when that is solved, we deal with the next symptom,' the *reductio ad absurdum* of a ridiculous *modus operandi*.)

'Some of the physicians we interviewed recalled being told as medical students that the more symptoms a patient complained of, the less validity any of them had.'[1] 'Validity' meaning, of course, sanity. For if one should be so unfortunate as to suffer from more than three symptoms one is classified as 'a fruit-cake' or 'a psycho-ceramic' (i.e. a crack-pot). These terms and far worse appeared on people's medical records and referral letters for many years; that is, back when they were kept secret. Unfortunately, those suffering from this '20th-century' type of illness do in fact have numerous symptoms because every system in the body can be affected.

Interestingly, looking again at the differences among French, English, German and American medical practice[2] we note that French doctors record an average of 10 symptoms per patient, the English 8.4 and the Germans 7.5, as against the American Freud-dominated 3. Undoubtedly French medical practice contributes to the longer life expectancy of the French, as well as their dietary habits. Those who are not French should perhaps be asking themselves why their health is far worse and why they do not live as long as the French. The answer may have to do with more than wine-drinking, which is after all not exclusive to the French.

One could guess that when one wields only a few drugs or referrals for surgery, physiotherapy, etc., the more symptoms the patient suffers the more awkward for the doctor. Whereas as noted, in France the doctor has so much more to offer. The numerous symptoms can be fitted into a pattern and the patient is treated in the variety of ways mentioned in the last chapter.

But getting back to those struck down with 20th-century illnesses, it was, at least in the English-speaking countries, never a case of 'I regret it, but our tests, our laboratory, are inadequate to determine what is wrong with you, and so am I. We'll do our best for you in the face of our ignorance.' Because Freud had said there were hidden things under the surface, in that dim and murky place which we call, with our pathetically superstitious and primitive understanding of the brain and logical human motivation, 'the mind'. And students at medical school **are actually taught to believe that up to 45% of their patients will say they are ill but will not actually be ill.** Here is the flowchart used at my local medical school:

Sickness
Any Month
Any 400 People Over 16
300 Have Symptoms
100 Go to Doctor or Equivalent

50 Objective Physical Disease	**50 No Physical Disease**
35 will clear without help	35 psycho-social
15 progressive disease need help	10 anxiety?
	5 admin, e.g. certificate

1 referred to specialist
2/5 to major hospital

According to this flowchart, only 15 out of every 100 who visit a doctor actually 'need help'. Too bad about the rest! The 35% will clear up, because most illness does. But then there's that 45% who claim to be ill but medicine has 'decided' are *not* ill. Among them would have been Charles Darwin and Florence Nightingale. With this kind of ingrained doctrinal prejudice what chance does one have with anything slightly unusual? For what this means is that the 15% who are acceptable are so because they have symptoms which are acceptable, and verifiable in the laboratory. They fit a known pattern.

For somehow, despite the fact that every few years another discovery causes the laboratory to enlarge its knowledge and testing abilities, at any one point in time it is considered that 'all that is worth knowing is known today.' Absurd! Unscientific! And yet this is how doctors never have to say the words, 'I don't 'know' or even 'We don't know.' How's that for a supposedly science-based profession? To have no room in their 'system' for anything new? So what right therefore do they have to label any other kind of practitioner with the damning word 'unscientific'?

Moreover, the chances are that those not in the acceptable 15% may eventually go on to experience far more serious ill-health than the seemingly trivial symptoms that brought them to the doctor's office in the first place.

The dismissal of the 85%, with placebos and platitudes, and at a price, is all extremely convenient for an inadequate medicine with entirely the wrong paradigm about illness and what constitutes human health. And I have established to my own satisfaction that one can be just about dead, but if the tests don't perform in the narrow way they're trained to expect, well then, 'you're not sick, dear.'

It was Freudian theory which gave medicine the excuse for the indescribable cruelty and indifference shown to the first waves of people in our century with environmental illnesses.

For starting as early as the 1950s in isolated parts of the world (building up around the sixties and seventies and now happening every day), people began to get ill in ways which seemed strange and unusual. Looking back on it and seeing it in its context it is plain to see why we got so ill. We used to call it 'The Disease of a Thousand Names' because all over the world the cause was not known and the effects were not accepted as 'real' illness, so in each place it was given a different and a unique name.

As noted in previous chapters there have been an estimated 80,000 plus, and growing all the time, man-made chemicals concocted since the Second World War, now in daily use.[3] They're just flung into the environment, into our soils and into our foods, along with all the toxic metals we dig up in ever greater amounts. And what we have produced for people to live in is a world which has never before existed except in small ways, such as in the living rooms of the well-off Victorians, absolute flukes, like the wallpaper which caused 'the green sickness'. But now it is the 'green sickness' on a gigantic scale.

We were and are subjected to so many things which are alien, with which our bodies, our immune and nervous systems are in no way designed to cope. There is no question that the overall cause of these many illnesses lies in what we have done to our air, water, our soils and foods, and the massive overload of toxicity which people of this planet have never before had to cope with.

To take one problem alone, that of toxicity from lead, let me quote one Dr Schroeder, author of *The Poisons Around Us*: 'Lead goes to the nervous system. That tired run-down feeling, nervousness, depression, apathy, lack of ambition, frequent colds and other infections, and mild psychoneuroses may be the result of lead in the air.'[4]

Sometimes it was an isolated poisoning, such as those who found themselves under a plane spewing deadly poison *supposedly on a neighbouring property*. Or there could have been an accidental intake of something very toxic. My friend Patricia dates her umpteen-year illness, neurological and every other kind of 'ogical', from the time she put an organo-phosphate poison into saucers around the house to be rid of a plague of crickets. She did this with the best of advice. And I know a young man who had everything in life ahead of him but who did some car spray-painting. He has been almost totally incapacitated for the last 15 years.

Then there are the women whose silicon breast implants leaked into the rest of their bodies. And, unfortunately the leaked silicon sometimes crossed the placenta and/or was transferred in breastmilk to their children, many of whom suffer the characteristic fatigue of the environmentally poisoned, as do their mothers.

Sometimes the poisoning can even be purposeful. We should be aware that there is never an end to those who use poisons to vanquish their enemies. In Asia they put pesticide in a drink if they wish to poison someone. There are numerous other handy poisons to use in this way.

But the most visible victims have been those who became ill in large numbers, all in that new and terrible way. First there were the Vietnam War veterans. Many were sick, and many died young, from exposure to a highly toxic herbicide used against the Vietnamese, Agent Orange. The fact that the US Government spent $40 million per year on this defoliant gives us some idea of the enormous amounts that were used.[5] Has anyone done studies on Vietnamese health?

Recent research has found that there is 10 times the rate of Spina Bifida in the offspring of these veterans than in the general population, along with many other problems.[6] Apparently this is because Agent Orange was a dioxin which can cross the DNA barrier. (See Chapter 21 on pesticides.) Also it is said that an experimental malaria drug was used on these hapless soldiers; the combination could have been too much for many.

More recently it has happened to Gulf War veterans in their thousands. Dr Gary Null reports that Dr Garth Nicolson, Professor and Chairman of the Department of Tumor Biology, Professor of Pathology and Internal Medicine at the University of Texas Medical School, estimates that 100,000 Americans have become sick from Gulf War Syndrome, with possibly over 7,000 soldiers killed by the Syndrome. He is including family members affected, such as the deformed infants born of the soldiers. Apart from a few who picked up some unusual bacteria which were defeated by antibiotics, most cases remain 'a mystery'. There were so many possibly toxic things they could have been poisoned with: the oil fire smoke, the kerosene-burning tent heaters, the nerve gas, as well as those 'experimental anti-botulism vaccines' they found out later they had been guinea pigs for; also they were injected with numerous other vaccines.

My San Francisco friend, Judith, speaks also of 'detonated chemical arsenals and pesticide-loaded uniforms'. It is also said that in its infinite wisdom the US Government banned the use of alcohol among the troops, out of 'deference to Arab culture'. This highly principled approach left the troops with nothing to get stoned on but their anti-chemical warfare drugs, which apparently gave them a real 'buzz'. What else these drugs did to them can only be guessed at.

With the latest report from the journal *Our Toxic Times* it begins to look as though if it were not the individual chemicals they were exposed to then it was the combinations, the synergistic effects that were so toxic. For example, a Duke University Medical Center study using different chemicals with poultry found that:

chickens exposed to individual chemicals showed no outward signs of illness or debilitation ... but chickens exposed to any two chemical combinations exhibited varying degrees of weight loss, diarrhoea, shortness of breath, decreased activity, stumbling, leg weakness and a reluctance to walk, impaired flying or tremors. The combination of all three chemicals produced the most severe signs resulting in total paralysis or death in some chickens.[7]

Apparently both a 1995 Israeli study and a 1996 Scottish study elicited similar results.

The illness is quite bad enough for these veterans, but serious birth defects are showing up in high rates among their babies – 30%, which is 10 times higher than the number of birth defects in the general population. They are being diagnosed with Goldenhar's Syndrome, a condition whereby children may miss vital parts such as ears, eyes and brain; or they may have enlarged or deformed hearts and internal organs which can be upside-down in the body.

Betty Mekdeci, Director of the Association of Birth Defect Children, links these deformities to the multiple and experimental vaccines forced on the soldiers, for the reason that the fathers of three of the deformed children were given the multiple vaccinations in preparation for war service but did not for some reason get to the Gulf. They were held back, possibly to be sent to war later, and did not get there.

Reinforcing this view is the fact that France has no sick soldiers or deformed children. France was also the only country which did *not* immunize their troops with experimental vaccines.

Since that brief war, many who fought in it have been rendered seriously ill for years with no relief in sight. One day we will regard the Gulf War as an environmental/health nightmare both for those who participated in it and for its intended victims, of whom of course we hear nothing.

In Auckland, New Zealand, in the 1980s there was a huge fire in a chemical company. Many of the firemen who battled those flames and inhaled those fumes were thereafter ill for years and years. Many are still sick today.

I spoke recently to one who told me sadly that every one of those firemen (over 20 of them) who became ill and chronically ill for many years, eventually paid the price of his marriage. It is difficult for any relationship to survive the long-term illness of one, to endure day after day the sufferings and demands of another.

But this illness has an added burden. In the face of medical ignorance and denial, and the lack of support which goes with those things, in the face of the lack of community support which follows on when that medical 'seal of approval' is lacking, and eventually the doubtings of family and friends, any two partners are under an additional burden, the burden we could call 'suspected hypochondriasis'. For any support given at first is gradually withdrawn. When people do not understand they prefer to believe that the problem does not exist.

And all of us sick in this way have similar symptoms. The people with AIDS have them too, only for some reason they do not appear to be nearly as incapacitated until the end. For all involve serious impairments of the immune system, but of different kinds.

However, those war veterans in NZ and the US, and the firemen in New Zealand were told at first, in fact for years, that they were suffering from 'mass hysteria'. The rest of us, of course, were suffering from plain old 'hysteria' all on our own.

Also in New Zealand in the 1980s there was 'an outbreak' in a little town called Tapanui. Numerous people in that small place all got sick at once. So of course it had to be a virus. And the media happily called it 'Tapanui Flu'. Only it was no such thing. Even the concerned doctors who tried to care for the people affected had no idea as to the cause because they had no idea where to look, having taken to heart the wrong paradigm about human illness, just like all the rest.

But an intelligent friend of mine who lived a few hours away was not so mightily brain-washed. Hearing reports of this 'strange viral illness' she went straight to the place just out of town where the water came in from the mountains. And there she saw that the area around the piping intake had recently been sprayed, probably with 245T in those days. There was a dead blackberry bush over the intake. Every New Zealander knows from an early age what the results of such spraying looks like. There is a characteristic orangey-brown dead colour, and not a speck of green anywhere. It is seen so often on the sides of our roads. So she knew what caused 'Tapanui Flu'.

There were no other 'outbreaks' anywhere in the vicinity, in fact anywhere else in the country. It has never been seen or heard of since. A strange way for such a virulent 'virus' to behave. I mean if it could cut through a whole town so easily, why didn't it go elsewhere? Why didn't the people of the nearby town of Gore, where the people of Tapanui did their shopping, become afflicted? None of them did. But not so strange when you consider that most of the time people are more careful where they spray. They are usually not so stupid or so mad as to spray into the water supply. But somebody did at Tapanui. And they got away with it because the doctors could think only in terms of viruses. All those dreadfully ill people should of course have been compensated, and never were, because it was not 'a virus'. But then how many of us have been compensated?

Moreover, the people of Tapanui should have been medically 'treated' quite differently, just as should the Gulf War Veterans, the NZ firemen and all the rest of us. When we get ill in this particular way we should immediately be *detoxified*. But modern medicine cannot grasp that concept, let alone know how to do it.

There was also a horticultural area in New South Wales, Australia, with a similar sudden 'viral' problem where a lot of people got ill. And I have heard rumours that even the local doctors thought it possibly due to spray damage. But of course no one makes a fuss about it because we know who wouldn't like it, and there could be serious legal problems. Why are not more people angry over the power of these manufacturers and users who can wreck numerous people's lives, render them ill and helpless for years, and get off scot free? It is, of course, orthodox medicine with it 'unknown virus' theories that makes this all possible. And the fact that the people most concerned are generally too ill to fight for themselves.

One of the most famous 'outbreaks' of this strange 'viral illness' occurred at Britain's Royal Free Hospital in the 1950s, with some victims left seriously ill for the remainder of their lives. It simply mowed down many of the medical staff, but touched not one patient.

Once again, such a strange 'virus' to be so discriminating! That is considering the weaker are more likely to pick up strange viruses. There was, of course, and has been ever since, talk of 'mass hysteria'. Now if it had affected the patients that would have been easier. But it was the staff thus affected.

It is my guess that there were different kitchens for patients and staff. Or that they ate in different shifts. And that something very toxic was dropped into the stew, or whatever, that the staff ate.

One can see how it could have happened. Here's a possible scenario: Nurses tend to be hell-on-wheels about flies, having in their training days been shown those gruesome blowups of flies doing disgusting things on our food. So it is not hard to envisage the Matron of the Royal Free Hospital arriving in the kitchen, or kitchens, with the words, 'I don't want to see a single fly in here. If I do, off with your heads!' or words to that effect. Matrons can be formidable creatures. And were especially so in those days.

Then one day, just as a meal is about to be served, the young lass who peels the vegetables and washes the dishes spies a fly hovering around the food. 'Oh Gawd! What if Matron should come? She often does about this time.' Panic! Quick, the fly spray!

In those days they did not have aerosol sprays. They had a tin of fly spray with what looked like a bicycle pump attached to it. It was unwieldy and difficult to hit the target. Supposing this young, fairly innocent lass chases the fly around the kitchen squirting as she goes and mostly missing it. The spray is floating down, some of it settling into the food. Then the fly settles down, right on the edge of the giant stew pot! Squirt squirt!

She didn't know any better. Something like this had to happen somewhere, didn't it? At some time in some place? When you consider the hundreds of thousands of humans working in hundreds of thousands of hospitals, and the numbers of years we have had hospitals, just by chance even, considering the infinite failings of human beings, something like this had to happen.

I've been talking about these dramatic episodes of mass poisonings to point out what can happen in a big way. But mostly there have been individuals poisoned in different ways, who got even shorter shrift from the doctors. Most victims have no idea how they got so ill. Because the effect can be cumulative rather than sudden.

Besides all the obvious toxins and the lack of decent food from our wasted and poisoned soils there are the vaccinations, the drugs, the antibiotics, the invasive procedures. All just loaded on to people with nary a thought as to the consequences. It is mostly the gradual overload principle, the drip drip drip until the barrel overflows. The barrel gradually fills up with various insults to the immune system, then one day a car accident, the birth of a child, a mere case of influenza, things that seemingly have no bearing on the subsequent events. But that additional stressor, no matter how mild, is just too much and one goes under. And in 'going under' one perhaps stays under for life. Others manage to rally after some years and get back to what looks like health, but they will always be vulnerable.

So those with the weakest livers, the weakest detoxification systems, went first. After all, through aeons of evolution there was *no time* in our past development when any ancestor had to cope with the enormous load of toxic substances and procedures so entirely foreign to the natural way of life we were evolved to live. And therefore a powerful detoxification system was not necessary. If you had one it would have been a random thing. A bit like having a motor capable of doing 200 miles an hour: you seldom need to use it, or never get much chance to 'let it out'. But in the 20th century these differing strengths of the immune system and liver, etc., the differing abilities to detoxify, would count for a great deal and affect the outcome of certain health situations, perhaps in the differing lengths of time it takes people to succumb.

Also, the childhood experiences: the mercury, the fluoride and so on, crossing the placental barrier from mother to growing infant, and then the vaccinations, the antibiotics, the almost entirely devitalized foods we give our children to eat;

also of course, the lack of Essential Fatty Acids and the non-nutritious fats and oils which have replaced them. All of these add to the toxic load on the modern human immune system.

And then I subscribe to another theory about victims of these illnesses. Children who endure very tense, unloving or abusive childhoods because of poor parenting develop shaky immune systems because they are constantly producing and subjected to unnatural levels of adrenalin (the 'fight or flight' hormone) at an early age.[8] This constant surging of the adrenalin can weaken the developing hormonal, immune and nervous systems, and possibly the detoxification systems. In my childhood the government sent medical teams around to all the schools. By the time I was five I had an enlarged thyroid gland and was sent home with a letter about treatment. I still have that enlarged thyroid today; in addition I have developed antibodies against my own thyroid.

Children brought up like me are therefore sitting ducks for such illnesses as the tuberculosis I contracted at the age of 10, and the later severe illness in adulthood. And recent research shows that children with these difficult childhoods are three times more likely than the average to eventually show up in the suicide statistics.[9]

A South African doctor came to New Zealand about the same time as the early waves of environmental illness hit the country. He alone among doctors actually took the time to talk to these patients. A whole 30 minutes I believe it was. And he said at a doctors' convention, one I also addressed, that all of those patients had had unhappy childhoods.

At the time I was irritated by this theory and dismissed it as the usual psychological poppycock. In fact I was furious with him because I knew it would just reinforce the doctors' opinion that the patients were not ill but 'screwed up'. But since then I have had numerous years to think about it and to study. Now I think he was right, but not in the way he meant; probably not in the Freudian psychological way of causation. I believe it was that tension and adrenalin which damaged our immune systems when we were quite young. Because our bodies never after that cope with stress well. And that makes us ripe for environmental illnesses.

Not all victims will have unhappy childhoods, though. I know a few who had happy ones but who were hit by sprays in a big way, and were thereafter ill for the rest of their days. For a massive dose of certain poisonous substances could perhaps overwhelm even someone with a fairly strong immune system, given enough poison. Enough of course, and you die.

And I know others who have been ill ever since that monkey virus polio vaccine with which the children of New Zealand were betrayed. Some of them may have had happy childhoods. Then there is a very strong and upright military man I know, now mostly on the horizontal, who while in the army brought up several platoons of men to take the polio vaccine. And each time he arrived with another platoon, they gave *him* some more vaccine, and he didn't know enough to say 'No'. He ended up with about six doses. Unfortunately he has had to pay with about 25 years of a ruined life.

And what has the medical profession done, what have governments done about this sickness now widespread throughout society, found in both sexes at every age and stage in life and in every class or level of education? What have they done? Well, for the most part you could say they've done nothing. Nothing sensible. They prescribe antidepressants. As usual we are to be grateful when the disease gets a classification at the US Centers for Disease Control, which it has now. But how is this classification being used?

A recent orthodox theory (Professors Graham A W Rook and Alimudden Zumla of the University College London Medical School writing for the *Lancet*) on what happens with these syndromes is that there is a switch in the balance between the Th1 and the Th2 cytokines in the immune system. Under toxicity and stress the balance may switch to the Th2 side of the system, which can, without the balancing Th1, wreak havoc in the body, with 'an increased frequency of allergic events, mood changes, depression' and the inevitable chronic exhaustion.[10] The professors state that this imbalance may be 'long-lasting. Also that the syndrome will vary between individuals and will also depend on other genetic and environmental factors.' Of particular interest was the fact that they recommended a moratorium on the compulsory vaccination policy, particularly for the Gulf War veterans.

However, the main body of medicine cannot even accept that once the immune system is so compromised then the ever-present yeast will come up strongly ... often with the aid of antibiotics. So that these '20th-century illnesses' are nearly always complicated by an overgrowth of Candida albicans and, worse still, sometimes Candida in the deadly myceliae form. I have seen them, thread-worm-like, undulating casually through one drop of my blood magnified and projected on to a screen.

Of course because of the 'hint of hysteria' surrounding these illnesses, those doctors who contract the illness themselves, and there are quite a few out there, either remain quiet or they launch into the game of 'hunt the virus' which could at least give the strange illness a semblance of 'respectability'. But in 20 years they have not found a virus, because it is not a virus which is causing all this. Just as you probably do not become ill for years with AIDS and die with the Human Immunodeficiency Virus, because no virus ever behaves in that way; so you do not lie around for 40 years, as Nightingale and Darwin did, with 'Acquired Immune Malfunction' because of 'a virus'.

But of course 'a virus' is more respectable, and falls within the orbit of ortho-dox medicine, and *has* made AIDS (and could make the modern version of 'the green sickness') so much more acceptable to it. We noted in the last chapter as to *why* a virus is more acceptable and why most doctors appear to have not the slightest interest in environmental matters. The entire fiasco will be included by future generations in 'the dark ages of medicine' as the ultimate in human ignorance.

I myself have lost 20 years of my life, and just about everything else along with it, owing to this kind of environmental illness.[11] Had Freud been perhaps 1% less ambitious and the medical profession perhaps 1% less obtuse, lazy, indifferent and concerned with their egos than with human suffering and the state of the environment in general, the story of our century and the disaster that has occurred might have been quite different. For had the millions of people who got ill in ways the medical profession could not understand been taken seriously, the alarm bells should have been ringing at least by 1980. There might have been time to save the human race, the planet. But nothing much was done, because apart from those doctors who themselves became ill in such a fashion, few took these '20th-century illnesses' seriously, and for all the reasons which we've looked at: the massive greed, corruption and carelessness which are part of modern medicine and, of course, of most governments. Also, of course, Freud the Fraud gave them the perfect way out of having to come to grips with these illnesses.

Dr Michael L Culbert DSc, editor of the journal *The Choice*, reported on a Pentagon study of Gulf War Syndrome in 15,000 veterans. Dr Stephen Joseph MD had asserted on behalf of the Pentagon that 4% of the sick veterans were suffering from infectious diseases, while 21% had psychological problems.[12]

Thus it is possible that the two medical fallacies, the Pasteurean and the Freudian, took care of one-quarter of the problem. They have no answer for the other 75% suffering from the syndrome.

It is also a fact that those who attempt to investigate the illness get into difficulties with the establishment. Dr Garth Nicholson, mentioned earlier in this chapter, has declared 'There is a huge cover-up of immense proportions,' and also that since his research into the illness became known, 'I'm being harrassed by federal agents.'[13]

Dr Nicholson is one of the most highly published and most frequently cited scientists in the biomedical literature today, but since he has been working on the Desert Storm illness he has been finding himself blocked at the publication level, his grant applications interfered with, his mail, phone calls and faxes repeatedly intercepted. He says,

It means that for years and years biological warfare has been going on in this country despite treaties that forbid it ... We have possibly uncovered one of the messiest controversies and cover-ups since Watergate, and this one makes Watergate seem like a tea party.

Dr Gary Null, writing in the *Townsend Letter for Doctors* about the victims of Gulf War Syndrome, said this:

Both the families and the veterans have suffered because of the government's lack of concern about their service people's post-war ailments. Since, until recently, the department of defence did not acknowledge the existence of any war-caused illnesses, soldiers who claim that they have the syndrome have been denied proper medical attention and have in some cases been instructed to leave the military. In pain, neglected by their country, and mistakenly diagnosed with psychiatric ailments, many veterans have tragically turned to suicide to cope with a problem that no one seemed to understand or care about.[14]

It is all a most terrible and familiar story to people attempting to deal with these victims. Those of us ill and dying and taking our miserable lives from terrible sicknesses incurred by the vast and careless toxicity now widespread in our environment should have been listened to, thanked, fully compensated and given the care and respect due to those giving the rest of the world, by our sufferings, the message of a dying planet. But we were not listened to at all. We were cursed and reviled and thrown out into the wilderness to cope God knows how, so many of us.

What does a sick person do when given the label 'hypochondriac'? What does one do when one cannot even stand up long enough to get oneself a meal? Let alone go out to earn the money to provide it? And to be told, 'There's nothing wrong with you'? How does one persuade others that one needs help when the medical profession has not deigned even to give one an acceptable label, as was the case until recently?

The story of those who struggle to survive with environmental illnesses in our time is a story of utter infamy. Those with '20th-century illnesses' are victims of the callousness and inefficacy of modern medicine, of orthodoxy's false view of health.

In addition, the medical inability to deal with this illness gives to those people desperate to feel superior the right to call ill people 'hypochondriacs'. For in our sick society, when you have no label and you have no medical support to speak of, that is what you are. And when people use that word they do not have to feel an iota of compassion, they can pass on by with a clear conscience, because after all you're not really sick, you're just lazy and self-obsessed.

Yes, for certain, that word 'hypochondriac' is the most obscene in the English language. I have talked at length to thousands of people sick in this particular way, and I have never once met 'a hypochondriac'. I have met only very ill people struggling bravely to be well, for that is all any of us on the face of the earth wants. But this word 'hypochondriac' is handed to people by a profession supposedly dedicated to caring for the sick but which would condemn some truly sick people to infinitely more suffering than is necessary, merely because from the depths of their indoctrinated ignorance they cannot understand such an illness, because their training enables them to see scarcely a tree or two of the whole forest.

⚠️

34: AIDS

'Caused by the Human Immunodeficiency Virus; death is successfully postponed by a drug, AZT, but in the end the disease inevitably proves fatal.'

There is 'something very rotten in the state of Denmark' or rather in the US (as there is in most of the English-speaking world). Well, we already know this from most of the chapters so far. But in addition there are a number of unanswered questions to do with what exactly AIDS (Acquired Immune Deficiency Syndrome) is. Moreover, the drug used by doctors to treat it appears to be a certain killer. In fact there are those who believe that it is the drug AZT which kills people with HIV (the Human Immunodeficiency Virus), and not the AIDS itself.

Dee Smith is one sufferer from AIDS, diagnosed in the acute stages and now willing to speak out about her experience. Her husband also had AIDS. He died in 1995 after spending $78,000 on medical bills in three years. He, unlike Dee, was a believer in conventional medicine. Dee Smith is not.[1]

She (described as 'upbeat and vivacious') survives, he does not. In fact, none of her friends of the 1980s with diagnosed AIDS who followed the orthodox medical path, which means AZT, is alive today.

She alone, who has stuck to natural healing methods all along and at a tiny fraction of the cost of her husband's treatment, today appears as a person with no disease at all. In fact she looks upon AIDS as chronic rather than fatal, provided it is treated correctly.

At the same time as 'the AIDS virus' was officially announced, in what has derisively been called 'Science by press release', a vaccine was promised within two years. The cure would be found. But what in fact was found was the failed chemotherapy drug, AZT. Immediately two enormous pharmaceutical companies, Burroughs Wellcome and Novapharm Incorporated, went to court to do battle over which was to garner the rich harvest from AIDS,[2] and the stocks of the winner shot up magnificently. The profits from AZT have been in the billions.

However, a recent European study has shown that AZT does not provide any benefit in prolonging the quantity or improving the quality of an AIDS patient's life.[3] According to Dr Jules Klotter, the study showed that AZT not only does not prevent AIDS, but that **25% more of the group taking AZT died than did those in the untreated control group**. And according to the largest US federally-funded study of male homosexuals at-risk for AIDS (the MAC study), not one long-term survivor has used AZT.[4] Another similar study concluded that 'AZT appears to be the most toxic drug ever approved for continual use in the United States.'[5]

One of the greatest of the dissenters on the subject of AIDS and HIV is the world authority on retroviruses, Professor Peter H Duesberg of the University of California Department of Molecular and Cell Biology. This is what he has to say of AZT:

AZT is a random killer of infected and non-infected cells. AZT cannot discriminate among them. It kills all cells. AZT is a chain terminator of DNA synthesis of all cells, no exceptions. It wipes out everything. In the long run it can lead only to the death of the organism, and the cemetery. AZT is a certain killer.[6]

Of course, as is true of all pharmaceutical drugs, AZT would be directed against the symptoms of the disease rather than the cause, which, whatever else it is, is a failing immune system. But on the package inserts that go with the drug AZT the truth-telling 'side-effects' are listed as follows: Cancer (Lymphoma), Hepatitis, Dementia, Mania (madness frenzy), Seizures (epileptic), Anxiety, Anaemia, Leucopoenia (Standard laboratory evidence of immune suppression), Impotence, Severe Nausea, Chest Pain, Insomnia, Ataxia (loss of balance), Depression, Muscle Atrophy (wasting)[7]; this is only half of the list of what can be caused by taking AZT.

This list sounds like a death sentence. In fact these health catastrophes caused by AZT sound exactly like – well, exactly like AIDS. Is this what AIDS is? The side-effects of a drug prescribed for HIV? Would you take it? Only those desperate to live, and thoroughly dependent upon their doctors, would dream of taking this appalling drug. And it is a fact that many of the group of dissenting scientists, some of them with international reputations, believe that AIDS is caused by long-term drug abuse (epidemic in the US), and AZT.

The latest 'miracle cure' for AIDS, Protease Inhibitors, may also be doomed. I will quote directly from my San Francisco friend, Judith Lopez, a writer, an artist, and a researcher in this field:

Protease Inhibitors work, supposedly, by blocking the retroviral protease and preventing the replication of HIV in the body.

Problem 1: HIV is never replicated. It is completely dormant. So why use a drug to block it? Problem 2: Like AZT, Protease Inhibitors are extremely toxic. In high doses they can actually block the proteases necessary for human LIFE (i.e. human digestive aspartyl protease cathespin D, in the intestine). They can also inhibit the liver from detoxifying other drugs, such as AZT, allowing these drugs to build up to lethal levels. In other words, Protease Inhibitors may make AZT even more toxic. It's all very reminiscent of the glory days of AZT ... remember how it was shown to increase people's T-cell counts? Everyone was cheering, people felt just great. Except the T-cell counts didn't do a thing to cure the patients; they died anyway. Similarly there are no studies to show any clinical benefits from the P.I.s, just a lot of publicity and hype.

On the basis of all this flim-flam, 'AIDS' is now being redefined as a treatable, non-fatal condition. Which it always was. And could be now, if they'd just stop with the fatal, poisonous 'treatments'.

Looks as though my friend Judith agrees with Dee Smith. Moreover, reports from a recent AIDS conference bear out Judith's assessment of Protease. True to form, the promoters of Protease Inhibitors were proud to announce that viral counts had been dramatically lowered by it. However, they refused to answer an honest question with regard to how the patients on this drug were faring. It sounds as though it could be a case of, 'The operation was a success, but the patient died.'

And there's more. On June 12, 1997, the FDA was forced to issue a warning on the formerly fully-approved Protease Inhibitors. As early as four days after beginning these drugs there may be a sudden blood sugar increase, which event had been life-threatening in six cases and had hospitalized 21. Over 40 people had to stop taking these drugs because of severe blood sugar abnormalities.

However, a recent report from *Positive Health News* (produced by the dedicated Mark Konlee) speaks more positively about a Protease 'cocktail'.[8] (See the end of the chapter for his recommendations.) But he also describes numerous individual successes among those using specialized nutrients only. Is it possible that the declining death rate is due rather to the fact that many people with AIDS are beginning to reject the whole drug approach? That they are beginning to be aware that the taking of some of these drugs may be a death sentence? Konlee emphasizes that some combinations can be lethal, but that others may help. The treatment of AIDS is indeed a minefield.

On the possibility of an AIDS vaccine, Judith Lopez has this to say:

A vaccine is supposed to trick the body into making antibodies against a disease. But how is AIDS diagnosed? By finding antibodies to HIV. No one has explained why one's own antibodies signal a fatal disease, while those created by a vaccine will confer protection. Or how they will tell the difference between the two. The logic of this eludes me.

The other question, the one querying the hypothesis that it is the Human Immunodeficiency Virus that causes AIDS, is a lot harder to come to grips with. And yet it is a fact that over 60% of the original AIDS patients used to create this hypothesis were, it is claimed, HIV-negative[9] – that is, out of 4,000 patients with AIDS, 2,400 and more had no sign of HIV.[10]

In addition to all the people with diagnosed AIDS who have no HIV, there are over 1 million Americans who are healthy and yet HIV-positive. In fact, according to Professor Duesberg, over 13–14 million people on this planet have HIV and are perfectly healthy. He believes that HIV is a harmless passenger found in large numbers of healthy people, just as there are many other 'harmless passengers' we all carry. In summary, he says, **'HIV is not the cause of AIDS.'**[11]

There is also the seemingly inexplicable fact that in Africa, AIDS occurs primarily in people who turn out to be HIV-negative. In 1992, Britain's most prestigious medical journal, the *Lancet*,[12] carried the following report: Among 227 Ghanaians diagnosed as having AIDS, based on clinical symptoms, it was found after multiple laboratory tests that 59% were negative for both HIV-1 and 2.

In 1993, a study of 122 tuberculosis patients in Nairobi, Kenya, found 69% of the patients to be HIV-negative. The authors of the report commented that 'the differences that exist between HIV-positive and HIV-negative patients are minor.'[13] And this is significant because TB is an official AIDS-related condition.

In another report, in a 1994 *Journal of AIDS*,[14] found that of 913 suspected AIDS/HIV-infected patients from towns with the highest number of reported cases in Kenya, 71% were HIV-negative.

How then could Dr Robert Gallo say, and continue to say, that AIDS *is caused by* HIV? He is now a multi-millionaire owing to his patents on the test for HIV.

However, more recently, Luc Montagnier of the Institute Pasteur, the original spotter of the virus, declared that the virus is 'a peaceful virus' and that it cannot possibly cause AIDS by itself.[15] In truth, since the April 1984 announcement that AIDS is caused by HIV there has not been a single scientific research publication that claims to prove that HIV causes AIDS. There is, as such, no documented evidence for the hypothesis.

Other scientists, such as Professor Duesberg and others, have been saying this for years. Duesberg claims that HIV is totally harmless. He calls it 'a pussy-cat' and insists that AIDS is caused by recreational drugs, multiple transfusions, malnutrition and AZT.

It is a fact that groups of haemophiliacs studied (that is, men with a severe blood-clotting disorder), some with and some without HIV, have the same mortality and morbidity – that is, death and sickness rates. Other transfusion recipients of HIV are similar. So as long as the HIV-positive haemophiliac sufferers do not take HIV medication they are unlikely to go on to get AIDS.

Efforts have been made to inject HIV into monkeys. Over 150 chimpanzees have been infected but after 10 years all remain healthy.[16] Furthermore, if it is an infectious disease or a sexually-transmitted one, why do we see it confined to specific risk groups? In the US, 90% of those with HIV are male; in Europe 86%. We do not see AIDS in prostitutes unless they are *also* intravenous drug users. Moreover, *no one in the entire health care scene has caught AIDS from their patients or vice versa*.

The news story of the HIV-positive dentist scared everyone, but the fact is that in almost every dental practice in America there will be 0.4% dentists registering positive for HIV. For that is the incidence of HIV in the population. So as this is the only such scare story, when one would expect it to be frequent, was this a case of the media playing up what was already there, and that any patients affected did not get it via their dentist?

Dr George Milowe reports that *if* HIV is transmitted through sexual contact, it is 'a highly inefficient means of transmission. In one study of 25 HIV-positive men, one man was found to have one HIV cell in 1 million sperm cells, while in the other 24 men, no HIV was found at all in their sperm.'[17]

Moreover, that exponentially increasing pandemic we were promised never occurred. The World Health Organization predicted 30 to 40 million cases by the year 2000, but in fact, regardless of the numbers of newly diagnosed cases, the deaths from AIDS are actually declining every year.[18]

The insistence that HIV is the cause and precursor to AIDS is also emphatically refuted by Dr Robert Wilner in his book, *Deadly Deception: The Proof that Sex and HIV Absolutely Do Not Cause AIDS*.[19] This book was reviewed by Frank Prescott in an article entitled, 'A Medical Doctor puts his life on the Line to Prove that Sex and HIV do not cause AIDS'.[20]

Dr Wilner states that

nearly 500 of the world's top scientists are now challenging Gallo's hypothesis that HIV causes AIDS, and the list is growing daily. Every statistic, every valid scientific observation, and even the test of time now go to prove Gallo wrong.

In short, Dr Wilner believes that what we know as 'AIDS' is 'the greatest fraud in medical history'.[21]

There are several other books on this subject, such as: Dr Robert Root-Bernstein's *Rethinking AIDS: The Tragic Cost of Premature Consensus*[22] and Dr Michael L Culbert's, DSc, *AIDS: Hope, Hoax, and Hoopla*.[23]

The Bechampian view of AIDS has been expressed by Luc Chaltin ND:

It is doubtful that the HIV virus can cause the deadly AIDS disease on its own. Infection with any virus is not enough to cause disease or its fatal evolution because this evolution depends not exclusively on the nature of the infective agent but primarily on the overall health of the patient.[24]

Dr Joseph Sonmabond, clinician and scientist, is another critic. He says this:

The harm in the whole notion of presenting speculation as fact, means that if the specula-tion proves to be untrue, the research and work on whatever is *truly* going on is being neglected, and this can be translated into the loss of tens of thousands of lives.

There is another whole school of thought which declares that AIDS is caused by a monkey virus transmitted in a polio vaccine. That is, in vaccines cultured in monkey kidneys. Scientific findings point to AIDS as a new disease, manifest in humans for the first time around 1960. Early cases all seem to be traced to Kinshasa, capital of Zaire (formerly the Belgian Congo) and other nearby areas.

This was in fact the area used as a field-test for a trial polio vaccine in 1959. Over 70,000 were vaccinated in that year. Can it be a coincidence that the Central African States most intensively immunized are also those most affected by AIDS?[25] It is possible that the weakening effect of multiple vaccines plus inadequate nutri-tion may have been enough to cause widespread immune system failure?

Several extremely respectable scientists are of the opinion that this might be where it all began. Professor Melnick, scientist and polio researcher: 'I find this theory plausible, and one of the several possible explanations for the still unsolved mystery of how the modern AIDS epidemic originated.'

However, there is another contender for the AIDS 'prize'. On the 5th of November 1987, the staid *Times* (London) newspaper exploded with the headline: SMALLPOX VACCINE 'TRIGGERED AIDS VIRUS'.

This was followed by:

The AIDS epidemic may have been triggered by the mass vaccination campaign which eradicated smallpox. The World Health Organization, which masterminded the 13-year campaign, is studying new scientific evidence suggesting that immunization with the smallpox vaccine Vaccinia awakened the unsuspected, dormant Human Immuno-deficiency Virus infection (HIV).

The *Times*, so thoroughly respectable and careful in its reporting, went into enor-mous detail – the numbers vaccinated, in what parts of Africa, and the numbers of

AIDS cases. Apparently 'the more than 2 million carriers, and 50,000 deaths ... are concentrated in the countries where the smallpox immunization programmes were most intensive.'

There was also a quote from Robert Gallo:

The link between the WHO programme and the epidemic in Africa is an interesting and important hypothesis. I cannot say that it actually happened, but I have been saying for some years that the use of live vaccines such as that used for smallpox can activate a dormant infection such as HIV.

Somewhat allied to this theory is the one about AIDS, Ebola and other 'emerging' new illnesses being deliberately lab-created biological agents designed specifically to destroy the immune systems of selected populations in time of war, or as a silent attack on an 'enemy' at any time. Dr Leonard A Cole, Associate Professor in Science, Technology and Society at Rutgers University, has written two books putting together the evidence for the creation of such biological agents: *The Eleventh Plague* and *Clouds of Secrecy.*[26]

After the First World War, the world reacted with intense revulsion against the weapons of chemical warfare such as mustard gas (which, in a modified form, eventually came to be used in chemotherapy against cancer). Instead, in the interests of 'national security' the US developed and tested numerous biological agents which could kill, maim and sicken in time of war. The problem was, and is, that if such weapons are to be 'useful' they have to be tested both for methods of application and for their effects. One has to read these two books for information on how this has been done.

Perhaps one of the most dangerous aspects of such 'science and technology' is that many of these weapons, both chemical and biological, have been sold to Iraq and other countries. According to Dr Cole, between 1984 and 1989 more than 80 agents (including botulinum toxoid, dengue virus and the West Nile fever virus) were **shipped from the US to Iraq** (some even by the US Centers for Disease Control), which does rather cast a note of hypocrisy over the recent affronted searches conducted in that country.

The Federation of American Scientists has recently set up the Program to Monitor Emerging Diseases (ProMED) to survey various disease outbreaks, which seems to offer the only hope for the containment of these diseases.

There are some who believe that the vaccine administered to 320,000 Africans between 1957 and 1959 contained live simian immunodeficiency virus (SIV). A similar vaccine was given to 98 million Americans. In this may lie a possible explanation[27] for the explosion of cancer, new infective agents, the '20th-century diseases' and other new immunological and neurological disorders among the Baby Boomers born between 1941 and 1961.

Meanwhile, speculation would have it that AIDS as a 'weapon' may have been used experimentally in the Belgian Congo with the Africans as guinea pigs. As noted, early AIDS cases can almost all be traced either to Kinshasa or to places not far from where the vaccine was field-tested. But there is another interesting facet: In Africa there is an equal gender distribution of 'AIDS', whereas in the West it is almost wholly found in the male sex.[28] Are we truly dealing with the same illness in both these places?

Other possibilities: Dr Raymond Peat is of the opinion that up until the 1940s young adulthood was the healthiest phase of life, and he would remind us that septicaemia, a severe bacterial infection, was associated with the declining immune deficiency of old age. But by the 1960s septicaemia was killing many young adults, in spite of the susceptibility of the germs to antibiotics. And some of those who were saved with antibiotics went on to more severe diseases, such as Pneumocystic carii, a lethal type of pneumonia. Dr Peat believes that AIDS was a recognized syndrome for many years, and that it was known to be increasing long before the 1980s. There are several chapters in this book which suggest a possible cause. But then, of course, along came AZT.

Dr Peat believes that the virus could be a 'co-factor' in the disease – that is, only one factor among several necessary to cause the total syndrome/disease. He speaks of

an increasing burden of immunosuppressive factors [some of which we have looked at in this book] which are causing an exponentially rising curve of immunodeficiency diseases, and that, arriving at a certain point on that curve, the HIV virus would help to push the rate of increase upward.

But the crunch point is that anything to do with a virus or a mycoplasm would infect its victims across the board, without regard to gender or way of life, **which clearly has not happened, at least not in the West**.

What is undeniable is that AIDS, whatever it is in its late stages, begins with immune system failure. In the 1950s there were sudden increases in the exposure of populations to several powerfully immunosuppressive factors: Radioactive fallout (widespread in the US, especially of strontium 90, which concentrated its damage near the bone marrow), medical X-rays, dioxins and other chlorinated carbon compounds, insecticides and herbicides, the upsurge in vaccination, the increased promotion of the use of hydrogenated liquid vegetable oils and margarine as food, and the use of lead as a gasoline additive. All had become important immunosuppressive factors by 1960.

Those who contracted 'AIDS', whatever it is, had been the children born in the 1950s to 1963 during the period of nuclear testing. Recreational drugs contribute to immunosuppression, just as excessive amounts of alcohol will. The immune system, like any system, can become ineffective or sick, and it is possible that a sick immune system could make some problems worse.

Professor Duesberg has pointed out that most of the present AIDS cases can be explained by various known causes other than HIV.

Others concur:

Duesberg is right in emphasizing that we have to think of immune deficiency in a broader context, of eliminating all the immunosuppressive factors, and understanding the real nature of the immune system ... the increased incidence of septicaemia among young adults suggests that phagocytosis is deficient.[29]

As George Bernard Shaw noted (see Chapter 27), phagocytosis is an important function of our immune system. We all have a roaming army of largish cells on the lookout for enemies. When they find something that shouldn't be there, they envelop it, carry it off and dispose of it; whereas antibiotics kill but do not clean up after themselves. Thus the disposal of the dead bacteria (plus the good bacteria we don't really want to lose) constitutes a further burden on the body, probably the reason some of us feel low during and after taking a course of antibiotics.

Since 1980 when symptoms and diseases from recreational drug use were first recorded, a long list of serious sequelae from such drug taking was compiled. And these sequelae match the symptoms for AIDS. In fact, between 1981 and 1984, before the hypothesis that HIV was the cause of AIDS, scientists, including some from the Centers for Disease Control (CDC), were looking to a link between drug use and AIDS. Epidemiologists and toxicologists believed the common denominator shared by nearly all AIDS sufferers was the use of drugs, either intravenous or aphrodisiac, and psychoactive agents like 'poppers'. Peter Duesberg and David Rasnick point out that:

the American drug epidemic of the last two to three decades coincides exactly with the AIDS epidemic, both chronologically and epidemiologically. Moreover, recreational drugs can cause immunodeficiency and all the AIDS-defining diseases listed by the CDC.[30]

In particular there was the specific correlation between nitrate inhalants (poppers), popular among some groups of male homosexuals, and the Kaposi's sarcoma which primarily afflicts male homosexual sufferers from AIDS and which caused these drugs to be banned. Unfortunately there are yet other drugs associated with AIDS which are not yet banned.

Most tellingly, Dr Milowe points out that:

Repeated rectal sex is a much more efficient way of transmitting the virus than vaginal intercourse (by a factor of 2–10 times). The use of nitrate inhalants and other oral aphrodisiac drugs facilitates anal intercourse, in part by relaxing the anal sphincter. The passive sexual partner in anal intercourse has a 2.75 to 4.4 times higher AIDS risk than the insertive partner. If HIV were the cause of AIDS, both partners should have equal AIDS risks. *Active and passive partners do have equal incidences of other sexually transmitted diseases.* Yet the passive partners take from 2 to 8 times more drugs than the active partners, in order to facilitate anal intercourse. Thus, this abuse of nitrite drugs correlates well with the development of AIDS.[31]

Another writer, Stephen C Byrnes, believes that benzene, found in lubricants, is a possible cause or contributing factor in AIDS.[32]

Despite all these diverse kinds of evidence, once the HIV virus had been 'discovered', any doctors or scientists who question mainstream medicine's beliefs about AIDS, its causes and treatment, no longer receive grant funding for their projects. Today, some of America's greatest medical minds have found that their entire working lives have dried up, come to an end, owing to the withdrawal of all the kinds of resources they had received before they expressed dissension. In some cases they have even lost *their jobs.*

There has been formed in the US the Group for the Scientific Reappraisal of the HIV/AIDS Hypothesis. And they point to the usual progress, throughout human history, of 'TRUTH':

1 It is ridiculed.
2 It is violently opposed.
3 It is finally accepted as self-evident.

Clearly we are in stage 2. The truth about the earth being round comes to mind. It will be interesting to see if we get to stage 3, and how long it will take.

Professor Duesberg maintains, 'The hallmark of a poorly-framed hypothesis is that it brings no results. And that is the current situation.' It is indeed. And not just for AIDS.

One thing that all agree on is that AIDS is a multi-billion dollar industry. The whole thing is referred to by some as

'The AIDS fraud': A cobbled together definition consisting of a number of other diseases, all previously known, but said to be AIDS, in the occasional presence of a virus which does not behave in any way like any other disease-producing virus known to science, and does not meet even one of the four standard medical criteria (which are known as Koch's postulates) for a disease-causing organism. (Nor do any of the '20th-century illnesses' conform to Koch's postulates.) If ever there were a case of the Emperor's New Clothes being invisible, with nothing to hide his nakedness, this could be it. [33]

Even the influential American financial weekly *Barron's* had a headline, **'No Magic Cure: The War on Aids Produces Few Gains, Except on Wall Street'**. [34]

Larry Kramer, long-term HIV carrier since 1978, says 'There is no doubt that this is the Great Medical Tragedy of all time, and the Greatest Government Scandal of all time.'

Dr Howard B Urnovitz PhD, a microbiologist who believes that contaminated vaccines are behind AIDS, says, 'In AIDS and now in Gulf War Syndrome, asking the US government to solve this problem is like asking the suspect to investigate the crime. The degree of truth is proportional to the level of government denial.' [35]

Perhaps AIDS is the final outcome of both the unhealthy way of life we are most of us forced to live, in a world where we truly nourish neither our world nor ourselves, and the failed paradigm of modern medicine. For the single-cause, single-disease, single-drug approach which is the cornerstone of modern medicine simply does not work with AIDS.

But then too, modern medicine has not only lost the 'War against AIDS', it has lost the wars against cancer, heart disease and almost all other chronic diseases. It is long past time for a new paradigm, a new approach to 'health care' (as against 'disease care'), both preventive and curative.

To learn more about the scientific 'rethink' of the HIV/AIDS Hypothesis, send US$20 for a one-year subscription for the monthly publication *Reappraising AIDS* to: 7514 Girard Ave, 1-331, La Jolla, CA 92037, US.

For Mark Konlee's recommendations on treatment, based on the extensive experience of PWAs (People with Aids):

The Protease Inhibitor Norvir (retinavir) is by far the most effective ... in preventing and remitting nearly all opportunistic infections ... It must be kept refrigerated. D4T (Zerit) and 3TC (Epivir) are the safest and most effective in combination with protease inhibitors. Rescriptor (delavirdine) is the most therapeutic of the two NNRTIs...

For the best drug combination therapy Konlee recommends 'Norvir plus Rescriptor; Norvir plus D4T; Norvir plus 3TC.'

Mark Konlee also believes, as I do, that there is no such thing as 'a drug side-effect'. There are only 'adverse reactions' to drugs. Clearly if a drug makes one feel worse it should be discontinued immediately. And for his latest findings on AIDS and its treatment, order his quarterly *Keep Hope Alive*: PO Box 27041, West Allis, WI 53227, US (price: US$15 per year).

35: POSITIVE THINKING

'Just think positively all the time,
and all will be well.'

This book is about lies and misinformation. And potentially lethal lies and misinformation. You must admit by now we're surrounded by it.

The first liar in human history might have been a Neanderthal caveman who, in answer to a query from a fellow tribesman (also his rival for the hand of the lovely Gloobie), shouted in reply:

'The tiger went thataway ...,' when in reality the tiger was the other way, in fact just behind his rival and about to pounce...

The point is that if we had not been programmed to 'think negatively' at times, to be watchful, to imagine the worst, to be on the alert for danger, we would not have survived as a species. After all, we could have been outrun by many of the predatory animals roaming the earth. To beat them we had to be smarter. And we had to be realistic. Only a kind of wary watchfulness prevented us from being devoured by the tiger coming over the hill; that tiger our caveman would have seen himself and avoided, had he not been distracted with thoughts of the lovely Gloobie. He was, of course, thinking most positively when the tiger brought him down.

In other words, 'Were it not for our intrinsic capacity to feel sad, we might not be around to lament the fact that we are not always ecstatic.'[1]

Today we've eliminated the predatory animals from our lives, but that doesn't mean the old instincts have died too. Moreover, there are still the cars to dodge and, increasingly, a brain-maddened percentage of the human race to watch out for.

So perhaps we've always needed to be somewhat on the alert. Perhaps the home is considered a haven or a castle because it should be the one place we can truly relax, a fortress against outsiders. But, as most of us know, the home too can be just another battleground if we're competitive, too alert for signs of danger there. We need the right minerals and trace elements, we need confidence and trust to be able to let our guards down cheerfully for each other. We need to be able to trust, and have that trust rewarded.

But even the minerals won't help when the 'positive thinkers' are on the prowl. It's getting so in some circles you can't even say 'It looks like rain' without some blithe spirit, some positive thinker, looking disapprovingly at you as they quickly come in with, 'Oh, but the sun will shine again! It always does!'

Well *that* I knew, didn't I? The disapproving glance implies that I've ruined everybody's day by 'thinking negatively'. Moreover, I am clearly spiritually lacking, too.

I think the ultimate one was when I called, 'Safe Journey!' to friends as they drove off into the rush-hour traffic, only to be accused of 'negative thinking' the next time we met. There is carnage on our roads! To me to say something like that is like saying 'I care about you, I care whether you survive or not. Be alert! Take care of yourself.'

It is as though 'positive thinking' is a kind of mantra that will protect one from harm. We must not say a negative thing because it programmes us 'negatively'. I believe this is mostly nonsense, because our brains are not stupid, and as I have said we are already programmed to worry and calculate danger in the deepest part of the brain, whether we like it or not. And it gets worse. Some even believe that 'if you say it, you can make it happen.' This would of course give us as much power as the gods of old.

It is a long way from the old idea that salvation or 'peace of mind' could be obtained through looking outwards (or rather upwards) to one's God. After that we had the emphasis on 'primary relationships replacing religion, clan and mere survival as the foundations of our lives ... with many coming to see communication as the cornerstone of that foundation'.[2]

More recently, many have come from this point to believe that 'salvation' may be brought about by an adjustment of the psyche, by counselling and psychoanalysis. And when those fail, drugs. For 'human problems are no longer seen as normal variations or unseemly twists of fate. We now view them as the products of internal psychological maladjustments.'[3] And the way to keep from such 'maladjustment' is to keep thinking positively.

But it is in fact impossible to think in positive images for long. You can, for example, have one picture in your mind of your ideal house. There it is, glowing in all its positive perfection, only one picture. But the things that can go wrong! Now there are a thousand pictures: a leaky roof, windows that need washing, dry rot and damp rot, lawns that need mowing, trees that need pruning, and on and on –

and this is only the outside. What about all the inside problems? All the work there?

Thus it is with everything! One picture of perfection. One positive image. And endless pictures of what can go wrong. And we have to deal with all of them. So what is happening today is cruel, cruel, cruel. We are told to 'think positively', an impossible dictum, and it is implied that there is something wrong with us if we cannot.

In practice, it is not just that one is not supposed to say a negative thing *en passant*, but the cult of positive thinking cuts out one whole aspect of conversation that creates solidarity between people. Deborah Tanner, Professor of Linguistics at Georgetown University, calls this conversational gambit 'ritual complaining'.[4] It establishes friendship through mutual trust. What it does is say: 'We are each of us struggling with life. But you won't judge me even though I'm complaining because you are complaining also.' Each person complains a little, mutually supporting each other in the process, and then they get on with the rest of the conversation.

There's a delightful little story in Ellen Langer's book, *Mindfulness*[5] wherein three older women are sitting on a park bench. The first one gives a long groan, whereupon the second heaves up a sigh. Then the third one reproves them: 'I thought we weren't going to discuss the children today.'

But positive thinkers, using an ideologically-driven conversational style, will steel themselves against even this brief ritual moaning. They may thus appear cold, withdrawn and judgemental. For the refusal to engage in this harmless conversational ritual marks them as conveying the message, 'I am superior to you. *I don't complain.*' They regard any negativity as somehow contaminating, as potentially dragging them down into some mire of despondency, depression and thwarted 'spiritual growth'. It is as though they personally have no resistance to withstand this mire! Because apparently the brain records everything uniformly, and takes it to heart. The brains of such positive thinkers apparently cannot discriminate between real trouble and having the odd moan. This brain is a locked in knee-jerk computer! If what they believe is true I don't know how anyone has ever survived wars, depressions, death and dissolution, not to mention abusive childhoods, through the ages.

But it gets worse. There's another irrational belief that usually goes with it. People 'choose' their lives in advance, their abusive parents or partners, their cancers and so on. They 'choose' them in order to aid their 'spiritual' development. Mind you, those who actually have to bear these burdens do not generally go along with this idea. But it is believed by those fortunates without too many disasters in their lives. It means you don't have to offer a helping hand to victims because they 'chose' it, and you certainly don't listen to their 'negativity'. Because it's all to the good for their 'spiritual development'. And of course this particular

New Age philosophy goes very well with New Right economics. In combination they have created a sick and selfish society.

But no matter how determinedly we may strive to avoid the negative, we humans are not truly able to avoid **a fascination** with it. For example, there have been people who have tried to bring out a 'Positive Newspaper', printing only good news. These are rather thin publications! Moreover they always fail spectacularly, because it seems no one **really wants** 'nothing but good news'.

The newspapers full of gossip and horror are successful. And when we consider the world's great art and literature it seems that we are inevitably drawn to the darker side of life. The Pollyannas, the Little Nells of this world cannot long keep our attention. It is not really the good pale Clarissa Harlowe who preoccupies us.[6] We are waiting, always waiting with impatience and possibly 'drawn breath' for the dark, the evil, the sex-driven Lovelace, who fascinates us.

Whether it is 'great art' or Victorian melodrama, it is always the same. It is not pictures of English country lanes that we dwell on in the art gallery. It is the horrific vision of Bosch's hell one lingers over, spellbound. And we see this again in the dark symbol of the crucifixion, a sombre symbol of a sombre religion. Is it really true that in those pagan matriarchal days of old, religious rites were all of flowers and dancing? Have we lost something? Or was it just a dream?

For our preoccupation is with violence and death. Perhaps it is again that evolutionary, biological imperative. Mihaly Csikszentmihalyi[7] has estimated that the average child today witnesses over 70,000 murders on television and films before reaching adulthood. Before these technological marvels there were games of Cowboys and Indians, 'Torture' (a game from my childhood devised by the neighbourhood boys), war games and other such cruel 'sports'.

It does not have to mean that we are inherently depraved, because despite this obsession with depravity few actually inflict the violence and cruelty to which we are drawn. It is probably something that goes very deep along with that wary watchfulness. Just as in the ritual mutual moaning, perhaps if we bring these things into the light of day, **only then** are we dealing with our fears. We are saying, 'There it is in a make-believe situation. I am dealing with this. Therefore it will not become real in my life,' or 'I will be able to cope with it, because I have here done so.'

I am not now condoning this preoccupation with the darker side of life. We love the light also. I am saying that it is a fact. Perhaps 'positive thinking' is an attempt to pretend that we are what we're not.

There is another aspect of television to consider. That is, all those false images of happiness and the preoccupation with the highlights of people's lives, the dramas. Then too, the people we tend to identify with are ultra-articulate at every moment of their television lives, never at a loss for words. After all, they have the best writers (and the best make-up artists). And any problem is usually temporary. So that the more we watch these superhuman beings, the more inadequate we feel. Sometimes we mumble, we bumble along, unable to solve every problem.

But under this pervasive influence, television, the whole of society ends up trying to live as do those screen images which hold up impossible models. In the privacy of our homes we know we cannot measure up to this ideal world. For we know that decent occupations and good relationships are hard to come by. Most of all, television tends to make us want more, more, more of everything, and to be dissatisfied with whatever we have.

George Orwell said 'Men can only be happy when they do not assume that the object of life is happiness.'[8] And Dr Larry Dossey, author of an article entitled 'In Praise of Unhappiness', points out that the American Declaration of Independence (a document put together by perhaps the most perceptive minds on the American continent in that day) insists on the right to *pursue* happiness, but it does not maintain that happiness *per se* is a human right. And we have heard from other wise people that happiness is the journey we make, not so much our arrival at the destination.

If one is not on a journey, one is not growing. And growing seems to be a way to a more satisfactory life. For example, the struggle against odds to get a particular qualification can challenge one, uplift one, inspire one and carry one onward. The actual piece of paper you get can be almost a letdown. You need another goal now you have that piece of paper. Or, if we cannot go on the journey we long for, we need to find smaller journeys.

So where's the danger? Isn't this rather mirthless and determined positive thinking harmless? No, it isn't. This 'cult of positive thinking' is directed at self and self alone. It turns people inward, it renders people indifferent to the sufferings of others. In terms of society in general, there is the loss to society of concerned individuals who care about others almost as much as they do about themselves.

And moreover, this overriding preoccupation with Self, a part of the Freudian legacy, the 'psychiatrization' of society, involves a constant taking of one's inner temperature, a constant search for 'normality' and 'tranquillity'. So that the inevitable 'negative' thoughts and our inability to dispense with them entirely can cause a great deal of anxiety among some.

'What is wrong with me that I can't think positively all the time, like other people?' ('Other people', of course, put up a good front.) 'There must be something wrong with me. I am mentally, emotionally and spiritually inadequate. In short I must be "depressed".' For the idea of perpetual positive thinking holds up an unrealistic, impossible-to-realize ideal in life, an untenable goal. It is as though we are to deny the human condition, the fact that humans alone on this planet are aware of death, of the fact that we will all die one day. In both small and large ways, **things will go wrong**. And even if they don't, we will sometimes fear that they will.

Then too, a small percentage of people today seek to inure themselves from all suffering by detaching themselves from reality, of clinging to the idea that nothing matters. And they may do this through the belief that they have thousands of future lives to look forward to. So it does not matter about this one. This approach is, in effect, yet another 'opiate of the people' guaranteed to create an acceptance of whatever injustices abound (until perhaps they happen to this person with a thousand lives).

But I believe there is no evidence, no guarantee that I will have numerous lives, so I'd like to make the most of this one, just in case. And the joke is, of course, that one could base a whole life on the presumption of many lives ahead, and never be disappointed, because one will never know if there is only one life after all.

But worst of all, as we noted in the discussion on Freud, the loss of the focus on society in favour of the focus on self has had the disastrous repercussions we see around us in every way, every day.

To individuals, unless one does reach that state of detachment from reality some would strive for, there is a down and dangerous side to the lie of 'positive thinking'. The danger lies in what it does to gullible people, which is most of us. As noted, we seem to have what Dr Dossey refers to as a 'biological predilection for negativity'.[9] There are such things as 'negative thoughts' and they are often quite valid, reasonable thoughts. They will surface now and then, even in the mentally healthy. They are unavoidable. And of course if one is eating lots of hydrogenated oils and margarine, and has a mouth full of mercury amalgam; if you're full of toxic pesticide residues and the daily dose of fluoride, MSG and so on, how on earth can you be perpetually cheerful?

Even in moments of the utmost triumph a tinge of melancholy may emerge. 'Well, I've made it. But will I be able to keep this up?' In the midst of a crowd, a sudden ineffable feeling of loneliness: 'Who are all these people, and what am I doing here? Does any of them give a damn about me?' There is in addition a yearning for perfection, always a yearning for what we have not. Perhaps moments of sadness emerge even with someone one is very close to, even in one's most intimate moments. The French call it 'le petit mort', often followed by 'la tristesse', an acceptance that there is both happiness and unhappiness in life. Or, as one waggish folk saying would have it: *First the ecstasy. Then the laundry.*

We are, of course, conditioned to think in terms of magic pills for everything. And so to the doctor for help, a pill to make us 'think positively'. The necessity to think positively all the time is a great boon to the pharmaceutical industry these days. Truckloads of psycho-pharmaceuticals are thus consumed.

But in many cases, as we have seen, Prozac and other 'anti-depressants' will not solve the problem. For drugs fail to help people to deal with the life experiences that can cause depression. We need clear heads to be able to cope. Some allege, although it has not yet been conventionally proven, that Prozac may even diminish one's already scant supply of minerals and contribute to factors causing one to become suicidal. All drugs diminish one's nutrients, as explained in the chapter on prescription drugs.

Moreover, there are also studies beginning to surface which indicate that we will actually lose our marbles a little faster on these brain-bludgeoning drugs. They in fact do not help one to think more clearly. They muddy the waters. From the evidence, it is possible that an unrecorded percentage of people who take their lives have done so under the influence of failed 'positive thinking' and drugs.

Perpetual positivity is a snare and a delusion. For life just isn't like that, and it's possible to die in the attempt to make it so. We have to accept that we will be unhappy at times, that it is part of the human condition. In earlier times people would take care of life crises with the help of families, friends or their religious advisors. Today, with the extensive loss of community which is perhaps the worst part of modern life, and the idea that our minds need adjusting, we feel the need for psychotherapy and drugs.

What we truly need is an acceptance that there will always be pain and sorrow, for it is a part of being human, a part of the human condition. Perhaps the price of the awareness of oneself as a separate being in time and space, the price of that enormous gift of life, of human consciousness, is to know pain, to be lonely, to suffer. For we cannot have one without the other.

So it can perhaps be seen that this business of 'positive thinking' is a lot more complex and difficult than is seen on the surface.

Are there ways to be happier? I say 'Yes.' For many years I have read the thoughts of numerous wise people. And I have been through a great deal myself, starting with a cruel childhood, tuberculosis at the age of 10 and, from then on, an indifferent and sometimes disastrous state of health, making of life a perpetual struggle. And mistakes a-plenty along the way. Three times in my life I have been close to death, very close.

And yet I persist in believing that a sense of humour and proportion are more important for getting us through life than an enforced mode of 'positive thinking'.

But we need more even than these to get us through. Apart from that sense of humour (or a sense of the ridiculous), apart from an awareness that life is not 'a bowl of cherries', that it is messy and difficult for most of us, I believe there are four things we have to do to get the best out of life:

1. CHERISH THE MOMENT

How does one explain the unexplainable? It is useless but I'll try. As I have mentioned before, I get up in the morning and go to my window. See what is beyond, and on a good morning feel the sheer and unutterable joy just in being alive. 'Bliss!' I say to myself.[10]

I head for the kitchen and make a cup of rather weak tea ... the tiny ritual of handling my old brown, most beloved teapot, the familiar tea caddies. Again, 'What Bliss! Tea!' Small things. Tiny things. But I can feel the joy rising in me.

Then I review the day ahead. 'I will work on chapter so and so, visit X in hospital, and must not forget to ring Y. And now my sleeping angel needs a cup of tea to get him going, so he can beat the traffic.' All moments of joy to contemplate. I call these 'moments of awareness'. And the idea is to extend these 'moments' so that much of life will be full of them. This is something quite different from the Freudian self-obsession with 'How'm I doing?' This is awareness of one's surroundings, of existence, of the gift of life.

I suppose this can come in part from getting the minerals and trace elements right in the brain, and from acquiring, perhaps, the right philosophy, the learning to cherish small things. If we can but see them as wonderful artefacts or moments stolen from time and space. When it works it can fill one with joy.

2. THE NEED TO DO WORTHWHILE WORK

At every age, and for all of our lives, we need to do worthwhile work. Whatever we can do, we need to do it, even if it is very little. We must try not to work at something destructive, destructive of the planet, of others and of ourselves. After all, this work can be for one-third of our lives to all of our lives, and it permeates every part of us. Perhaps someone has to make H Bombs, plastic flowers and pesticides to earn a living? But let it not be those of us who yearn for better things.

3. THE NEED TO RECOGNIZE THE VALUE OF HAVING REALISTIC GOALS

This means assessing our personal strengths and weaknesses and what we can realistically expect from life. It is good to extend ourselves, to strive for better things, but I suspect most of us strive for what is beyond the bounds of possibility, which brings us into disappointment and grief. Our goals in life should be both short term and long term, with those goals up for reappraisal as circumstances change.

4. THE ABSOLUTE NECESSITY OF DEDICATING ONESELF TO SOMETHING LARGER THAN ONESELF

Preferably a cause of great importance. This may be involved with one's religious beliefs, one's commitment to society, and/or one's conviction that we can each make a difference in solving the problems around us. Through devoting even an hour or two a week to a great cause, one has the companionship of others similarly dedicated and we have the feeling of doing something worthwhile.

'Happiness is to take up the struggle in the midst of the raging storm and not to pluck the lute in the moonlight or recite poetry among the blossoms'.[11]

Sam Keen, author of *Fire in the Belly*, believes that if we look out upon the world with all its suffering and cruelty, 'man's inhumanity to man', and *feel no rage, we are no longer human, we are no longer truly alive.*

A visitor to New Zealand said recently, 'New Zealanders are too polite. They hate dissension, disagreement, differences of opinion. They refrain from arguing about ideas. And then they get in their cars and become homicidal maniacs!'

I believe he was both right and wrong. Because he's probably talking about two different groups of people. However, looking back at the history of the last 20 years, I would say that New Zealanders are sleepwalkers ... sleepwalking towards disaster. I prefer the enraged approach myself. Dylan Thomas advised, 'Rage! Rage! Rage against the dying of the light!' Surely our light is dying. Should we not be enraged?

For when we do pit our little strength against the wrong with others, that strength can be multiplied exponentially. Doing things for ourselves alone will not in the long run satisfy! We have to find the 'cause' that suits us. If in doubt, what greater cause than the one of restoring our planet to health, or the local environment, saving them from the further ravages of those who do not care? Moreover, almost every chapter in this book describes a problem that can be solved if people are prepared to work together on it.

Margaret Mead said, 'Never doubt that a small group of thoughtful citizens can change the world. Indeed, it's the only thing that ever has.'

As to 'positive thinking', life is a matter of ups and downs, light and shade, good and bad.

Life is a tide that goes out and joyfully comes in again. Life is being aware that somewhere in the world 400,000 children die every day, and doing something about it if you can.

The most important point to me is that anything we may feel that is what we call 'happiness' *is a kind of byproduct* from the several states of awareness and activity I have mentioned above.

The bravery, the nobility of the human spirit at its best lie not with those who attempt through mantras and drugs and delusions to avoid all unhappiness. They lie in those who do what they can to improve the lot of others, who face adversity with courage, who endure and endure, sometimes against all odds, because they know that feelings of melancholy and unhappiness are the lot of all of us. And it is my belief that you can have that marvellous feeling of absolute *bliss*, of exquisite *joy*, only if you also experience the downside of life, the contrasts in life. Why numb oneself into an even kind of nothingness when there is so much bliss and so much joy still to be experienced?

All the best to you!

EMERGENCY ADVICE

There is none better than the alcoholic's prayer for both believers and non-believers:

> Grant me the Serenity to accept
> the things I cannot change,
> The Courage to change the things I can
> And the Wisdom to know the difference.

If you're lucky, your local Alcoholics Anonymous may be able to supply a beautiful colour rendition of this, for a small donation.

Also: **THIS TOO WILL PASS.**

Both of these have helped me through some bad times.

CONCLUSION

We shall require a substantially new manner of thinking, if mankind
is to survive … No problem can be solved from the same
consciousness that created it.
Albert Einstein

When I began this book, I knew the health situation was not good. Now that I have done a little research I stand appalled. For, at least in the English-speaking world, one can truthfully say that the world has been made convenient for the few to make a lot of money out of endangering the health and shortening the lives of the rest of us.

Those perceptive people from the future will see that in our time we were most of us at the mercy of what one could term 'The Almighty Triumvirate'. That is, the three multi-billion dollar industries: the technologized food industry, the pharmaceutical/medical complex, and what I call the polluting industries.

1 We cannot totally create our own food supplies, as we did of old. But we can choose those foods which create health, in particular the right fats and oils, and vegetables and fruits we grow ourselves. That is, we should grow them using real compost-fed soils, or buy them from others who grow organically. Apparently these contain up to 50% more nutrients than ordinary fruits and vegetables.

2 We must avoid if possible the 'high-tech' medicine created by the pharmaceutical industries and the doctors who are used as front-line 'drug and vaccine peddlers'. We should save orthodox medicine for emergencies, and otherwise seek advice from those doctors and others who use methods which can truly create health.

3 The polluting industries – the manufacturers of pesticides and all those substances that endanger health, the petrochemical industries, the heavy metal industries along whose front line we must unfortunately include most dentists, and those which create dangerous waste products such as fluoride – all these must be avoided if we wish to stay well and live long, healthy and happy lives.

Unfortunately this enormously wealthy and powerful triumvirate can afford to spend millions of dollars on 'public relations' aimed at convincing us that all is well with their activities and that we should continue to enrich them. They have a powerful influence over various media. And this is the reason we are told at least once a year that 'a cure for cancer is on the way.' Unfortunately it never eventuates, or not yet. Meanwhile at least once a month there is a renewed attack on natural health care in the form of misinformation about the alleged dangers or inefficacy of herbs and supplements; meanwhile few people seem to be aware of the very real dangers in taking many prescribed pharmaceutical drugs.

This triumvirate is, for the most part, a three-pronged attack on our money, our health and our lives.

But the good news is that there is no doubt that the Western world is now engaged in one of the greatest struggles in human history: the struggle for a rational health care system, the struggle between those who put money and power before human health and those who want a better way. Considering what is at stake, the struggle is ongoing and intense.

It is only a matter of time before sanity wins. But unfortunately it could be a very long struggle, as the power is all on the side of the triumvirate. How long it will take to defeat it depends on all of us.

Over and over again throughout history, gross misconceptions have become a part of everyday life, have directed people's lives. They cannot be shaken unless by a revolution in thought. It is this revolution we are seeing today, a revolution that pits those who see the environment we live in as unimportant, and see disease as an invasion of the body to be cut out, burned out or bombarded with noxious substances ultimately poisonous to the body, as against those of us who see disease as the result of a weakened body which needs nourishing and strengthening to recover, in the context of an improved environment, one in which we were designed to flourish.

We used to have a concept known as 'cannon fodder'. That is, ordinary people were put up against cannons in battle to fight and often lose their lives in wars initiated by the aristocracy, by the big boys, to resolve their little piques and feuds. Thus the big boys arranged their wars; the arms manufacturers made their fortunes many times over; only the 'cannon fodder' paid the price. It is not quite so easy to round up 'cannon fodder' today. But judging by the situation in health today there is another kind of 'fodder'. We are, most of us, 'food fodder', 'medical fodder' and above all 'dollar fodder'.

However, by exercising care in our spending choices we can, both as individuals and then en masse, influence the course of both our own lives and the direction in which society is to go. Because every penny we spend goes to maintain, enrich and support the continuance of those who supply us. And thus it is that every penny we spend carries a grave responsibility.

We started with a question about sending men to the moon and beyond. What good was it to achieve this 'pinnacle' of scientific achievement if those men are to suffer from clogged arteries, blood that is liable to form clots, impaired immune systems and brains already declining from the many poisons and nutrient deficiencies in their lives?

The jury has long ago delivered its verdict on the reasons why so many of us die of heart disease, cancer and many other degenerative diseases. The reasons have been there in the most esteemed and well-read medical journals in the English-speaking world for many years. They are there whenever we compare our situation in the English-speaking countries with those in most other cultures.

The main reason we die of heart disease and cancer must be laid at the door of our ruined soils and depleted foods, the hydrogenation of our fats and oils, the homogenization of milk, the refinement away of essential nutrients, the 'sugarization' of our world and other such perversities. For it is well beyond doubt that it is the abnormal clots forming in our blood and the clogging of our arteries on the one hand, and the suppression of the immune system (our defence against cancer and other diseases) on the other, which are today the main causes of death in the West.

But all the other things we have looked at – the pesticides which damage all life and are now everywhere, the fluoride in our water and food, the mercury and the root canal-treated teeth in our mouths, the total pollution of our environment – all will play their part. And there is no doubt in my mind that lives have been lost and health has been ruined by vaccines, in greater numbers than from the illnesses they claim to prevent; that the nutrient-poor, corrupted and deformed food we eat can and does shorten and deplete our lives. Moreover, the almighty triumvirate works together to crush any viable opposition to the making of their fortunes.[1] And this corruption and carelessness with people's lives in the health field is fully echoed in the political world. In fact, the failure in health is symptomatic of a much wider failure.

It is a long way from the governments of the Netherlands and Denmark, who will not permit the degenerate form of margarine to be sold to their people; from the governments of Sweden, Denmark, Austria and Germany, who have forbidden any further amalgam to be placed in their people's mouths; to the governments of, say, New Zealand and the US, who knowingly permitted a corrupt vaccine to be injected into their children, who allow in the name of 'free enterprise' foods that are known to be harmful to be sold to their people. It is not so far geographically, but morally these nations are light-years apart.

I have more questions to ask as to how the situation has arisen. What are governments *for* if not to concern themselves with the health and welfare of their people, *all of their people?* Do they exist to 'turn a blind eye' to all the sorts of things we have been looking at in this book? Do they exist to be ignorant of these important matters?

Unfortunately, most of the governments of the Western world in this, the last quarter of the great shambles we call the 20th century, appear to be there for the benefit of a small percentage whose main occupation seems to be the making of money for their own personal self-indulgence and status. These governments do not appear to feel any but the most cursory responsibility for the welfare of their peoples.

We must confront the problem: We have governments which, long after the knowledge as to harm has been established, permit pollution of our world on a grand scale. They allow the poisoning of our water supply, permit dentists to continue putting the second most deadly and poisonous substance on the planet in our mouths, permit our milk to be distorted in such a way that it can cause heart attacks, while on television it is perfectly OK for people to dance around telling us that we will stay vibrant and healthy if we eat their dubious margarine.

In my view these are crimes against people, and as such should not be permitted.

And what should be the role of the medical profession? Most members of this profession are extremely well-rewarded for their role as 'guardians of the people's health'. The problem is that only a few of them are able to surmount and overcome their 'medical education', which amounts to a long-term brain-washing enterprise in favour of the methods that support a gigantic 'disease industry', a money-making industry, an industry which operates with apparently scant regard for real health. And this disease industry is linked by ties of money and power with those other disease industries, the pharmaceutical and food technology industries. One has to say that all the evidence points to the fact that most doctors are 'drug and vaccine peddlers' being used by the pharmaceutical industries for their billion-dollar purposes.

The evidence for all this has been in now for at least the last 25 years. But have our governments responded appropriately? Certainly not in most English-speaking countries. Have our doctors advised us appropriately? They have not. And the question we should be asking ourselves is, why not? Above all, the over-riding question must be: **Who is taking care of our health?**

I would submit that, for most of us, truly no one is taking care of our health. And since no one is, we owe it to ourselves to become as informed as possible on all the questions raised in this book. There are numerous excellent books written on the subject matter of almost every chapter, as indicated in the references. We must act as individuals to prevent our lives being cut short by the dangers we have been considering. We *should* also act *together* to get much better governments.

When those people from the middle of the next century look back on us they will see that our century struggled on throughout its years, particularly from the mid-century on, with Freud's faulty picture of the mind and Pasteur's faulty picture of the body and how it works.

Freud was not only responsible for an inaccurate picture of how the brain works, but by the middle of the century 'the cult of Freudianism' had resulted in a widespread self-obsession, an inward-looking preoccupation that ultimately led to selfishness and the decline in the sense of community with others.

This preoccupation with 'personality', 'ego' and 'personal development' has in fact overshadowed the need to alter social systems. It has led to what one could call 'the pablumizing of reforming zeal', a zeal which existed in the first half of the century and which led to far greater things than has the preoccupation with self and its accompanying flight from reason in the second half of the century.

We have already noted what the 'Pasteurization of Medicine' has led to. And once one understands the two great forces of Freud and Pasteur, we can understand why the 20th century has been such a disaster, both for us and for the planet. The century being almost over, all we can do is to try to repair as much of the damage as we can so that our children and grandchildren will inherit a saner world.

Perhaps most of all, it is becoming increasingly apparent that no country in the world can afford the ever-escalating costs of supporting a disease-care industry. It is simply unsustainable in practical terms. In the long run a truly preventive health care system would be vastly more affordable. But until we put an end to governments of expediency, governments with short-term goals and limited vision, it will never happen. And entire countries will be crushed under the weight of insupportable tax burdens, or 'health' insurance costs, while at the same time the increasing ill-health of its citizens will make paying for the 'disease-care' system more and more difficult.

Already the infant death rates, that primary indication of the worth of a health care system and human concern, are rising in once proud countries. For example, New Zealand, which once had the lowest infant death rates in the Western world, now has among the highest in the Organisation for Economic Co-operation and Development (OECD). In the rush for money and self-congratulatory greed, this trend has not even been noted.

In the US and elsewhere people are voting with their feet and returning to the traditional gentle healers: the herbalists,[2] the naturopaths, the acupuncturists, the homoeopaths, those who do bodywork and so on. They seek out those few health practitioners and doctors who have been able to break through the Freudian and Pasteurean fallacies. But unless this dissatisfaction becomes more widespread and is transferred to the political arena, I can see it dragging on for 10 or 20 years. That is, 10 or 20 years during which, to put it mildly, our children and grandchildren will not be receiving a good start in life.

But it is my hope that readers of this book will see, not only the horrors of the modern world, but also the positive side of what has here been written. There *are* numerous dedicated and intelligent doctors and many, many others who have put their careers, their comfortable lives on the line, and there *is* a clear way out of the horrors, if we will only choose it.

The truth is we already know how to achieve a viable 'health-care' system. We found it out late in the 19th century and early in this one. But in the welter of shiny propaganda and the mighty power of advertising for billion-dollar industries we have forgotten it all. 'The bonds we are unaware of are the most binding of all.'[3] If humanity is to survive, the lessons once learned will have to be learned all over again.

The truth is actually very simple and goes back even further. Hippocrates said it thousands of years ago. The only things that work for the long-term health care of people are as follows:

Clean, unpolluted air, water, and food grown on bountiful soil, full of the life-bringing nutrients we all of us need.

These are the basic necessities of life.

And should be a basic right of all humans at birth.

TODAY WE HAVE NONE OF THEM!

In addition, we need a decent basic income, good housing and education for all, with the emphasis on major educational programmes in preventive health care.

Only this way can we work towards the greatest good for the greatest number of the people in our countries. And only this way will we have some chance of preserving our home, this planet. It is clear that not until we take an entirely fresh look at the question of human health in its environmental context will a system of real health care emerge. And only then will the problem cease to seem insurmountable.

Titanic, a vast and expensive ship with all the latest technology, launched with great hopes early in our century, was declared to be unsinkable by virtue of its separate watertight compartments – the idea being that any possible problem could be confined to those separate compartments and would not therefore affect the rest of the ship.

Titanic has therefore become a fitting symbol for our century, because we have conducted our affairs as though we can confine any problems, as though we can damage one part of our bodies without it affecting the rest, that we can spray or bomb place A without it affecting place B, that we can favour one group and that other groups will remain as is.

But just as *Titanic* could not confine its watery problems to a few compartments, so have we also failed to do so. The wretched *Titanic* is thus a fitting symbol for our 20th century.

I would like to hope and believe that much could be salvaged in the life boats, but before then, a great deal of ballast must be jettisoned.

I think perhaps, on a question as important as this, we need to listen to a towering voice from the past. Here is Maurice Maeterlinck (1862–1949) speaking to us across the years:

At every crossway on the road that leads to the future, each progressive spirit is opposed by a thousand men appointed to guard the past. Let us have no fear lest the fair towers of former days be sufficiently defended. The least that the most timid among us can do is not to add to the immense dead weight which custom drags along.

Let us not say to ourselves that the best truth always lies in moderation, in the decent average. This would perhaps be so if the majority of men did not think on a much lower plane than is needful. That is why it behooves others to think and hope on a higher plane than seems reasonable. For the average, the decent moderation of today, will be the least human of things tomorrow. At the time of the Spanish Inquisition, the opinion of good sense and of the good medium was certainly that people ought not to burn too large a number of heretics. Extreme and unreasonable opinion obviously demanded that they should burn none at all.

Let us think of the great invisible ship that carries our human destinies upon eternity. Like the vessels of our confined oceans, she has her sails and her ballast. The fear that she may pitch or roll on leaving the roadstead is no reason for increasing the weight of the ballast by stowing the fair white sails in the depths of the hold. They were not woven to molder side by side with cobblestones in the dark. Ballast exists everywhere; all the pebbles of the harbour, all the sand of the beach, will serve for that. But sails are rare and precious things; their place is not in the murk of the well, but amid the light of the tall masts, where they will collect the winds of space.

Well then, let us unfurl our fairest of fair white sails; high, high up on the tall masts, and let the fresh winds catch and fill them. We could do no better with our lives.

REFERENCES

INTRODUCTION

1 Olarsch and Stockton, *Townsend Letter for Doctors* August/September 1996: 114.
2 US Social Security Administration Actuarial Study No. 87, September 1980.
3 In Dr J D Weisman, MD, *Choose to Live* (Penguin Books, 1988).
4 *The 20-Day Rejuvenation Diet Program* (New Canaan, CT: Keats Publishing Co, 1997).
5 *New Zealand Herald* July 7, 1998. (The NZ population is approximately 3.9 million.)
6 Rachel Carson, *Silent Spring* (London: Readers Union, 1962).
7 Dr Robert W Bradford, DSc, 'Pseudoscience Masquerading as Medical Fact', in *Townsend Letter for Doctors* October 1996: 93.
8 *Guardian Weekly*, December 14, 1997: 17.
9 911 Tyler Street, Port Townsend, WA 98368-6541 US; 24-hour fax 360-385-0699; http://www.tldp.com

CHAPTER 1

1 Dr Russell L Smith PhD and Dr Edward R Pinkney MD, *Cholesterol Conspiracy* (St Louis, MO: Warren H Green Inc, 1991).
2 Dr Elaine N Marieb PhD, *Human Anatomy and Physiology* (2nd edn; Benjamin Cummings Publishing Company Inc, 1992): G-5.
3 *Well Mind Association Newsletter*, Seattle, Washington, September 1997: 4.
4 Dr Alan R Gaby, 'Cholesterol Deficiency & Suicide', *Townsend Letter* December 1995: 21.
5 Rosetta Schuman, 'Where's the Fat?', *Townsend Letter* January 1993: 40–43 (42).

6 Rosetta Schuman, 'Cholesterol Mania', *Townsend Letter* April 1990: 229–33 (233).

7 Thomas J Moore, *Lifespan – Who Lives Longer and Why* (Simon & Schuster, 1993).

8 Schuman 1990: 233.

9 Schuman 1990: 229.

10 Sheldon Zerdon, *The Cholesterol Hoax; 101+ Lies* (Carson City, NV: Bridger House Publications, 1998).

11 C G Isles, *et al.*, *British Medical Journal* April 8, 1989: 920–24.

12 Schuman 1995, op cit.

13 *Journal of the Royal College of General Practitioners* April 1987.

14 Schuman 1990: 229.

15 *Medical History* Supplement No. 5, 185: 151–168.

16 Editorial, *Lancet* June 13, 1931.

17 *Transactions of the American Clinical and Climatological Association* 58, 1973: 100–122.

18 *World Review of Nutrition and Dietetics* 12, 1970: 1–42.

19 *American Journal of Clinical Nutrition* 20, May 1967.

20 Dr Wayne Martin, 'Cholesterol Theory: A Therapeutic Cul de Sac', *Townsend Letter* February/March 1995: 98–104 (102).

21 *Journal of the American Medical Association* November 7, 1996.

22 *Circulation* March 1968.

23 *Lancet* ii, 1968: 693.

24 *New Trition* 1984.

25 Dr Morton Walker DPM, *Townsend Letter* July 1997: 131.

26 Editorial, *British Medical Journal* October 6, 1973.

27 Dr Wayne Martin, 'Saturated Fats & Cholesterol not the cause of CHD', *Townsend Letter* August/September 1992: 715.

28 Dr Wayne Martin, 'The Miracle of Evening Primrose Oil', *Townsend Letter* November 1992: 991.

29 *Lancet* January 17 1987: 155–6.

30 J A Golier *et al.*, 'Low serum cholesterol and attempted suicide', *American Journal of Psychiatry* March 1995, 152: 419–423.

31 Dr H Engelberg MD, *Lancet* 339 (1991): 727–9.

32 A U MacKinnon, 'The origin of the modern epidemic of coronary artery disease', *Journal of the Royal College of General Practitioners* April 1987: 174–176.

33 Smith and Pinkney, *The Cholesterol Conspiracy*, cover copy.

34 Schuman 1990: 229.

35 Dr George Mann, *Coronary Heart Disease: The Dietary Sense and Nonsense* (NY: Paul & Co, 1993).

36 Robert Crayhorn BS, 'Is the Emperor Wearing Any Clothes?' *Townsend Letter* December 1994: 1414.

CHAPTER 2

1 NZ Heart Foundation information leaflets, dated August 1996; received February 1997.
2 Udo Erasmus, *Fats That Heal; Fats That Kill* (5th edn; Vancouver, BC: Alive Books, 1995): 8.
3 Erasmus: 3, 7.
4 Erasmus: 3.
5 Dr Joanna Budwig PhD, *Flax Oil as a True Aid Against Arthritis, Heart Infarction, Cancer and Other Diseases* (Vancouver, BC: Apple Publishing Company Ltd, 1994 [English edn]): 6.
6 Dr Elaine N Marieb PhD, *Human Anatomy and Physiology* (2nd edn; Benjamin Cummings Publishing Company, Inc, 1992): 848.
7 Erasmus: 210.
8 Ibid.
9 Dr Wayne Martin, *Townsend Letter* February/March 1995: 102–4.
10 B D Bowmer and E H Newsholme, 'Treatment of idiopathic polyneuritis by a polyunsaturated fatty-acid diet', *Lancet* March 18, 1978: 583–4.
11 Budwig: 3.
12 Ibid.
13 Budwig: 4.
14 John Finnegan, *The Facts About Oils* (Berkeley, CA: Celestial Arts Publisher, 1994).
15 Ibid.
16 John Finnegan, *Fats and Oils: A Consumer's Guide* (Malibu, CA: Elysian Arts, 1992).
17 Dr Wayne Martin, 'The Miracle of Evening Primrose Oil,' *Townsend Letter* November 1992: 990.
18 Dr George Tamari, 'To Prevent CHD and Cancer,' *Townsend Letter* May 1996: 71.
19 Judith A DeCava, *Townsend Letter* January 1997: 124.
20 Colquhoun & Bunday, 'A lack of essential fatty acids as a possible cause of hyperactivity in children', *Medical Hypotheses* 5, 1981: 673–9; Stevens *et al.*, 'Essential fatty acid metabolism in boys with attention-deficit hyperactivity disorder', *American Journal of Clinical Nutrition* 62 (4), 1995: 761–8.

21 Tamari: 72–3.

22 Dr Robert E Wilner MD, PhD, *The Cancer Solution* (FL: Peltec Publisher Co, Inc, 1994).

23 However, an article in the *Sunday Star Times* (July 12, 1998) would dispute this: Camille Cosby, American educator, claims that the University of Texas at Galveston 'conducted a controversial study on primarily black babies from 1956 to 1962. The researchers withheld an essential fatty acid from the babies' formulas that humans need for the growth of the whole body and nervous system ... several of the infants died during the course of the study.' I must add that many other infants are in this terrible situation as a result of ignorance rather than through deliberate experimentation.

24 *Effects of Fish Oils and Polyunsaturated Omega-3 Fatty Acids in Health and Disease*, National Library of Medicine, National Institute of Health, 1995.

25 Crawford and Marsh, *The Driving Force – Food, Evolution, and the Future* (NY: Harper & Row, 1989); Dr Michael Crawford, *What We Eat Today* (London: Neville Spearman, 1972).

26 Crawford and Marsh, op cit.

27 As for note 24.

28 John Finnegan, 'The Vital Role of Essential Fatty Acids for Pregnant and Nursing Women', in *The Facts About Fats* (Berkeley, CA: Celestial Arts, 1993).

29 Dr Donald Rudin MD, *The Omega-3 Phenomenon* (Sidgwick and Jackson, 1988).

30 Holman *et al.*, 'Deficiency of essential fatty acids and membrane fluidity during pregnancy and lactation,' *Biochemistry* Proceedings of the National Academy of Sciences, US, vol 88, June 1991: 4835–9.

31 Dr Joseph G Hattersley, 'Crib Death: Sudden Infant Death that isn't sudden at all,' *Townsend Letter* May 1996: 62–5.

32 Finnegan, op cit.

33 Rosetta Schuman, *Townsend Letter* January 1993: 41.

34 Rudin, op cit.

35 Erasmus: 210.

36 Finnegan: 40.

37 Dr Sherry Rogers MD, *Townsend Letter* January 1993: 936

38 *Townsend Letter* November 1996: 13.

39 Dr Alfred H Wertheim, *Townsend Letter* January 1996: 107.

40 *Townsend Letter* November 1996: 13.

41 Budwig: 10.

42 Ann Louise Gittleman, *Beyond Pritiken* (NY: Bantam Publishing, 1989).

43 *Townsend Letter* February/March 1996.

44 Mensink and Katam, 'TFAs and Lipoprotein Levels', *New England Journal of Medicine* 328 (7), August 16, 1990.

45 *Journal of Lipid Research* 33: 1493–1501.

46 *Clinical Science* 88 (4) April 1995: 375–92.

47 *Townsend Letter* October 1993: 936, and December 1993: 1212. (Chances are that even the coconut and olive oil margarine sold in New Zealand has been heated as for other margarines.)

48 Channing Laboratory, Harvard Medical School, *Lancet* March 6 1993: 581–5.

49 *Harvard Health Letter* Summer 1994.

50 *Lancet* April 28, 1956.

51 *Townsend Letter* August/September 1992: 716.

52 M G Enig *et al.*, 'Fatty acid composition of fat in selected food items with emphases on trans components', *JAOCS* 60 (10), October 1983: 1788–95; *New York Times* October 7 1992: 1.

53 *Townsend Letter* June 1992, 530.

54 Finnegan, op cit.

55 Leeches actually produce four active substances which counter different diseases. Bleeding, in moderation, causes our body to make fresh blood.

56 Rosetta Schuman, *Townsend Letter* January 1993: 41, 'Our space technology helped him walk on the moon, but our health technology could not prevent him from developing heart disease.'

57 Advice from a New Zealand Heart Foundation leaflet dated August 1996: 'Eat less fat, especially saturated fat.' 'Use small amounts of margarine instead of butter and other animal fats.' Margarine is recommended for children. Clearly the cardiologists who advise the Heart Foundation are not reading their own medical journals.

58 S Parthasarathy *et al.*, 'Low density lipoprotein rich in oleic acid is protective against oxidative modification: implications for dietary prevention of atherosclerosis'. *Proceedings of the National Academy of Science* 87, 1990: 3894–8.

59 'Coconut Oil', *Townsend Letter* June 1995: 155.

60 Dr John Finnegan, 'The Vital Role of Essential Fatty Acids for Pregnant and Nursing Women', *Townsend Letter* December 1995: 52–3.

CHAPTER 3

1 W A Price, *Nutrition and Physical Degeneration* (New Canaan, CT: Keats Publishing Co, 1945), cited by Dr Joseph G Hattersley, 'Crib Death: Sudden Infant Death that isn't sudden at all,' *Townsend Letter* May 1996: 62–5.

2 E E Zeigler *et al.*, 'Cows' Milk Feeding in Infancy: Blood loss from the gastrointestinal tract', *Journal of Paediatrics* 116, 1990: 11–18.

3 J C Annand, 'Hypothesis: Heated milk protein and thrombosis', *J. Atherosclerosis Res* 7, 1967: 797–801.

4 Walker, 'World Scientists Warn Humanity About Loss of Health & Ecology', *Townsend Letter* July 1993: 772.

5 Dr Kurt A Oster, MD *et al.*, *The XO Factor* (NY: Park City Press, 1995).

6 Walker, op cit.

7 Hattersley, 'Crib Death': 64.

8 A Lucas *et al.*, *Lancet* February 1, 1992; C I Lantry *et al.*, *Lancet* November 12, 1994.

9 Kurek *et al.*, 'A naturally occurring opioid peptide from cow's milk, beta-somorphine-7, is a direct histamine releaser in man', *Int Arch Allergy Appl Immunol* 97, 1992: 115–20.

10 Jules Klotter, 'The Dangers of Cow's Milk', *Townsend Letter* May 1995: 16.

11 Oster, op cit.

12 Ibid.

13 S Sternberg, *Science News* September 7, 1996: 151.

14 Oster, op cit.

15 *Medical Hypotheses* 7, 1981: 907.

16 Ibid.

17 Dr Nancy Appleton, *Healthy Bones: What you need to know about osteoporosis* (Garden City Park, NY: Avery Publishing Group Inc, 1990).

18 Ibid.

19 Ibid.

20 Ibid.

21 *20th Century Living* 14 (1), March/April 1990: 17.

22 US Dept of Health & Human Services, National Center for Health Statistics, US Mortality data tapes.

23 American Heart Association, *Heart and Stroke Facts* report, 1992.

24 I M Cox *et al.*, 'Red blood cell magnesium and CFS', *Lancet* 337, 1991: 757–60.

25 Dr Sherry A Rogers, *20th Century Living* 13 (6), November/December 1989: 16.

26 Appleton, op cit.

27 Dr Kathryn Fuchs PhD, 'Calcium Controversy', *Townsend Letter* August/September 1993: 906.

28 Dr Kathryn Fuchs PhD, *Women's Health Letter* March 1994.

29 Dr Susan Brown, *Better Bones, Better Body* (New Canaan, CT: Keats Publishing Co, 1996).

30 Dr J Gordon Millichap MD, *Environmental Poisons in Our Food* (Chicago: PNB Publishers, 1993).

31 Dr Raos E Mazariegos *et al.*, 'Consumption of soft drinks with phosphoric acid as a risk factor for the development of hypocalcaemia in children', *Journal of Paediatrics* 126, 1955: 940–2.

32 *Well Mind Association Seattle Newsletter* April 1992.

33 Dr Wayne Martin, *Townsend Letter* May 1995: 117.

34 *New England Journal of Medicine* March 6, 1993.

35 *Townsend Letter* May 1995: 117.

36 Martin, op cit.

37 Hattersley, 'Crib Death': 65.

38 'Microwave tragedy', *PPNF Nutrition Journal* 18 (nos 1 and 2), 1994: 1–5

CHAPTER 4

1   *Townsend Letter* January 1994: 62–3

2   *British Medical Journal* 1974: 436–40; *Lancet* 1979: 1313–15.

3   *Science* 208, 1980; *Journal of the American Medical Association* February 16, 1980: 6610–19.

4   *Stroke* 8, 1977: 301.

5   *New England Journal of Medicine* 299, 1978: 53

6   *Lancet* July 29, 1978.

7   *British Medical Journal* 296, 1988: 320–31.

8   *New England Journal of Medicine* July 20, 1989.

9   As for note 1.

10 *Journal of the American Medical Association* April 23, 1989.

11 *New England Journal of Medicine* January 20, 1983: 139–41

12 *Lancet* 1976: 48.

13 *Lancet* March 6 1993.

14 'Aspirin for Stroke – Kill or Cure?' *Townsend Letter* February/March: 125.

15 Dr William F Koch, *The Survival Factor*, 1960: 225.

16 Dr Otto Warburg, 'The Prime Cause and Prevention of Cancer', lecture delivered to the annual meeting of Nobel Prize winners, 1966.

17 As for note 14.

18 Dr Elaine N Marieb PhD, *Human Anatomy and Physiology* (2nd edn; Benjamin Cummings Publishing Company Inc, 1992).

19 Dr Wayne Martin, 'The Miracle of Evening Primrose Oil', *Townsend Letter* November 1992, 990–2.

20 Among the most important nutrients for people with diabetes are Chromium; and the herb Gymnema sylvestre which can actually lower blood

sugar levels (progress should therefore be carefully monitored). For a full discussion on diet and diabetes, see: Dr Ralph Golan MD *Optimal Wellness* (NY: Ballantine Books, 1995: 359–61).

CHAPTER 5

1 Dr Charles T McGee MD, *Heart Frauds: The Misapplication of High Technology in Heart Disease* (Medipress, 1993).
2 'Coronary artery bypass surgery – indications and limitations', *Lancet* 2, 1980: 511. (The death of Ernie Wise in March 1999, following a triple bypass in January, is an obvious example.)
3 Cited in Dr Elmer Cranton MD, *Bypassing Bypass* (Troutdale, VA: Medex Publishers Inc, 1990).
4 McGee, op cit.
5 Drs Ornstein and Sobel, *The Healing Brain* (NY: Simon & Schuster, 1987): 81.
6 Dr Ralph Ellis, *Townsend Letter* January 1997: 110–3.
7 Ibid.
8 'Chelation Therapy', *Townsend Letter* May 1992: 382–3.
9 McGee, op cit.
10 Ibid.
11 'Vitamin B_6 is Anti-Atheroma and Anti-Thrombic', *Townsend Letter* May 1992: 381–2.
12 Ellis: 112
13 Rosetta Schuman, 'Cholesterol Mania', *Townsend Letter* April 1990: 229–33 (233).
14 Dr Morton Walker *et al.*, *The Chelation Answer*
15 Cranton, op cit.
16 *New Zealand Herald* 11 February 1998: A19. Again, there are better ways.
17 'Kentucky Disciplines Chelation Physician', *Townsend Letter* January 1997: 110–12.
18 The total breast removal operation was in this category for six decades.
19 Auckland *Sunday Star Times* 11 October 1998.
20 Dr Joseph G Hattersley, 'Heart Attacks and Strokes: How to avoid them for pennies a day', *Townsend Letter* January 1992: 53–55.
21 Ibid.
22 Ellis: 112.

CHAPTER 6

1 Dr Keith W Sehnert MD, Minnesota, US, on the Internet, June 1997.
2 *Essentials of Environmental Toxicology* (Taylor & Francis, 1996).
3 Burton Goldbert, 'First Do No Harm', *Townsend Letter* October 1996: 8.
4 *New Zealand Herald* 17 March 1999: A20.
5 Dr Gary Null, 'Mercury Dental Amalgams', *Townsend Letter for Doctors* August/September 1992: 760–70.
6 Hal Huggins DDS, *It's All in Your Head: Diseases caused by Silver-Mercury Fillings* (4th edn; Life Sciences Press, 1990).
7 Sam and Michael Ziff DDS, 'The Medical Profession Should Rediscover Mercury', *Townsend Letter* November 1993: 1109–1111 (1110).
8 C K Blesius *et al.*, 'Dental Amalgam and Mercury', *Townsend Letter* October 1996: 86.
9 Ibid.
10 Gross and Harrison, 1989 and Dr C K Blesius *et al.*, *Biological Therapy* XIII (2), 1995 (Menaco Publishing).
11 Dr Gary Null, *Townsend Letter* August/September 1992: 760.
12 Dr Joyal Taylor DDS, *The Complete Guide to Mercury Toxicity from Dental Fillings* (San Diego, CA: Scripps Publishing, 1998).
13 Hahn *et al.*, 1990, in Blesius *et al.*, 'Dental Amalgam and Mercury', *Townsend Letter* October 1996: 86.
14 Personal communication from Dr Mike Godfrey, Tauranga, New Zealand.
15 Sehnert, op cit.
16 Keith W Sehnert MD *et al.*, 'Is Mercury Toxicity an Autoimmune Disorder?' *Townsend Letter* October 1995: 134–7.
17 Hahn, op cit.
18 Null August/September 1992, op cit.
19 *Archives of Environmental Health* 19, December 1969: 891–905.
20 Hahn *et al.*, 'Whole body imaging of mercury released in dental fillings in monkey tissues', University of Calgary, Alberta, Canada, August 3, 1990: 3256–60; J D Vimy *et al.*, 'Maternal-fetal distribution of mercury released from dental amalgam fillings', *American Journal of Physiology* 258, 1990: 939–45.
21 'My Fillings Left My Sons Handicapped', *Sunday Star Times*, May 17, 1998: C5.
22 Dr Thomas Ely MD, *Townsend Letter* June 1992: 528.
23 Dr Douglas E Swarzendruber PhD, 'Adverse Immunomodulating Effects of Heavy Metals in Dental Materials', *Int. J. Biosocial Med. Research* 12 (2) 1990: 134.
24 Null August/September 1992, op cit.

25 Blesius, op cit.

26 Wenstrup *et al.*, 'Trace element imbalances in isolated subcellular fractions of Alzheimer's disease brains', *Brain Research* 533: 125–31.

27 Tom Warren, *Beating Alzheimer's* (Garden City Park, NY: Avery Publishing Group Inc, 1992).

28 Tom Warren, 'Reversing Alzheimer's Disease', *Townsend Letter* June 1992: 530.

29 Ibid.

30 Healthy Options December/January 1996.

31 Dr Morton Walker DPM and Dr H Richard Casdorph MD PhD, *Toxic Metal Syndrome: How Metal Poisonings can Affect Your Brain* (NY: Every Publishing Group, 1995).

32 *Report of the International Conference on the Biocompatibility of Materials* 1988: 44.

33 Tom Warren, 'Beating the Diagnosis', *Townsend Letter* April 1997: 50.

34 Ibid.

35 Dr Robert Kimmel MD, Specialist in Preventive Family Medicine, *Townsend Letter* January 1992: 73.

36 *Townsend Letter* August/September 1992: 736.

37 Information sheets as supplied by Dentsply/Caulk, Ivoclar.

38 *Well Mind Association Newsletter* 1997, Seattle, Washington.

39 Personal communication from Dr Mike Godfrey, op cit.

40 Ziff, op cit: 1109.

CHAPTER 7

1 Dr George E Meinig DDS, FACD *Root Canal Cover-up* (Ojai, CA: Bion Publishing, 1993).

2 Ibid.

3 Ibid.

4 Dr Hal Huggins DDS, MS, 'Hazards of Root Canal', *Townsend Letter* October 1990: 659–60

5 M Fisher, *Death and Dentistry* (1940).

6 Tom Warren, 'Beating the Diagnosis', *Townsend Letter* April 1997: 55.

7 Meinig, op cit.

8 Tom Warren, 'Tom Warren Responds', *Townsend Letter* June 1997: 104. ('...Not a single scientist or dentist that I was able to talk with really believes that Biocalex 6.9 gives perfect asepsis.')

9 Warren, April 1997: 55.

10 Dr Richard Gerber MD, *Vibrational Medicine* (Santa Fe, NM: Bear & Co, 1988).

11 Second World Congress on Cancer, Sydney, 1995. Personal communication from Dr Michael Godfrey, Tauranga, New Zealand.

12 Dr Weston Price, *Dental Infections and Degenerative Disease* (1940).

13 *Townsend Letter* April 1997: 112.

14 From a Finnish study reported in the *British Medical Journal*, unspecified, cited in *Holistic Dental Digest* New York, and reproduced in *20th Century Living* 14 (2) March/April 1990: 19

15 Quoted in *20th Century Living* 14 (2) March/April 1990: note 14.

16 From a Finnish study (see note 14 above).

17 Ibid.

18 Ibid.

19 Ibid.

20 'A Case of Lethal Endodontis', *Townsend Letter* November 1992: 998–100.

21 Warren April 1997, op cit.

22 Ibid.

23 Huggins, op cit.

24 Ibid.

25 Meinig, op cit.

CHAPTER 8

1 Waves Forest, 'Oxygen and the Future of Life on Earth', *Townsend Letter* May 1993: 482–92.

2 Ibid.

CHAPTER 9

1 Linda Weiss, 'A Water Story', *20th Century Living* 16 (2) March/April 1992: 19–20.

2 Dr F Batmanghelidj MD, *Our Body's Many Cries for Water* (Falls Church, VA: Global Health Solutions, Inc, 1997).

3 Colin Ingram, *The Drinking Water Book: A Complete Guide to Safe Drinking Water* (Berkeley, CA: Ten Speed Press, 1991).

4 Ibid.

5 *20th Century Living* 13 (4) July/August 1989: 10.

6 Jeff Breakey, 'Pure Water – A Choice for Health', *20th Century Living* 11 (5) September/Octocber 1987.

7 Ingram, op cit.

8 Breakey, op cit: 9.

9 Rachel Carson, *Silent Spring* (London: Readers Union, 1962): 35.

10 Linda Weiss, 'Water, Water Everywhere, but Not a Drop to Drink', *20th Century Living* 14 (2) March/April 1990: 12.

11 Dr Morton Walker, DPM, 'Aluminium-contaminated Drinking Water, Milk, Tea and Cookware', *Townsend Letter* April 1993: 288–92.

12 D N Martyn *et al.*, 'Geographical relation between Alzheimer's disease and aluminium in drinking water', *Lancet* January 14, 1989: 59–62.

13 T P Flaten, 'An investigation of the chemical composition of Norwegian drinking water and its possible relationships with the epidemiology of some diseases', Institut for Norganisk Kjemi, Norges Tekniske Hogskole, Trondheim, 1986; T Vogt, 'Water quality and health – a study of possible relationship between aluminium in drinking water and dementia', *Sociale og okonomiske studier* 61: 1–99, Oslo Central Bureau of Statistics of Norway, 1986; A Jorn *et al.*, 'Regional differences in mortality from dementia in Australia; an analysis of death certificate data' *Acta Psychiat Scand.*

14 Walker, op cit.

15 L T Weaver *et al.*, 'Intestinal permeability in the newborn', *Arch Dis Child* 54, 1984: 236–41.

16 Janet Raloff, 'Drugged waters', *Science News* March 21, 1998.

17 Jules Klotter, *Townsend Letter* July 1999.

18 Ingram, op cit.

19 Breakey, op cit.

20 Weiss 1992, op cit.

CHAPTER 10

1 Eustace Mullins, *Murder By Injection* (Staunton, VA: 1988).

2 Ibid.

3 *Watershed* 3 (3), October 1997: 1.

4 Kaj Roholm, *Fluorine Intoxication: A Clinical-Hygienic Study* (London and Denmark: H K Lewis, 1937).

5 Dr R G Foulkes BA, MD, 'Fluoridation of Community Water Supplies: 1992 Update', *Townsend Letter* June 1992: 450–7 (450).

6   *NZ Soil & Health* February/March 1995.

7   Foulkes, op cit: 452–4.

8   Transcripts from 1983 Show Disagreements About Fluoride, *Townsend Letter* December 1989: 676–7.

9   As for note 6.

10 John Colquhoun PhD, BDS, *Fluoride* 23 (3), July 1990.

11 Jacobson, *Journal of the American Medical Association* 264, 1990: 501–2.

12 Heilman *et al.*, *Journal of the American Dental Association* July 1997.

13 A Machoy-Mokrzynska, 'Fluoride-Magnesium interaction', *Fluoride* 28 (4), November 1995: 175.

14 *Journal of the American Medical Association* 65, 1961: 694–710.

15 Machoy-Mokrzynska, op cit.

16 Charlotte H Sogaard *et al.*, Twenty-first conference of the *International Society for Fluoride Research*; Budapest Hungary, August 25–28, 1996; as reported in *Fluoride* 1996.

17 B A Duresmith *et al.*, *Jnl Clinical Endocrinology, Endocrinology & Metabolism* 81 (1), 1996: 269–75.

18 Danielson, 'Hip Fractures in Utah's Elderly', *Journal of the American Medical Association* 268, 1992: 746–48, for one.

19 *Osteoporosis*, 1987.

20 D S Kumari, *Biochemistry International* 23 (4), March 1991.

21 *JAMA* 264, 1990: 500–2.

22 *Fluoride* 29 (2), May 1996: 62.

23 Jules Klotter, 'Shorts', *Townsend Letter* June 1992: 534.

24 *Fluoride* 29 (2), May 1996: 111–13.

25 *University of Ottawa Medical Journal*, 1967.

26 Rosetta Schuman, 'Go tell it on the mountain', *Townsend Letter* July 1994: 732.

27 *Neurotoxicology and Teratology* 17 (2), 1995.

28 Dr P Mullenix *et al.*, *Fluoride* 29 (2), May 1996.

29 *Fluoride* 28 (4), November 1995: 89.

30 Mauret *et al.*, *Jnl NCI*, 1990.

31 'A Brief Report on the Association of Drinking Water Fluoridation and the Incidence of Osteosarcoma Among Young Males', *Environmental Health Service*, NJ Department of Health, November 8, 1992.

32 Dr J M Howard, Biolab Medical Unit (UK) reported in *Interaction, Journal of 'Action for ME'* 14, Autumn 1993.

33 As for note 5: 454.

34 Research Report, *Fluoride* 29 (2), May 1996: 89–94.

35 *Fluoride* 14, 1981: 123–28.

36 *Nature* 322, July 10. 1986.

37 *Fluoride* 23 (3), July 1990.

38 Newbrun, *Journ PH Dent* 49 (5), 1989, and A J P H Kumar, May 1989.

39 John Colquhoun PhD, BDS, *Fluoride* 23 (3), July 1990.

40 Foulkes, 'The "Cost" of Fluoridation', *Townsend Letter* November 1993: 1086–7.

41 *Seattle Well Mind Association Newsletter*, January 94: 7.

42 Anne Anderson and Richard Foulkes, 'Re: Fluoride Pollution', *Townsend Letter* July 1993: 734–5.

43 Foulkes 1992: 452.

44 *Fluoride* 28 (4), November 1995: 179.

45 Bob Woffinden, 'Clear and present danger', *Townsend Letter* June 7, 1997: 27.

46 *Sunday Times*, London, June 15, 1997.

47 Elizabeth Baker, *The Unmedical Miracle, Oxygen* (Indianola, WA: Delwood Communications Inc, 1993); David Nudelman, 'On Hydrogen Peroxide', *Townsend Letter* July 1993: 754.

48 As for note 44.

49 Ibid.

50 Philip Sutton DDS, *The Greatest Fraud: Fluoridation* (Lorne Publishing, 1996; PO Box 22, Lorne, Victoria 3232, Australia).

CHAPTER 11

1 Dr Harold E Buttram, MD, 'Overuse of Antibiotics ...', *Townsend Letter* November 1991: 869.

2 'Estimated Annual Production and Consumption of Soft Drinks', *US Soft Drink Association*, 1985.

3 Dr W H Glinsmann MD, *et al.*, 'Evaluation of Health Aspects of Sugars contained in Carbohydrate Sweeteners', Center for Food Safety and Applied Nutrition, US Food and Drug Administration, 1986.

4 A R Sanchez *et al.*, 'Role of sugar in human neutrophilic phagocytosis', *American Journal of Clinical Nutrition* 973 (26.1): 180–4.

5 Nancy Appleton, 'Diet, Stress, and the Immune System', *Townsend Letter* August/September 1992: 728.

6 Wayne Martin, *Townsend Letter* July 1995: 79.

7 Nancy Appleton, '49 Reasons Why Sugar Ruins Your Health', *Townsend Letter* February/March 1993: 202.

8 A bibliography of the 49 references for these 49 points is appended here:

1 Sanchez, A *et al.*, 'Role of Sugars in Human Neutrophilic Phagocytosis', *American Journal of Clinical Nutrition* November 1973: 1180–4.

2 Appleton, Nancy, *Lick the Sugar Habit* (Garden City Park, NY: Avery Publishing Group Inc, 1988): 16.

3 Goldman, J *et al.*, 'Behavioral Effects of Sucrose on Preschool Children', *Journal Abnormal Child Psychology* 14 (4), 1986: 565–77.

4 Scanto, S and Yudkin, John, 'The Effect of Dietary Sucrose on Blood Lipids, Serum Insulin, Platelet Adhesiveness and Body Weight in Human Volunteers', *Postgraduate Medicine Journal* 45, 1969: 602–7.

5 Ringsdorfz, W, Cheraskin, E and Ramsay, R, 'Sucrose, Neutrophilic Phagocytosis and Resistance to Disease', *Dental Survey* 52 (12), 1976: 46–8.

6 Yudkin, J, Kang, S and Bruckdorfer, K, 'Effects of High Dietary Sugar', *British Journal of Medicine* 281, November 22, 1980: 1396.

7 Yudkin, J, Kang, S and Bruckdorfer, K, 'Effects of High Dietary Sugar', *British Journal of Medicine* 281, November 22, 1980: 1396.

8 Kozlovsky, A *et al.*, 'Effects of Diets High in Simple Sugars on Urinary Chromium losses', *Metabolism* 35, June 1986: 515–18.

9 Takahashi, E, Tohuku University School of Medicine, *Wholistic Health Digest* October 1982: 41.

10 Kelsay, J *et al.*, 'Diets High in Glucose or Sucrose and Young women', *American Journal of Clinical Nutrition* 27, 1974: 926–36.

11 Fields, M. *et al.*, 'Effect of copper Deficiency on Metabolism and Wrtali1r in Rats Fed Sucrose or Starch Diets', *Journal of Nutrition* 113, 1983: 1335–45.

12 Lemann, J: 'Evidence that Glucose Ingestion Inhibits Net Renal Tubular Reabsorption of Calcium and Magnesium', *Journal of Laboratory and Clinical Medicine* 70, 1967: 236–45.

13 Taub, H (ed), 'Sugar Weakens Eyesight', *VM Newsletter* 5, May 6, 1986.

14 *University of California, Berkeley Wellness Letter* 6 (3), December 1989: 4–5. A quote from Dr Richard Wurtman, a neurobiologist at MIT.

15 Dufty, W: *Sugar Blues* (NY: Warner Books, 1975).

16 Dufty, W: *Sugar Blues* (NY: Warner Books, 1975).

17 Lewis, J: 'Health Briefings', *Fort Worth Star Telegram*, June 11, 1990. Reported to the Society for Pediatric Research in Anaheim, CA, on May 9, 1990 by Yale medical researchers.

18 Lewis, J: 'Health Briefings', *Fort Worth Star Telegram* June 11, 1990. Reported to the Society for Pediatric Research in Anaheim, CA on May 9, 1990 by Dr Timothy Jones, a scientist from Perth, Australia.

19 Simmons, J: 'Is The Sand of Time Sugar?', *Longevity* June 1990: 49–53.

20 Abrahamson, E, and Peqet, A: *Body Mind and Sugar* (NY: Avon, 1977).

21 Glinsmann, W, Irausquin, H and Youngmee, K, 'Evaluation of Health Aspects of

Sugars Contained in Carbohydrate Sweeteners', Report of Sugars Task Force, 1986: 39. Food and Drug Administration, 200 C Street SW, Washington, DC 20204.

22 Keen, H, Thomas, B, Jarrett, R and Fuller, J, 'Nutrient Intake, Adiposity, and Diabetes', *British Medical Journal* 1, 1979: 655–8.

23 Yudkin, J, *Sweet and Dangerous* (NY: Bantam Books, 1974).

24 Yudkin, J, *Sweet and Dangerous* (NY: Bantam Books, 1974).

25 Darlington, L, Ramsey and Mansfield: 'Placebo-Controlled, Blind Study of Dietary Manipulation Therapy in Rheumatoid Arthritis', *Lancet* February 6, 1986, 236–8.

26 Powers, Lawrence, 'Sensitivity: You React to What You Eat', *Los Angeles Times* February 12, 1985.

27 Crook, W, *The Yeast Connection* (Jackson, TN: Professional Books, 1984).

28 Wheaten, K, 'The Sweet Road to Gallstones', *British Medical Journal* 288, April 14, 1984: 1103–4.

29 Yudkin, J, 'Dietary Fat and Dietary Sugar in Relation to Ischemic Heart Disease and Diabetes', *Lancet* 2, 1964: 4.

30 Cleave, T, *The Saccharine Disease* (New Canaan, CT: Keats Publishing Co, 1974).

31 Erlander, S, 'The Cause and Cure of Multiple Sclerosis', *The Diet to End Disease* 1 (3), March 3, 1979: 59–63.

32 Cleave, T, *The Saccharine Disease* (New Canaan, CT: Keats Publishing Co, 1974).

33 Cleave, T and Campbell, G, *Diabetes, Coronary Thrombosis and the Saccharine Disease* (Bristol: John Wright and Sons, 1960).

34 Behall, K, 'Influence of Estrogen Content of Oral Contraceptives and Consumption of Sucrose on Blood Parameters', *Diss. Abstr. Int. B.* 43, 1982: 1437.

35 Glinsmann, M, Irausquin, H and Youngmee, K 'Evaluation of Report of Sugars Task Force, 1986 Food and Drug Administration, 200 C Street, SW Washington, DC 20204.

36 Appleton, N, *Healthy Bones* (Garden City Park, NY: Avery Publishing Group Inc, 1990): 36–8.

37 Appleton, N, *Healthy Bones* (Garden City Park, NY: Avery Publishing Group Inc, 1990): 19.

38 Beck-Nielsen, H, Pedersen, O and Schwartz, Sorensen, 'Effects of Diet on the Cellular Insulin binding and the Insulin Sensitivity in Young Healthy Subjects', *Diabetes* 15, 1978: 289–96.

39 Keen, H, Thomas, B, Jarrett, R, and Fuller, J, 'Nutritional Factors in Diabetes Mellitus', in Yudkin, J (ed), *Applied Science* (London, 1977): 89–108.

40 Gardner, L and Reiser, S, 'Effects of Dietary Carbohydrate on Fasting Levels of Human Growth Hormone and Cortisol', *Proc. Soc, Exp. Bio. Mad.* 169, 1982: 36–40.

41 Reiser, S, 'Effects of Dietary Sugars on Metabolic Risk Factors Associated with Heart Disease', *Nutr. Health* 3, 1985: 203–16.

42. Hodges, R and Rebello, T, 'Carbohydrates and Blood Pressure', *Annals of Internal Medicine* 98, 1983: 838–41.

43 Behar, D, Rapoport, J, Adans, Berg C and Cornblath, M, 'Sugar Challenge Testing with Children Considered Behaviorally Sugar Reactive', *Nutritional Behavior* 1, 1984: 277–88.

44 Grand, E, 'Food allergies and migraine', *Lancet* 1, 1979: 955–9.

45 Simmons, J: 'Is The Sand of Time Sugar?', *Longevity* June 1990: 49–53.

46 Appleton, Nancy: *Lick the Sugar Habit* (Garden City Park, NY: Avery Publishing Group Inc, 1988).

47 'Sucrose Induces Diabetes in Cat', *Federal Pro.* 6, 1974: 97.

48 Cleave, T, *The Saccharine Disease* (New Canaan, CT: Keats Publishing Co, 1974): 131.

49 Cleave, T, *The Saccharine Disease* (New Canaan, CT: Keats Publishing Co, 1974): 132.

9 'Atkins, Fredericks, Harris, and Page Condemn High-Carbohydrate ("Low Fat") Diets', *Townsend Letter* August/September 1996: 105

10 Rosetta Schuman, 'Cholesterol Mania', *Townsend Letter* April 1990: 229.

11 Dr Abram Hoffer and Dr Morton Walker, *Orthomolecular Nutrition – New Lifestyle for Super Good Health* (1978).

12 Alfred Wertheim, 'What's Wrong with Sugar?' *Townsend Letter* July 1995: 85–6.

13 Appleton August/September 1992, op cit.

14 David Richard, *Stevia Rebaudiana: Nature's Sweet Secret* (Bloomingdale, IL: Blue Heron Press, 1996).

15 Appleton August/September 1992, op cit.

CHAPTER 12

1 Dr Weston Price, *Nutrition and Physical Degeneration* (La Mesa, CA: Price-Pottinger Nutrition Foundation, 1954).

2 *Townsend Letter* May 1996, 146.

CHAPTER 13

1 'Tobacco Firm Shows How Ammonia spurs Delivery of Nicotine', Alix M Freedman in the *Wall Street Journal*, October 18, 1995, as reported in the *Townsend Letter* April 1996: 9.

2 David Krogh, *Smoking: The Artificial Passion* (NY: W H Freeman & Co, 1991).

3 NZ TV 3 News, May 30, 1997.

CHAPTER 14

1   Truth in Labeling Campaign, PO Box 2532, Darien, Illinois 60561, US, or 312-642-9333. 'Trial Begins on MSG Near Death', *Townsend Letter* January 1996: 17.

2   'FDA fights labelling MSG: Consumers charge FDA manipulated, misrepresented report on MSG Safety', *Townsend Letter* January 1996: 15.

3   NOMSG, PO Box 367, Santa Fe, New Mexico, 87504. Fax 505-983-1733.

4   Dr Russell Blaycock MD, *Excitotoxins, The Taste that Kills* (Santa Fe, NM: Health Press, 1994).

5   Dr George Shambaugh MD in *NOHA* 1997, reviewed in the *Well Mind Association Newsletter* February 1997.

6   As for note 2.

7   Beatrice Trum Hunter, *New England Journal of Medicine* 27, February 1991.

8   Dr Derrick Lonsdale, 'Lack of Adverse Behaviour by Consumption of Sugar', *Townsend Letter* June 1994: 608–9.

9   *Journal of Applied Nutrition* 40 (1988): 85–94; *Clinical Research* 3 (1988): 489A; *Clinical Research* 36 (1988): 349A; Department of Health and Human Services: Summary of Adverse Reactions Attributed to Aspartame, April 20, 1995; *American Journal of Clinical Nutrition* 41 (1985): 171; *Lancet* 349 (1997): 362; *Neurology* 48 (1997): 549–50; *Archives of Internal Medicine* 156 (1996): 1027.

10 *Aspartame: Is It Safe?* (Philadelphia: The Charles Press, 1989); *Sweet'ner Dearest* (Sunrise Sentinel Press, 1992); *Defense Against Alzheimer's Disease* (Sunshine Sentinel Press, 1995).

11 wsisyg://Main.14/http://users.kcyb.com/rockitech/aidaparker/224/poisons.htr

12 *Townsend Letter* November 1993: 1074–5.

13 *Townsend Letter* June 1997.

14 Ibid.

15 *Journal of Neuropathology and Experimental Neurology* 55 (11), November 1996: 1115–23.

16 H J Roberts, 'Is Aspartame Safe?' *On Call* (Bulletin of the Palm Beach County Medical Society), January 1987: 16–20; N J Roberts, 'Neurologic, psychiatric and behavioural reactions to Aspartame in 505 Aspartame reactors', *Proceedings of the First International Conference on Dietary Phenylalanine and Brain Function*, Washington DC May 8–10, 1987: 477–81.

17 Ibid.

18 As for note 13.

19 As for note 2.

20 From Betty Martini of the anti-Aspartame group Mission Possible, as reported in *New Zealand Soil & Health* March/April 1998: 8.

CHAPTER 15

1 *NZ Listener* May 2, 1998: 26–30.
2 Morton Walker, 'Frankenstein Food', *Townsend Letter* May 1993: 422–5 (423).
3 Most of the soya now found in many processed foods is 'pesticide-resistant'. That means it can take any amount of spray to get rid of weeds/insects, but will not itself be affected. Biocide residues will therefore be high in this soya. The rest of my pudding is imaginary.
4 Walker, op cit: 423.
5 *SOMA Newsletter* October 1996 (Bondi Beach NSW 2026).
6 *New Scientist* January 1997.
7 Dr Peter Will, 'Genetically Altered Foods – Another Pitfall', *Well Mind Association Newsletter* March/April 1998: 2.
8 Walker, op cit: 423.
9 *Well Mind Newsletter* March/April 1998.
10 Walker, op cit: 424.
11 'The FDA Ban of L-Tryptophan: Politics, Profits and Prozac', *Social Policy* 26.1 (Winter 1995); Brian Leibovitz PhD, 'Nutrition at the Crossroads', *Journal of Optimal Nutrition* 1 (1992): 69–83
12 *NZ Listener* March 13, 1999.
13 'Artificial Life Forms Are Killing Us', *Townsend Letter* May 1995: 128.
14 *NZ Listener* March 13, 1999: 20.
15 M Polen, 'Playing God in the garden', *New York Times* Magazine October 25, 1998.
16 As for note 9.

CHAPTER 16

1 'The Problem of Poisonous Plastics', *Nexus* October/November 1996: 11–14. (Email: bdensley@newscorp.om.au)
2 *NZ Soil & Health* July/August 1998: 21–2.
3 Commercially-made infant formulas are, of course, worse in *every* way.
4 T Colburn, Myers and Dumanoski, *Our Stolen Future* (NY: Dutton/Penguin, 1996).

CHAPTER 17

1 New Zealand Director-General of Health Gillian Durham quoted in Denis Welch, 'A Jab in the Dark', *NZ Listener* August 23, 1997: 18–21 (18).

2 US Taskforce for Safer Childhood Vaccines, Ref.21CFR 600.3p, 13; December 1, 1994.

3 Harris L Coulter and Barbara Loe Fisher, *DPT: A Shot in the Dark* (NY: Harcourt, 1985): 2.

4 W C Torch, 'Diphtheria-pertussis-tetanus (DPT) immunization: A potential cause of sudden infant death syndrome', American Academy of Neurology 34th Annual Meeting, April/May 1982: A169–70.

5 Harris L Coulter, *Vaccination, Social Violence and Criminality: The Medical Assault on the American Brain* (Berkeley, CA: North Atlantic Books, 1990).

6 Dr Joseph G Hattersley, 'Crib Death: Sudden Infant Death that isn't sudden at all,' *Townsend Letter* May 1996: 62–5.

7 Dr Robert Riesinger, 'A final mechanism of cardiac and respiratory failure', *International Symposium on SIDS in Infancy* 1974. (Also Internet http://www.erols.com/drrobert/sids.html)

8 Harris L Coulter and Barbara Loe Fisher, *DPT: A Shot in the Dark* (NY: Harcourt, 1985).

9 Torch, op cit.

10 L Baraff *et al.*, 'DPT Immunization and Sudden Infant Death Syndrome', *Pediatric Infectious Diseases* 1983.

11 *Pediatrics* 101 (3), 11 March 1998.

12 Reported in *Campaign Against Fraudulent Medical Research Newsletter* Spring 1996.

13 Dr Archie Kalokerinos MBBS, PhD, *Every Second Child* (New Canaan, CT: Keats Publishing Co, 1981; Australia: Thomas Nelson, 1974).

14 For the protocols Dr Kalokerinos has used successfully in his practice, see *Vitamin C, Nature's Miraculous and Healing Missile* (Melbourne: Frederick Todd, 1993).

15 *What Your Doctor Will Never Tell You* December 1997: 6.

16 *International Vaccination Newsletter* December 1996.

17 'Just Who is Responsible?' *Sunday Star Times* March 1, 1998.

18 Welch, op cit: 20.

19 *Sunday Times Magazine* December 17, 1995; *British Medical Journal* 308, April 16, 1994: 1015–17.

20 Dawbarns Factsheet 'MMR and MR vaccines' (Email: dawbarns@paston.co.uk)

21 US Vaccination Adverse Reports, November 1, 1990 – July 31, 1992, as reprinted in *IAS N/L NZ* 6 (1) August 1993: 6.

22 Neil Z Miller, *Immunization – Theory vs Reality* (New Atlantean Press, 1995).

23 Dr Michel R Odent *et al.*, *Journal of the American Medical Association* 272 (8), August 24/31 1994: 592–3.

24 M H Williams, 'Increasing severity of asthma from 1960 to 1987', *New England Journal of Medicine* April 13, 1989: 1015–16.

25 *British Medical Journal* 287, September 17, 1985: 775–6.

26 *Lancet* April 29, 1995.

27 *New Zealand Medical Journal* May 24, 1996.

28 Robert P Wise *et al.*, 'Hair Loss after Routine Immunizations', *Journal of the American Medical Association* 278, 1997: 1176–8.

29 Health Studies Collegium Seminar, Tysons Corner, Virginia, March 4–5 1989.

30 A S Krolewski *et al.*, 'Epidemiological approach to the aetiology of type I diabetes mellitus and its complications', *New England Journal of Medicine* November 26, 1987: 1390–7.

31 Welch, op cit: 19.

32 *20th Century Living* 13 (4) July/August 1989: 15.

33 *International Vaccination Newsletter*.

34 Dr R Mendelsohn, *How to Bring Up a Healthy Child ... In Spite of Your Doctor* (NY: Ballantine Books, 1984): 20.

35 *Limits to Medicine: Medical Nemesis: The Expropriation of Health* (London: Marion Boyars, 1976).

36 R R Porter, 'The Contribution of the Biological and Medical Sciences to Human Welfare', Presidential Address to the British Association for the Advancement of Science, Swansea Meeting, 1971 (London: The Association, 1972): 95.

37 *Archives of Internal Medicine* 154, August 22, 1994 (16:1815-20).

38 *Northern News* November 30, 1996.

39 Welch, op cit: 20.

40 'Immunizations: Good or Bad?' *Well Mind Association Newsletter* Seattle WA, October 1993: 2.

41 Ibid.

42 Jamie Murphy, *What Every Parent Should Know About Childhood Immunization* (Boston: Earth Health Products, 1992): 118.

43 *Infectious Diseases* January 1982: 21.

44 J Trueta and R Hodes, 'Provoking and Localising Factors in Poliomyelitis', *Lancet* 1 1954: 998–9 [my emphasis].

45 R I Watkins, 'Salk Vaccine and the Nervous System', cited in E McBean, *The Poisoned Needle* (Health Research Publications, 1974).

46 Neil Z Miller, *Vaccines: Are They Really Safe and Effective?* (New Atlantean Press, 1992).

47 *Science* March 17, 1972: 1225–30.

48 *US Organic Consumer Reports* March 11, 1975.

49 'Vaccination Myth #6', *Family Christian Academy* Summer 1996: 17.

50 Patricia Savage, *Mothering* 13, Fall 1979.

51 Dr Guylaine Lancetot MD, *The Medical Mafia* (Here's the Key, Inc, 1995): 117.

52 *20th Century Living* 13 (1), January/February 1989: 7.

53 Dr Harold E Buttram MD and John Chriss Hoffman PhD, *Vaccinations and Immune Malfunctions* (Quakertown, PA: Humanitarian Publishing Co, 1982).

54 George Blanck *et al.*, 'Multiple insertions and tandem repeats of origan-mins simian virus 40 DNA in transformed rat and mouse cells', *Journal of Virology* May 1988: 1520–3.

55 S Kumar and L K Miller, 'Effects of serial passage of autographa California nuclear polyhedrosis virus in cell culture', *Virus Research* 7, 1987: 335–49.

56 Buttram and Hoffman, op cit.

57 Lancetot, op cit.

58 Immunisation Advisory Service publication.

59 M Eibl *et al.*, 'Abnormal T-lymphocyte subpopulations in healthy subjects after tetanus booster immunization', *New England Journal of Medicine* 310 (3), January 19, 1984: 198–9.

60 Laurie Garrett, *The Coming Plague* (NY: Farrar, Strauss & Giroux, 1994).

61 Senate Record, March 5, 1987; Committee on Select Revenue Measures.

62 Laurie Garnett, *The Coming Plague* (NY: Farrar, Strauss & Giroux, 1994): 52.

63 *Mothering* 11, Spring 1979.

64 Reviewing *Vaccination* by Vera Scheibner (published by Naturally Write, Mansfield DC Qld, Australia 4122, 1993), *Townsend Letter* October 1995: 114.

65 Lancetot, op cit: 35.

CHAPTER 18

1 Dr Henry Schroeder, *The Poisons Around Us* (Indiana University Press, 1974; reprint New Canaan, CT: Keats Publishing Co, 1994).

2 Schroeder: 43.

3 Schroeder: 48.

4 From D Maddock, 'Leaded versus unleaded petrols', *Australasian Health and Healing* 14 (1), 1994/95: 15–16.

CHAPTER 19

1 Margaret Wirkus, 'Warning: The Electricity Around You May Be Hazardous to Your Health', *ISSSEEM News Magazine* (International Society for the Study of Subtle Energies and Energy Medicine) 356, Fall 1993 (Goldco Circle, Golden, CO, 80401).
2 Peter Sierck, *Townsend Letter* July 1993: 754
3 Chloe Wadsworth MA, 'Electromagnetic radiation', *Townsend Letter* January 1993: 14–15.
4 Wirkus, op cit.
5 Noel O'Hare, 'Bad vibes', *Listener* September 27, 1997: 51.
6 *What Your Doctor Will Never Tell You* March 1998: 5.
7 O'Hare, op cit.
8 Sierck, op cit.
9 Michael Riversong, 'Electromagnetism and Environmental Illness', *ISSSEEM News Magazine* 356, Fall 1993.

CHAPTER 20

1 TV 1 News, April 22, 1998.
2 John Violanti, Rochester Institute of Technology, Alternative Medicine Connection, Arline Brecher, website address: http://www.arxc.com, *Townsend Letter* February/March 1996: 41.
3 *North Shore Times Advertiser* October 21, 1997: 5.
4 *NZ Listener* September 27, 1997.

CHAPTER 21

1 Rachel Carson, *Silent Spring* (London: Readers Union, 1962): 41.
2 Ibid.
3 Carson, op cit: 35.
4 Professor W William Hughes, *Essentials of Environmental Toxicology* (Taylor & Francis 1996): 13.
5 Meriel Watts, *The Poisoning of New Zealand* (AIT Press, 1994): 64.
6 R Saracci *et al.*, 'Cancer Mortality in Workers Exposed to Chlorophenoxy Herbicides and Chlorophenols', *Townsend Letter* May 1992: 377–8.

7   Dr Morton Walker DPM, *Townsend Letter* July 1993: 772.

8   *Journal of Pesticide Reform* 17, 1997.

9   *NZ Soil & Health* July/August 1998: 21–2.

10 *New Zealand Toxins Awareness Group Newsletter No 38* December 1997: 3.

11 *New Zealand Toxins Awareness Group Newsletter No 39* May 1998: 3.

12 D Bear *et al.*, 'Aggression in cat and human precipitated by a cholinesterase inhibitor', *Psychosomatics* 27 (7), July 1986: 535–6.

13 *Well Mind Association Newsletter* March 1996: 2.

14 *Self Help Cancer Cure Book* (produced by the Soil & Health Assn of New Zealand Inc, 1997).

15 Dr Victor Penzer MD, DMD, FASCD, 'Beware of Vermicides!' *Townsend Letter* May 1992: 376–7.

16 Pimentel *et al.*, 'Assessment of environmental and economic impacts of pesticide use', in Pimentel and Lehman (eds), *The Pesticide Question – Environment, Economics and Ethics* (NY: Chapman and Hall, 1993).

17 Ibid.

18 Robert Repetto and Sanjay S Baliga, *Pesticides and the Immune System: The Public Health Risks* (World Resources Institute, March 1996).

19 Repetto and Baliga, op cit: 4.

20 Repetto and Baliga, op cit: 9.

21 Repetto and Baliga, op cit: 13.

22 Repetto and Baliga, op cit: 14.

23 Repetto and Baliga, op cit: 15.

24 Repetto and Baliga, op cit: 19.

25 Repetto and Baliga, op cit: 21.

26 Repetto and Baliga, op cit: 41.

27 Repetto and Baliga, op cit: 45.

28 Repetto and Baliga, op cit: 48.

29 Repetto and Baliga, op cit: 52.

30 Repetto and Baliga, op cit: 56.

31 Repetto and Baliga, op cit: 57.

32 Repetto and Baliga, op cit: 61.

33 Repetto and Baliga, op cit: 62.

34 *Pesticides News* 37, September 1997.

35 *What Your Doctor Will Never Tell You* 1 (4), November 1997: 4.

36 Dr Alan Gaby, 'Human Canaries and Silent Spring', *Townsend Letter* October 1990: 668.

37 EarthSave Foundation, *Townsend Letter* May 1993: 408.

38 Michael Crawford and David Marsh, *The Driving Force: Food, Evolution, and the Future* (NY: Harper & Row, 1989) [my emphasis].

39 Theo Colborn & Coralie Clement (eds), *Chemically-induced Alterations in Sexual and Functional Development* (vol 21 of the series 'Modern Environmental Toxicology'; Princeton, NJ: Princeton Scientific Publishing Company, 1992).

40 Carson, op cit: 7.

41 As for note 34.

CHAPTER 23

1   *Well Mind Association Newsletter* Seattle, WA, September 1997: 6.

2   Martin L Gross, *Psychological Society* (NY: Random House, 1978): 18.

3   Gross, op cit: 25.

4   Gross, op cit: 24.

5   Dr Bradford Weeks MD, 'Why I became a psychiatrist', *Well Mind Association Newsletter* Seattle, WA, March 1996: 3.

6   E Fuller Torrey, *Freudian Fraud* (Harper Perennial, 1992): 7–8.

7   Ibid.

8   Gross, op cit: 4.

9   Ibid.

10 Gross, op cit: 5

11 Ibid.

12 Gross, op cit: 10

13 Gross, op cit: 3.

14 Gross, op cit: 16.

15 I must hasten to add that I am not here knocking embroidery, or any form of handiwork – only the fact that these ladies had little else in their lives. As for most of our history, it was an age of servants and female servitude at all levels.

16 This one's easy to figure out: Unless he was taking more cocaine than usual, he had probably developed a sensitivity to something he ate too often on his travels, possibly wheat. Deteriorating handwriting and intestinal troubles are signs of food allergy. But he had no access to or inclination towards that kind of knowledge, any more than do most of his medical and psychiatric fellows to this day.

17 Gross, op cit: 250.

18 Gross, op cit: 249.

19 Gross, op cit: 248.

20 A Hoffer and H Osmond, *The Chemical Basis of Clinical Psychiatry* (Springfield, IL: C C Thomas, 1960); A Hoffer, *Niacin Therapy in Psychiatry* (Springfield, IL: C C Thomas, 1962).

21 B Bower, 'New Culprits Cited for Schizophrenia', *Science News* February 3, 1996.

22 A Hoffer and H Osmond, 'Massive Niacin Treatment in Schizophrenia; Review of a Nine-Year Study', *Lancet* 1, 1963: 316–20.

23 A Hoffer, 'Treatment of Schizophrenia', *Townsend Letter* July 1995: 52–7.

24 K S Dalla, *et al.*, *Mol Cell Biochem* 878, 1989: 85–92.

25 Hoffer 1995, op cit: 56.

26 A Hoffer, 'The Vitamin Paradigm Wars', *Townsend Letter* June 1996: 56–60.

27 Gross, op cit.

28 Hoffer 1995, op cit: 52.

29 Hoffer and Osmond, op cit.

30 *Townsend Letter* May 1992: 426.

31 Hoffer 1995, op cit: 56.

32 Caution is urged with copper, and organic forms of all minerals are preferable.

33 Hoffer 1995, op cit: 53.

34 'An anecdote describing the treatment of one case of schizophrenia', *Townsend Letter* July 1997: 76–9.

35 I would differentiate severe mental illness from the everyday 'neurosis', which does not appear to have the major biochemical problem. But there could still be mineral deficiencies and other imbalances which contribute to the problem.

36 Dr Kristin Leutwyler, *Scientific American* March 1997: 13–14.

37 Torrey, op cit: 46.

38 *Townsend Letter* July 1994: 732.

39 Torrey, op cit: 257.

CHAPTER 24

1 *Well Mind Association Newsletter* Seattle, WA, February 1995: 2.

2 Ibid.

3 N R Cook *et al.*, 'An unexpected result for sodium – causal or casual?' *Hypertension* 25, 1995: 1153–4.

CHAPTER 25

1   Radio New Zealand news item, April 1998.
2   Finlay MacDonald, 'Happiness is ...', *Metro* December 1996: 68.
3   Margo White, *NZ Listener* March 7, 1998: 34–7.
4   *Sunday Star Times* July 1998.
5   Jules Klotter, 'Relighting the Inner Flame', *Townsend Letter* 1996: 66.
6   *What Your Doctor Will Never Tell You* I (1), March/April 1997: 3.
7   Dr Gary Null PhD, *Townsend Letter* February/March 1993: 178.
8   MacDonald, op cit.
9   Maureen Kennedy Salaman, 'Would you hire the FDA?' *Townsend Letter* May 1994: 535.
10 Ibid.
11 Null February/March 1993, op cit: 182.
12 Dr Gary Null, 'Safety of Prozac', *Townsend Letter* November 1993: 1095.
13 MacDonald, op cit.
14 Null November 1993, op cit.
15 Breggin & Breggin, *Talking Back to Prozac: What Doctors Aren't Telling You About Today's Most Controversial Drug* (NY: St Martin's Press, 1994): 40.
16 Null November 1993, op cit.
17 Dr Gary Null, 'The Hidden Side of Psychiatry', *Townsend Letter* January 1997: 89.
18 Null November 1993, op cit.
19 Dr Steven Bratman MD, *Beat Depression with St John's Wort* (Prima Publishing, 1997).
20 Null November 1993, op cit.
21 For legal reasons, some material published in the original New Zealand edition of this book has had to be deleted for this UK edition.
22 Dr Peter Breggin, interview with Dr Gary Null, November 9, 1994, as reported in 'The Hidden Side of Psychiatry', *Townsend Letter* January 1997.

CHAPTER 26

1   In many parts of the world a sneeze brings this automatic rejoinder from others. 'Gezundheit!' means 'Good health!' a sign of respect and concern. But also it is particularly appropriate when speaking of the FDA, because the origins of the custom lie in the medieval plagues of Europe, when the first sign from a victim was often a sneeze. 'Gezundheit!' was therefore an attempt to ward off the plague.

2 Editorial, 'The FDA's Double Standard Revealed by Its Deeds', *Townsend Letter* December 1992: 1123–4.

3 Dr Gary Null, 'Prozac, Eli Lilly, and the FDA', *Townsend Letter* February/March 1993: 185.

4 As for note 2.

5 Dr Peter Breggin, interview with Dr Gary Null, November 9, 1994, as reported in 'The Hidden Side of Psychiatry', *Townsend Letter* January 1997: 88.

7 Null, op cit.

8 Breggin, op cit.

9 Gambee and Hoffine, 'Fraudulent Medical Practices – Watch and Be Wary'; transcript: *Townsend Letter* February/March 1997: 84–94 (88).

10 Maureen Kennedy Salaman, 'Would you hire the FDA?' *Townsend Letter* April 1994: 327–31.

11 *Time Magazine* August 26, 1991: 45.

12 Irene Alleger, 'The Fleecing of America by the Pharmaceuticals', *Townsend Letter* August/Sept 1996: 129.

13 As for note 2.

14 'Letter to Editor', *Townsend Letter* July 1990: 460.

15 Breggin, op cit.

16 Therese Emmanuel and Steven Mehler, 'Dr Stanislaw Burzynski, a Pioneer in Alternative Cancer Treatment, Faces 290 Years Imprisonment on the FDA's Trumped-up Charges', *Townsend Letter* February/March 1997: 130.

17 Ibid.

18 G Witford and B Morrow, *Environmental Health Group Newsletter* (Cavan, Ontario LOA 1CO, Canada) in *Townsend Letter* February/March 1997: 134.

19 Dr Jules Klotter, 'FDA vs Natural Food for Pets', *Townsend Letter* January 1997: 21.

20 'A Grim Truth in a Democratic Society', *Newsletter* August 1994. (Independent Citizens Research Foundation for the Study of Degenerative Disease, Inc. PO Box 97, Ardsley, New York 10502.)

CHAPTER 27

1 *New Zealand Herald* August 20, 1998.

2 Television One (New Zealand) November 25, 1997.

3 *New Zealand Herald* June 26, 1995.

4 *Public Citizen* July/August 1990: 24.

5 Olarsch & Stockton, *Townsend Letter* August/September 1996: 114.

6   *Time* January 8, 1990.

7   *USA Today* January 4, 1990.

8   Maureen Kennedy Salaman, 'Would you hire the FDA?' *Townsend Letter* April 1994: 327.

9   Maureen Kennedy Salaman, 'The FDA's Double Standard Revealed', *Townsend Letter* December 1992: 1124.

10 *Journal of the American Medical Association* April 15, 1998.

11 Kennedy Salaman 1992, op cit.

12 Robe B Carson quoting Victor Penzer in 'Common Denominators in Cancer Remedies; Implications and Inferences', *Townsend Letter* August/September 1991: 629.

13 'Western Medicine or Homeopathy?' *Townsend Letter* May 1994: 452–5.

14 *Jnl Anthroposophic Medicine* 9 (3).

15 L Ovesen, 'Drugs', *New England Journal of Medicine* 18, 1979: 278–98; D A Roe, *Drug Induced Nutritional Deficiencies* (Westport, CT: Aci Publishing Inc, 1978): 228–38.

16 D A Roe, 'Diet-drug interactions and incompatibilities', April 1990: 217–9.

17 The charts on pages 206–07 are adapted from L Ovesen, 'Drugs', *New England Journal of Medicine* 18, 1979: 278–98, as printed in *Townsend Letter* April 1990: 219.

18 Polly Horn reviewing Hartmut Heine's *Matrix and Matrix Regulation*, 1991, in *Townsend Letter* May 1997: 134.

19 Dr E T Krebs Jr, DSc, 'An Aspirin a Day and Nosebleeds', *Townsend Letter* June 1991: 431.

20 Udo Erasmus, in *Fats and Oils* 1986: 193.

21 I was in dire straits at the time. It is unusual.

22 Dr Alan Gaby, 'Arthritis treatment: Who are the quacks?' *Townsend Letter* February/March 1993: 142.

23 Dr Timothy Gerrity, University of Illinois College of Medicine, January 23, 1983.

24 'Set back for lidocaine', *Cortlandt Forum* November 1990: 22.

25 Dr Russell L Smith PhD and Dr Edward R Pinkney MD, *The Cholesterol Conspiracy* (St Louis, MO: Warren H Green Inc, 1991).

26 Bill Sardi, as reported in 'Anti-cholesterol Drug Cuts Heart Attacks, But ...', *Townsend Letter* May 1996: 88–9.

27 Folkers *et al.* 'Lovastatin Decreases Coenzyme Q Levels in Humans', *Proceedings of the National Academy of Science* 87, November 1990: 8931–4.

28 'Cholesterol Lowering Drugs Disrupt Biochemistry', *Townsend Letter* November 1997: 116.

29 'Rx Comparison: HRT vs Remifemin in Menopause', *Townsend Letter* June 1996: 80.

30 G A Colditz, *et al.*: 'The use of estrogen and progestins and the risk of breast cancer in postmenopausal years', *New England Journal of Medicine* 332, 1995: 1589–93; J B Heinrich, 'The postmenopausal estrogen/breast cancer controversy' *Journal of the American Medical Association* 268, 1992: 1900–2; K K Steinberg, 'A meta-analysis of the effect of estrogen replacement therapy on the risk of breast cancer', *Journal of the American Medical Association* 265, 1991: 1985–90; B K Armstrong, 'Oestrogen therapy after the menopause. Boon or bane?' *Medical Journal of Australia* 148, 1998: 213–4; W D Du Pont and D L Page: 'Menopausal estrogen replacement therapy and breast cancer', *Arch Int Med* 151, 1991: 67–72.

31 *New England Journal of Medicine* August 16, 1990.

32 *Lancet* October 1997.

33 Marc Lippman *et al.*, 'Effects of estrone, estradiol and estriol on hormone-responsive human breast cancer in long term tissue culture', *Cancer Res* 37 (6), 1977: 1901–7.

34 'Important News About Breast Health for Women 40–50', *Townsend Letter* June 1997: 138.

35 As for note 29.

36 Robe B Carson, 'Common Denominators in Cancer Non-Remedies and in Human Longevity', *Townsend Letter* January 1992: 51.

37 David J Orman, letter, *Townsend Letter* May 1993: 469.

38 *Townsend Letter* August/September 1991: 15, ref 23; January 1992: 15, ref 11.

39 *Townsend Letter* January 1997: 54.

40 Dr Raymond Peat PhD, 'Estriol DES, DDT', *Townsend Letter* January 1997: 54.

41 *Townsend Letter* June 1998: 78.

42 Peat, op cit: 56–7.

43 Dr Alan Gaby MD, 'Modern Medicine is Too Complicated', *Townsend Letter* August/September 1993: 864.

44 *Annals of Internal Medicine* 1992: 117.

45 Kennedy Salaman 1994, op cit.

46 Kennedy Salaman 1992, op cit: 1123–4.

47 GAO/HEHS-95-152, *Prescription Drugs and the Elderly* July 1995.

48 Dr Robert S Mendelsohn MD, *Confessions of a Medical Heretic* (Warner Books, 1979): 186–7.

49 Dr Toni Jeffreys PhD, *The Mile-High Staircase* (Hodder & Stoughton, 1982): 40.

50 An old word for pharmacists.

51 Dr Richard Clarke Cabot, *Journal of the American Medical Association* 47, 1906: 982.

52 Samuel E Stumpf, *Annals of Internal Medicine* 64, 1966: 460.

53 George Bernard Shaw, *The Doctor's Dilemma* 1913.

54 *Townsend Letter* May 1994: 454.

55 Carson 1992, op cit: 48–53.

56 *Townsend Letter* January 1992: 12.

57 Dr Alan R Gaby MD, 'Literature Review & Commentary', *Townsend Letter* August/September 1990: 523.

58 Dr Alan R Gaby MD, 'Drug Money Influences Medical Opinions', *Townsend Letter* June 1997: 118.

59 Professor Edzard Ernst, *Auckland Daily News* March 24, 1999: 4.

60 Dr N M Kaplan MD, 'Dietary aspects of the treatment of hypertension', *Annual Review of Public Health* 7, 1986: 501–19.

61 *New England Journal of Medicine* 328, 1993: 959.

62 *Townsend Letter* January 1997: 54.

63 Dr Jeffrey S Bland PhD, *Townsend Letter* October 1993: 998.

64 Kennedy Salaman 1994, op cit.

CHAPTER 28

1 G Cowley *et al.* 'In pursuit of a terrible killer', *Newsweek* December 10, 1990: 66–8.

2 P Skrabanek, 'False premises and false promises of breast cancer screening', *Lancet* August 10, 1985: 316–20.

3 Ellen Hodgson Brown JD, *Townsend Letter* July 1993: 743–5.

CHAPTER 29

1 Dr Alan R Gaby MD, 'Does Wearing a Bra Cause Breast Cancer?' *Townsend Letter* May 1996: 29.

2 Arline Brecher, 'Alternative Medicine Connection', http://www.arxc.com, *Townsend Letter* February/March 1996: 42.

3 S Singer and S Grismaijer, *Dressed to Kill: The Link Between Breast Cancer and Bras* (Garden City Park, NY: Avery Publishing Group Inc, 1995).

4 NZ TV 3 News, May 8, 1998.

CHAPTER 30

1   Judith Brady, *One in Three: Women with Cancer Confront an Epidemic* (Pittsburgh, PA: Cleis Press, 1991).

2   *NZ Herald* May 30–31, 1998: A15.

3   *Townsend Letter* June 1996: 73 (figure for 1995).

4   Auckland Cancer Information Centre, July 1997; no statistics beyond 1993 available.

5   As for note 3.

6   Dr Robert M Kradjian MD, *Save Yourself from Breast Cancer* (NY: Berkeley Publishing Group, 1994).

7   E H Brown JD, *Townsend Letter* July 1993: 745.

8   Liane Clorfene-Casten, *Breast Cancer: Poisons, Profits and Prevention* (Monroe, ME: Common Courage Press, 1996 [tel. 207-525-0900]).

9   Dr Sherry Rogers MD, *Townsend Letter* May 1997: 124.

10 Dr Wayne Martin, *Townsend Letter* January 1992: 58.

11 *Townsend Letter* May 1992: 361.

12 *Journal of Urology* 1982.

13 Martin, op cit: 57–8.

14 Kradjian, op cit.

15 Editorial, *Lancet* 341, February 6, 1993.

16 Dr Joseph Beasley MD, *The Betrayal of Health* (NY: Time Books/Random House, 1991) or *The Kellog Report* 1989.

17 Dr Hardin B Jones, *Cancer Control Journal* 5 (3/4): 147.

18 Beasley, op cit.

19 Al Schaefer, 'Dr Warner's Time Has Come', editorial, *Townsend Letter* February/March 1997: 114.

20 Ibid.

21 Dr Joanna Budwig, as reported in *Townsend Letter* August/September 1991: 626.

22 Dr Ralph Moss, *Questioning Chemotherapy* (NY: Equinox Press, 1995).

23 Lee Hitchcox, *Long Life Now: Strategies for Staying Alive* (Berkeley, CA: Celestial Arts, 1997).

24 Schaefer, op cit.

25 *British Medical Journal* March 28, 1992; *Science News* 144, April 25, 1992: 266–7.

26 Jules Klotter: 'What your Doctors won't tell you about cancer' Malibu Videos 1993, in *Townsend Letter* December 1993: 1,254.

27 Dr Barbara Joseph MD, *My Healing from Breast Cancer* (New Canaan, CT: Keats Publishing Inc, 1996).

28 Klotter, op cit.

29 Barbara Holt, *Newsletter of the New Zealand Breast Cancer Action Group* 18, 1997.

30 Kradjian, op cit.

31 F P Fouche, 'Freedom of the Negro races from cancer', *British Medical Journal* June 30, 1923: 1,116.

32 *British Medical Journal* July 7, 1923: 45; *BMJ* July 14, 1923: 86; *BMJ* July 21, 1923: 130–1.

33 Dr Albert Schweitzer, *On the Edge of the Primeval Forest* (NY: Macmillan, 1931).

34 Dr Wayne Martin in correspondence with Professor Manual Navarro of Santo Tomas University in Manila.

35 'Beware of the Ox', *Lancet* April 27, 1994: 791.

36 Dr David Horrobin and Dr Stephen Seely, 'Diet and breast cancer: the possible connection with sugar consumption', *Medical Hypotheses* 11.3 (July 1983): 319–27.

37 Dr Raymond Peat PhD, 'Estriol, DES, DDT', *Townsend Letter* January 1997: 56.

38 Auckland Cancer Information Centre, July 1997 (no figures available after 1993).

39 Kradjian, op cit.

40 *New England Journal of Medicine* 332, 1995: 1589–93.

41 *NZ Soil & Health* (NZ) October/November 1994: 2.

42 *Lancet* March 6, 1993: 581–5.

43 Joseph, op cit.

44 Lisa and Chuck Winther, 'What Your Doctor Won't Tell You About Cancer', Malibu Videos 1993 – see note 26.

45 Therese Emmanuel and Steven Mehler, 'Dr Stanislaw Burzynski, a Pioneer in Alternative Cancer Treatment, Faces 290 Years Imprisonment on the FDA's Trumped-up Charges', *Townsend Letter* February/March 1997: 130.

46 Ellen H Brown JD, 'Cancer Treatment', *Townsend Letter* July 1993: 744.

47 As for note 3: 74 (figure for 1995).

48 Dr Ralph W Moss, *The Cancer Industry*.

49 Moss, *Questioning Chemotherapy*, op cit.

50 Ibid.

51 Klotter, op cit.

52 Kradjian, op cit.

53 Schepper *et al.*, *Lancet* 348, 1996: 1149–51.

54 According to Wayne Martin, CoQ10 should be taken at the same time as fat or oil if it is to be utilized. Good fat or oil, of course!

55 'Stop Breast Cancer in its Tracks', *Townsend Letter* May 1997: 124–5; *European Journal of Cancer* 28A (4/5), 1992: 784–8; *Life Sciences* (54) 18, 1994: 1299–1303.

CHAPTER 31

1 Virginia Woolf (1882–1941), *Moments of Being* (Hogarth Press, 1976).
2 Dr Harold E Buttram MD, 'Overuse of Antibiotics ...' *Townsend Letter* November 1991: 867–72.
3 K Melby and T Midvedt, 'Effects of some antibacterial agents on phagocytosis', *Acta Pathology and Microbiology, Scandinavia Section B* 88, 1980: 103–6.
4 *British Medical Journal* 7, December 1991; *Journal of the American Medical Association* December 18, 1991.
5 Kuvaeva *et al.*, 'Microecology of the gastrointestinal tract and the immunological status under food allergy', *De Nahrung* 28 (6/7): 189.
6 Buttram, op cit: 869.
7 Dr Morton Walker DPM, 'You Can Eliminate Parasites', *Townsend Letter* February/March 1997: 64–9 (64).
8 W John Diamond MD, 'Salmonellosis', *Biological Therapy* June 1992.
9 ' "Silver" Tooth Fillings Implicated in the Spread of Antibiotic Resistant Bacteria', *Townsend Letter* July 1993: 756.
10 Letter signed by Maxine Hayes MD, MPH, Assistant Secretary/Acting Health Officer, Washington Department of Health.
11 M J Seelig, 'Role of antibiotics in the pathogenesis of Candida infections', *American Journal of Medicine* 40, 1966: 887–917; M J Seelig, 'The rationale for preventing antibacterial-induced fungal overgrowth', *Medical Times* 96 (7), 1968: 689–710; M J Seelig, 'Mechanisms by which antibiotics increase the incidence and severity of Candidiasis and alter the immunological defences', *Bacteriological Review* 30 (2), June 1968.
12 C Voiculescu *et al.*, 'Experimental study of antibiotic-induced immunosuppression in mice', *Comp Immune Microbial Infect Dis* 6 (4), 1983: 2991–9; and J P Trowbridge, *The Yeast Syndrome* (Bantam Books, 1983): 42–54.
13 Dr C O Truss MD, *The Missing Diagnosis* (Birmingham, AL) and Dr W G Crook, *The Yeast Connection* (1986) and *Chronic Fatigue Syndrome and the Yeast Connection* (Professional Books, 1992).
14 K Iwata and Y Yamamoto, Proceedings of the 4th International Conference on the Mycoses, June 1977, PAHO, *Scientific Publication* No. 356.

15 Dr Steven S Witkin PhD, 'Defective Immune Responses in Patients with Recurrent Candidiasis', *Infections in Medicine* May/June 1985: 129–32.

16 Buttram, op cit: 868.

17 'Candidiasis: An Initial Indication of a Positive Treatment Approach', *Townsend Letter* July 1995: 68.

18 Dr Harold E Buttram MD, 'A Review of Potential Therapies in Care of the Hyperactive Child', *Townsend Letter* October 1996: 112–14.

19 Dr Mary A K Matossian, *Poisons of the Past: Molds, Epidemics and History* (Yale University Press, 1989).

20 Truss, op cit 13.

21 Buttram 1991, op cit: 867.

22 Marc Lappée, *When Antibiotics Fail* (Berkeley, CA: North Atlantic Books, 1986).

23 Ibid.

CHAPTER 32

1   *Journal of the American Medical Association* December 12, 1996.

2   Dr Robert Wilner MD, *Deadly Deception* (Boca Raton, FL: Peltec Publishing Co, 1994).

3   Dr Luc de Schepper MD, PhD, 'Western Medicine or Homeopathy ... which one is the real Science?' *Townsend Letter* May 1994: 452–5 (454).

4   Robert Bell, *Impure Science: Fraud, Compromise and Political Influence in Scientific Research* (Wylie, 1992); William Broad and Nicholas Wade, *Betrayers of the Truth* (Century, 1982), also about fraud in science.

5   Christine Russell, 'Louis Pasteur and the Question of Fraud', *Townsend Letter* October 1993: 960.

6   G Lancetot, *Medical Mafia* (Here's the Key Inc, 1995).

7   Bell, op cit.

8   Wayne Martin, 'The Miracle of Evening Primrose Oil', *Townsend Letter*, November 1992, 992.

9   However, 'The unexplained is the unexamined', *Well Mind Association Newsletter* Seattle, WA, May 1997: 2.

10 E Douglas Hume, *Bechamp or Pasteur – A Lost Chapter in the History of Biology* (C W Daniel).

11 Lendon Smith, *Feed Your Body Right* (NY: M Evans & Co, 1994): 25.

12 Christopher Bird, 'Cats, Insects and Rosebushes', *Townsend Letter* April 1993, 294–9.

13 Since verified with a positive Mantoux test and X-rays which reveal substantial but healed TB lesions.

14 Irene Alleger, 'The Holistic Tradition of the West', *Townsend Letter*.

15 Martin J Walker, *Dirty Medicine* (Slingshot, 1993).

16 Jules Klotter, review of *Dirty Medicine*, 'Lies and Misdirection', *Townsend Letter* May 1994: 415.

17 Lyn Payer, *Medicine and Culture: Varieties of Treatments in the United States, England, West Germany, and France* (NY: Henry Holt, 1988).

18 PB 286/929, United States Office of Technology Assessment 9/78.

19 Dr William B Kannel MD, *Internal Medicine World Report* January 1–14, 1995.

20 *Townsend Letter* June 1997: 114.

21 *Townsend Letter* August/September: 1996.

22 Dr Alan R Gaby MD, *Townsend Letter* December 1990: 879.

23 Bird, op cit: 295.

24 *Lancet* 341, February 6, 1993.

25 D Eisenberg, 'Unconventional Medicine in the US', *New England Journal of Medicine* 328, 1993: 246.

26 Dr Julian M Whitaker MD, *Townsend Letter* July 1997: 110–14.

27 John Robbins, *Reclaiming Our Health: Exploding The Medical Myth And Embracing the Source of True Healing* (H J Kramer, 1997).

28 Morton Walker DPM, *Townsend Letter* July 1997: 131.

29 Dr Robert S Mendelsohn MD, *Confessions of a Medical Heretic* (Warner Books, 1979): xiii.

30 Jean Tissot, *Constitution des Organismes Animaux et Vegetaux, Causes des Maladies Qui les Atteignent* (Paris 1926–46).

31 Thomas Kuhn, *The Structure of Scientific Revolutions* (University of Chicago Press, 1962).

CHAPTER 33

1 Nicholas A Ashford and Claudia S Miller, *Chemical Exposures* (NY: Van Nostrand Reinhold, 1991: 74).

2 Lyn Payer, *Medicine and Culture* (NY: Henry Holt, 1988).

3 Professor W William Hughes, *Essentials of Environmental Toxicology* (Taylor & Francis, 1996): 13.

4 Schroeder, *The Poisons Around Us* (Indiana University Press, 1974): 49.

5 Radio New Zealand, May 25, 1998.

6 *New Zealand Herald* March 31, 1998.

7 'Gulf War Study Investigates the Dangers of Combined Chemical Exposures' September 1996, *Chemical Injury Information Network* PO Box 301, White Sulphur Springs MT 59645–0301.

8 'Persistent, repeated elicitation of the flight or fight response disrupts nearly every body system influencing *immune disorders*, heart disease, gastro intestinal disease and hypertension', in Ornstein and Sobel, *The Healing Brain* (NY: Simon & Schuster, 1987): 69.

9 *New Zealand Herald* March 31, 1998.

10 Tom Valentine, 'Vaccines Linked to Gulf War Syndrome', *Spotlight* August 25, 1997: B6.

11 Fortunately 'the Universe' is beginning to make amends these days.

12 Dr Michael L Culbert DSc, 'Gulf War Syndrome', *Townsend Letter* November 1995: 18–19.

13 Ibid.

14 Dr Gary Null, *Townsend Letter* April 1998: 54.

CHAPTER 34

1 Janice Tait, 'AIDS: Alternative Medicine and the Whole Person', *Townsend Letter* July 1996: 48–52 (51).

2 *Medical Tribune* October 1992: 3.

3 Dr Luc de Schepper MD, PhD, 'CFIDS & Homeopathy', *Townsend Letter* July 1994: 768.

4 Jules Klotter, 'Bypassing Censorship', *Townsend Letter* August/September 1997: 130.

5 Dr George Milowe MD, 'Does HIV Cause AIDS?', *Townsend Letter* April 1995: 111.

6 Dr Peter Duesberg, *Pharmac Ther.* 55, 1992: 201–77.

7 Klotter, op cit.

8 Mark Konlee (ed), *Keep Hope Alive* Report No 16, Spring 1998: 2 (available from: PO Box 27041, West Allis, WI 53227, US).

9 Tait, op cit: 48.

10 Milowe, op cit: 109–11.

11 Dr P H Duesberg, 'AIDS epidemiology: inconsistencies with human immuno-deficiency virus and with infectious disease', *Proceeding of the National Academy of Science* 88 (1991a): 1575–9.

12 *Lancet* 340, October 17, 1992: 971.

13 *American Review of Respiratory Disease* 147 (1993): 958.

14 *Journal of AIDS* 7.8 (1994): 876.

15 Milowe, op cit: 109.

16 Milowe, op cit: 110.

17 Ibid.

18 Milowe, op cit.

19 Dr Robert Wilner MD, *Deadly Deception* (Boca Raton, FL: Peltec Publishing Co, 1994).

20 'A Medical Doctor puts his life on the Line to Prove that Sex and HIV do not cause AIDS', *Heal* special edition (1995): 14–17.

21 Tait, op cit: 48. (To be fair, we'd actually have to take a poll to decide between this and the myth of cholesterol!).

22 Dr Robert Root-Bernstein, *Rethinking AIDS: The Tragic Cost of Premature Consensus* (NY: The Free Press, 1993).

23 Dr Michael L Culbert DSc, *AIDS: Hope, Hoax, and Hoopla* (Chula Vista, CA: The Bradford Foundation, 1989).

24 Luc Chaltin ND, *The American Chiropractor* April 1992.

25 Dr Joseph Sonmabond, *Journal of International Vaccine Network* December 1996.

26 Dr Leonard A Cole, *The Eleventh Plague: The Politics of Biological and Chemical Weapons* (NY: W H Freeman & Co, 1997); *Clouds of Secrecy: The Army's Germ Warfare Tests Over Populated Areas* with a Foreword by Senator Alan Cranston (Savage, MD: Littlefields, Adams Quality Paperbacks, 1997).

27 *The Vaccine Reaction* 2 (1), April 1996: 4 (National Vaccine Information Centre, 512 W Maple Avenue, #206, Vienna, VA 22180, US).

28 Milowe, op cit: 109–11.

29 Tait, op cit.

30 Peter Duesberg and David Rasnick, 'The Drug-AIDS Hypothesis', *International Journal of Medicine* February 1997.

31 Milowe, op cit: 111 [my emphasis].

32 Stephen C Byrnes, 'Benzene, Lubricants, & AIDS', *Explore!* 8 (1). See also *Overcoming AIDS with Natural Medicine* (Centaur; 2909 Winam Ave, #2; Honolulu, HI 96816, US).

33 John Bryant, 'Science & "antiscience",' *Townsend Letter* August/September 1994: 907.

34 *Barron's* December 16, 1991.

35 Dr Howard B Urnovitz PhD, Addressing the Eighth Annual Houston Conference on AIDS in America.

CHAPTER 35

1   I am indebted to Dr Larry Dossey MD, 'In Praise of Unhappiness', *Alternative Therapies in Health and Medicine* 2 (1), January 1996 (101 Columbia, Aliso Viejo, CA 92656), for some of the ideas in this chapter.
2   Deborah Tanner, *That's Not What I Meant* (Virago Press 1992): 97.
3   Dr Martin L Gross, *Psychological Society* (NY: Random House, 1978): 7.
4   Tanner, op cit: 40.
5   Ellen Langer, *Mindfulness* (Harvill, London 1989).
6   Samuel Richardson (1689–1761), *Clarissa Harlowe*, a novel in seven (!) volumes.
7   Mihaly Csikszentmihalyi, *The Evolving Self* (NY: Harper Collins, 1993).
8   George Orwell cited in T Miller, *How to Want What You Have* (NY: Henry Holt, 1994).
9   As for note 1.
10 'Bliss was it in that dawn to be alive ...' Wordsworth.
11 Ding Ling, *The Sun* 1995.

CONCLUSION

1   Martin J Walker, *Dirty Medicine* (Slingshot Publications, 1993).
2   Every few months more clinical trials establish the effectiveness of specific herbs and supplements.
3   *Townsend Letter* October 1994: 1101.

INDEX

Appleton, Dr Nancy 30, 90, 91, 94
arsenic 32, 268
arteries, clogging of 2, 3, 5, 20, 30, 306
    and chelation therapy 46–8
    cow's milk effects 28–9
arthritis:
    from dairy products 31, 32
    EFA lack 17
    ginger root for 34–5, 209
    high-heeled shoes link 225
    root-filled teeth link 69
aspartame 104–7
aspartic acid 103
aspirin 37–42, 204
asthma 127
Attention Deficit Disorder 15
autism 125
autoimmune diseases 54–5, 127–8
avoidance, of health hazards xiv
AZT 282–5, 289

bacteria, resistant (superbugs) 242–3,
        246–7
Barnard, Dr Neil 31
Bass, Dr C.C. 67
Beasley, Dr Joseph 228, 237
Bechamp (bacteriologist) 253–4, 255,
        259, 266
Beecher, H.K. 45
beef 33–4
Bevis, Martha 79
Billings, Dr Frank 64
biochemical view, of mental illness
        171–9
bipolar illness 174, 175–6, 180–1
Bird, Dr Christopher 263
birth defects 55, 272–3
black cohosh 212
Bland, Dr Jeffrey xii
Blastocysts homis 242

Blaylock, Dr Russell 107
blood clots 3, 306
borage oil 42
bottled water 75–6
bovine growth hormone (BGH) 109,
        113
bra wearing 65, 224–5
brain:
    development, and EFAs 16–17, 27–8
    effects of toxins 152–3
    mercury in 56
brain chemicals 9
brain-washing 262–3
Breakthrough 41–2
breast cancer 209–10, 226–33, 237
    and bra wearing 224–5
    HRT link 211–12
    mammograms 221–3
    olive oil prevention 13
    and pesticides 157
    sugar link 90–1
    in thin women 65–6
    tooth infection link 64–5
breast implants 272
breastmilk 17, 27, 35–6, 123
    mercury in 54
    pesticides in 151, 155, 157
    silicon in 272
Brecher, Arline 161
Breggin, Dr Peter 187–8, 189, 192
Breuer, Dr Joseph 167
Bross, Dr Irwin 236
Brown, Dr Susan 32
Budwig, Dr Joanna 14, 23, 229
Burket, Dr Lester 67
Burkett, Denis 231
Burzynski, Dr Stanislaw 195–6, 235
Butler, Dr Paul 117
Butler, Hilary 138, 139
butter 6–7, 14, 21, 23

De Schepper, Dr Luc 203
Dean, Dr Trendley 78
deaths, premature xi, 9
degenerative diseases 11, 17, 31
deliquency 33
Demand Switch 146
Densley, Barry 118
dental fluorosis 81
dentistry:
    mercury amalgam fillings 51–61, 64,
        66, 232
    root canal work 62–9, 232
deodorants, aluminium in 65
depression 182–90
DES 214–15
DHEA 1
diabetes 25, 28, 41–2, 83, 89, 105
Diesendorf, Prof Mark 84
diet:
    and cancer 231–2
    and longevity 259
digestive flora 241, 249
dioxin 151–2
diptheria vaccination 129–31
dipyridamole 39
disease-care industry 251, 258, 261–2,
        264, 292, 308
DNA 110, 115, 117
Dobbs, Geoffrey 85
doctors see medical profession
Dorfler, Dr Walter 110
Dossey, Dr Larry 298, 299
DPT vaccine 122–7
dreams, interpretation 167
dried milk 27
drinks, diet 105–6
drug abuse 202, 285, 286, 290
drugs, prescribed 201–20, 233, 251,
        292–3
DTPH3 vaccine 122

Dubos, René 137
Duesberg, Prof Peter H. 283, 285, 290,
        291
Dugdale, Dr A.E. 8

Ebola 288
EDTA chelation therapy 46–8
EFAs see essential fatty acids
Einstein, Albert xiv
elderly, drug treatment 215–16
electromagnetic fields 144–7, 183–4
Ellis, Dr Ralph 45, 48–9
Elsas, Dr Louis 105
EMFs see electromagnetic fields
Emmanuel, Therese 195
employment 184–5
encephalitis 123, 125, 132
encephalomyelitis 124
encephalopathy 123
Enderlin (bacteriologist) 255
Engelberg, Dr Hyman 9
Enig, Dr Mary 21
environmental pollution 232, 268,
        271–3, 289–90
epilepsy 174
Erasmus, Dr Udo 11, 13, 205
Ernst, Dr Edzard 218
Eskimos 6, 15
essential fatty acids (EFAs) 13, 15–19,
        22, 41–2, 122, 183, 232
Evening Primrose oil 24, 41, 42
extra-cellular matrix 204–5

faith healing 44
farmers, pesticide effects 155–6
fat:
    isolated 14
    vital functions and 12–13, 16–17
fats 11–24
    highly refined 15

monosaturated 13
polyunsaturated 2–3, 8–9, 13–14, 219, 231, 232, 233
saturated (animal) 1–7, 9–10, 50
unsaturated 2
FDA 191–200
fear 297
fibre 231
Finlayson, Dr Rodney 4
Finnegan, Dr 17, 21
fish 16, 86
fish oil 8, 24, 41, 42
Fisher, Dr Martin 63
Fitzsimons 113
5-HTP 113, 190
flax seed oil 17, 23–4, 41
Fleming, Sir Alexander 246, 248, 258
flu vaccines 137
fluoride 77–88, 306, 307
fluoxetine *see* Prozac
focal infections 64, 67, 68
foetus, pesticide effects 151–2, 155
Folkers, Dr 211
food:
   genetically-engineered 108–17
   highly refined 5, 18–19, 306
   irradiation 115
   pesticide residues 153
food allergies 109
Food and Drug Administration (FDA) *see* American Food and Drug Administration
food technology industry 191, 260, 265–6, 304
Forest, Waves 71
formaldehyde 145
Forman, Dr Jonathan 83
Foulkes, Dr Richard G. 78–9, 85, 86
Framingham project 4, 82
France, healthcare 259–60, 266, 269–70

free radicals 1
Freeman, Dr Hugh 174
Freud, Sigmund 163–71, 178, 183, 308
Freudian fallacy 169–71, 178, 183, 251, 260, 262, 265–6, 269, 270, 271, 279, 308
Friedman, Milton 184, 191, 203

Gaby, Dr Alan R. 1, 158, 208–9, 215, 218, 262–3
Gallo, Dr Robert 285, 286, 288
Gambee, Dr 193
Gamma–linolenic acid (GLA) 42
garlic 41
Gaublomme, Dr Kris 128, 140
gender, and synthetic oestrogens 118–19
genetic defects 55
genetic predispositions 230–1
genetically-engineered food 108–17
Germ Theory of Disease (Doctrine of Specfic Aetiology) 254
German measles vaccine 139
Gerrity, Dr Timothy 40
giardia 73
GM food *see* genetically-engineered food
goals:
   need for 298
   realistic 301–2
Godfrey, Dr Mike 55, 60
golf 160–1
Gottschalk, Dr Louis 162
governments, welfare responsibilities 306–7
green sickness 268, 271, 279
Greenberg, Dr Bern 134
Greewald, Dr Peter 231
Griesinger, Wilhelm 172
Grismaijer, Soma 224
growth hormones, in animal feed 27

Maeterlink, Maurice 310

magnesium 30–3, 39, 41, 81–2, 83, 183–4, 187, 190

malaria 137

male births 118–19, 152

Malhotra, Dr S.L. 6

mammograms 221–3, 233

Manders, Dr Wolfe 112–13

Mann, Dr George V. 9–10

margarine 5, 9, 11–22, 40, 50, 306, 307

Marsh, David 158

Martin, Dr Wayne 6, 8, 13, 21, 37, 39–40, 41

Martini, Betty 106

Matossian, Dr Mary 245

mattresses 123

Maudsley, Henry 172

ME (Chronic Fatigue Immune Dysfunction Syndrome) xiii, 32, 267–8, 271–81

Mead, Margaret 302

measles vaccine 126, 127, 131–2

meat 33, 231

medical profession 205–8, 250–66, 269–71, 304, 307

Mediterranean diet 5

megavitamin therapy 174–6

Mehler, Steven 195

Meinig, Dr George 7

Mekdeki, Betty 273

Melnick, Prof 287

men, tight jeans 224

Mencken, H.L. 167

Mendelsohn, Dr Robert S. 129, 139, 140, 265

meningitis 133

menopause 32, 212

mental health 8–9, 17, 33, 162–79, 182–90

mercury poisoning 51–61, 64, 66, 150, 232, 306, 307

meridians 65

milk 25–36, 50, 81, 82, 233
    see also homogenized milk

Miller, Dr Samuel Charles 67

Miller, Neil Z. 132, 136

Millichap, Dr J. Gordon 32

Milowe, Dr George 286, 291

minerals 90, 150, 187, 295

mobile phones 146, 148

moment, cherishing 301

monosodium glutamate 101–7

Montagnier, Luc 285

Moss, Dr Ralph W. 236

mouth washes 69

MSG 101–7

Mullenix, Dr Phyllis 83

Multiple Sclerosis (MS) 17, 54

Murray, Dr Michael T. 211

Murray, Prof John 87

Myocardial Infarction 3, 4–5, 9, 181

N-acetyl cysteine 61

National Diet Heart Study 7

negativity *see* positive thinking

Neill, Joe 106

nervous system diseases 83, 106

Nicolson, Dr Garth 272, 279

nicotine 99

Nieper, Dr Hans 66

Nightingale, Florence xiii, 252, 267–8, 270, 278

Null, Dr Gary 186, 188–9, 192, 272, 280

nut butters 24

nutrient deficiencies:
    and mental illness 171–9, 183
    and prescription drugs 204

oils, hydrogenated *see* hydrogenated fats and oils

olive oil 5, 13, 14, 21, 23, 41, 50

Raloff, Janet 74
Rasnick, David 290
religion 299
Renner, Dr John 193
rheumatic heart disease 4
rheumatoid arthritis 208–9
Riesinger, Dr Robert 123
Rifkin, Jeremy 116
Ritchie, Dr David 132
Riversong, Michael 146
Robbins, John 264
Roberts, Dr H.J. 105, 106
Rockefeller, John D. 258
Rogers, Dr Sherry A. 30, 32, 238
Roholm, Kaj 78
Rook, Prof Graham A. 278
root canal work 62–9, 232, 306, 307
Root–Bernstein, Dr Robert 286
Roshal, Dr M.A. 83
Rostend, Jean 140
Royal Free disease 275–6

safflower oil 14
St John's Wort 182, 187, 190
Salaman, Maureen Kennedy 186
Salk, Dr Jonas 134, 139
salmonellosis 242
salt 180–1
Samuels, Jack 102
Samuelsson, Dr Bengt 41
Sardi, Bill 210
scarlet fever 131
Schaefer, Al 228
Schauss, Dr Alexander 33
schizophrenia 168, 172–6
Schroeder, Dr Henry 142, 271
Schuman, Rosetta 2, 47, 50, 83
Schweitzer, Albert 231
seed butters 24
Seelig, Dr Mildred 243, 245, 256

Seely, Dr Stephen 90, 231
Sehnert, Dr Keith W. 55
selenium 82
self-limitation, in illness 44
self-obsession 183, 298, 308
Semmelweiss, Dr F. 252–3
serotonin 9, 113, 177
sesame oil 24
sexually transmitted diseases 246
Shaw, George Bernard 217
shock 124
Shull, Dr Fred 194
SIDS 17, 27, 119, 122–4, 138
Sierck, Peter 146
silicon breast implants 272
Simian Virus 40 133
Sinclair, Dr Hugh 33
Singer, Sidney 224
SIV (Simian Immunodeficiency Virus)
    137, 288
skim milk 27, 29
skin disease 17
slimming, and EFA need 18, 22
smallpox vaccine 134, 287–8
Smith, Dee 282, 284
Smith, Dr Edward M.B. 155
Smith, Dr Russel L. 1, 2, 10
smoking 5, 8, 50, 99–100
soft drinks 33
Sonmabond, Dr Joseph 287
soya milk 32
soyabeans 109, 113, 212
Spanish flu 248
species barrier, crossing 110, 135
spending choices 305–6
Stevia rebaudiana 93
Stewart, Dr Marion 95
Steyne, Prof Douw G. 80
Streptococcus fecalis 68
stress, and cholesterol 1

stroke 38, 39, 40, 48, 50
Strom, Dr Brian 215–16
strontium 90 289
sugar 50, 89–94, 231
suicide 8–9, 162, 176–7, 182, 185–7, 189, 300
sunflower oil 14, 15
supplements 213, 218–19
suppositories 249, 260
Sutton, Philip 88
Swartz, William E. 115
symptoms 203, 257, 269–70
of mercury poisoning 57
tahini paste 24
tamoxifen 212, 229–30
Tanner, Deborah 296
Tapanui Flu 274–5
see also ME
Teicher, Dr Martin 187
television, false images 297–8
Telleen, Carl K. 66
testicular cancer 118–19
thalidomide 214
thinking, positive 294–303
THMs (trihalomethanes) 73
Thudichum, Dr J.W. 172
tick powder 152–3
Tissot, Jean 265
Titanic, as symbol 309–10
tonsillectomies 64
tooth decay 77, 78, 84–5
Torch, Dr William 123
Torrey, Fuller 171
trace elements 30, 295
trans fatty acids (TFAs) 19–22, 28, 40, 114, 122–3
transgenic pigs 111
tristesse 299
Truss, Dr Orion 178, 256
tryptophan 112–13, 190

tuberculosis 255
turtles 158
20th-century illnesses xiii, 128, 245, 257–8, 267–81

ulcerative colitis 127
Urnovitz, Dr Howard B. 292

vaccination see immunization
vaccines, production 134–6
vegetarian diet 33, 231
Vinca rosea 227
Virchow, Rudolf 254–5
vitamin B_6 50
vitamin C 61, 124
vitamin E 10, 23, 40, 41–2, 210

Walker, Dr Morton 26–7, 74, 108–9, 111–12, 265
Walker, Malcolm 116
Walker, Martin J. 259
Warren, Tom 56–8, 64–5, 68
water, need for 72
water distillers 76, 120
water quality 72–6
and fluoride 77–88
Wegener, Henrik 243
weight gain, mobile phones 148
Weiss, Linda 74
Werbach, Dr Melvyn R. 179
White, Dr Paul Dudley 2–3, 4
White, Margo 108, 182, 185
whooping cough 131
see also DPT vaccine
Will, Dr Peter 110
Willet, Dr Walter 20
Wilner, Dr Robert 251, 286
wine drinking 5–6
Winther, Chuck 234
Winther, Lisa 234

Witkin, Dr Steven S. 244
Witsenberg, Dr Bob 203
Wolf, Prof Stewart 5
Wolff, Dr Mary 157
work, worthwhile 301
Wurtzel, Elizabeth 186

Xanthine oxidase 29, 82

xeno-oestrogens 118–19

yoghurt 29, 249
Yudkin, John 89

Ziegelbecker, Dr D. 84
zinc 56–7
Zumla, Prof Alimudden 278

Natural Heart Health for Women

A Woman's Guide to Preventing
and Reversing Heart Disease Naturally
Linda Ojeda Ph.D.

Although the majority of women worry about the threat of breast cancer, heart disease kills more women than all types of cancer combined. This is the first major book to focus on heart disease and women. With a sympathetic yet informative style, Linda Ojeda looks at:

- how to create your own personal heart health plan with a risk profile questionnaire and specific dietary guidelines
- the causes and symptoms of heart disease and women, including the effects of hormones, pregnancy and the menopause
- how women can best combine good eating habits, exercise and stress reduction
- the importance of supplements from homocysteine lowering B vitamins and antioxidants, to food sources like soy, green tea and fibre
- the effects of HRT and oral contraceptives

Complete Book of Men's Health

Dr Sarah Brewer

This fully revised edition of the popular classic is an essential guide to the male body. This edition includes new discoveries in men's health – including Viagra and saw palmetto – and a wide variety of complementary herbal supplements specific to male conditions.

For too long men have ignored their health and fewer have gone to the doctor's if they were unwell, but recently the media has been putting the focus on men's health. This is the *only* comprehensive book to deal with all aspects of health and the male body including:

- relieving prostate problems with herbal remedy saw palmetto
- the verdict on Viagra and a look at herbal alternatives
- expert guide to monitoring your cholesterol
- simple exercises to combat stress
- men's depression and taking St John's Wort
- how to create balance with exercise and nutrition